T0131004

History of Critical Care Medicine

Editor

HANNAH WUNSCH

CRITICAL CARE CLINICS

www.criticalcare.theclinics.com

Consulting Editor
GREGORY S. MARTIN

July 2023 • Volume 39 • Number 3

ELSEVIER

1600 John F. Kennedy Boulevard • Suite 1800 • Philadelphia, Pennsylvania, 19103-2899

http://www.theclinics.com

CRITICAL CARE CLINICS Volume 39, Number 3
July 2023 ISSN 0749-0704, ISBN-13: 978-0-323-94011-5

Editor: Joanna Gascoine
Developmental Editor: Hannah Almira Lopez

Critical Care Clinics (ISSN: 0749-0704) is published quarterly by Elsevier Inc., 360 Park Avenue South, New York, NY 10010-1710. Months of issue are January, April, July, and October. Business and Editorial Offices: 1600 John F. Kennedy Blvd., Suite 1800, Philadelphia, PA 19103-2899. Customer Service Office: 6277 Sea Harbor Drive, Orlando, FL 32887-4800. Periodicals postage paid at New York, NY and additional mailing offices. Subscription prices are $274.00 per year for US individuals, $779 per year for US institutions, $100.00 per year for US students and residents, $305.00 per year for Canadian individuals, $976.00 per year for Canadian institutions, $348.00 per year for international individuals, $976.00 per year for international institutions, $100.00 per year for Canadian students/residents, and $150.00 per year for foreign students/residents. To receive student/resident rate, orders must be accompanied by name of affiliated institution, date of term, and the signature of program/residency coordinator on institution letterhead. Orders will be billed at individual rate until proof of status is received. Foreign air speed delivery is included in all *Clinics* subscription prices. All prices are subject to change without notice. POSTMASTER: Send address changes to *Critical Care Clinics*, Elsevier Periodicals Customer Service, 11830 Westline Industrial Drive, St. Louis, MO 63146. **Customer Service: 1-800-654-2452 (US). From outside of the US, call 1-314-447-8871. Fax: 1-314-447-8029. E-mail: journalscustomerservice-usa@elsevier.com (for print support) or journalsonlinesupport-usa@elsevier.com (for online support).**

Reprints. For copies of 100 or more of articles in this publication, please contact the Commercial Reprints Department, Elsevier Inc., 360 Park Avenue South, New York, NY 10010-1710. Tel.: 212-633-3874; Fax: 212-633-3820; E-mail: reprints@elsevier.com.

Critical Care Clinics is also published in Spanish by Editorial Inter-Medica, Junin 917, 1er A, 1113, Buenos Aires, Argentina.

Critical Care Clinics is covered in *MEDLINE/PubMed (Index Medicus), EMBASE/Excerpta Medica, Current Concepts/ Clinical Medicine, ISI/BIOMED,* and *Chemical Abstracts.*

Contributors

CONSULTING EDITOR

GREGORY S. MARTIN, MD, MSC
Professor, Division of Pulmonary, Allergy, Critical Care and Sleep Medicine, Research Director, Emory Critical Care Center, Director, Emory/Georgia Tech Predictive Health Institute, Co-Director, Atlanta Center for Microsystems Engineered Point-of-Care Technologies (ACME POCT), President, Society of Critical Care Medicine, Atlanta, Georgia, USA

EDITOR

HANNAH WUNSCH, MD, MSc
Department of Critical Care Medicine, Sunnybrook Health Sciences Centre, Professor of Anesthesiology and Critical Care Medicine, Department of Anesthesiology and Pain Medicine and Interdepartmental Division of Critical Care Medicine, University of Toronto, Toronto, Ontario, Canada

AUTHORS

DIANA ANDERSON, MD, MArch
Instructor of Neurology, Boston University School of Medicine, VA Boston Health Care System, Boston, Massachusetts, USA

LAURENT J. BROCHARD, MD
Professor of Medicine, Keenan Research Centre, St Michael's Hospital, Unity Health Toronto, Interdepartmental Division of Critical Care Medicine, University of Toronto, Toronto, Ontario, Canada

SHEELA PAI COLE, MD, FASE, FASA
Clinical Professor, Department of Anesthesiology, Perioperative and Pain Medicine, Stanford University, Stanford University School of Medicine Palo Alto, California, USA

BRONWEN CONNOLLY, MSc, PhD, MCSP
Wellcome-Wolfson Institute for Experimental Medicine, Queen's University Belfast, Belfast, United Kingdom

JAMES DOWNAR, MDCM, MHSc (Bioethics)
Division of Palliative Care, Department of Medicine, University of Ottawa, Department of Critical Care, The Ottawa Hospital, Ottawa, Ontario, Canada

E. WESLEY ELY, MD, MPH
Critical Illness, Brain Dysfunction, and Survivorship (CIBS) Center, Division of Allergy, Pulmonary, and Critical Care Medicine, Department of Medicine, Vanderbilt University Medical Center, Geriatric Research and Education Clinical Center (GRECC), Veterans Affairs Tennessee Valley Health System, Nashville, Tennessee, USA

H. BARRIE FAIRLEY, MB, BS (Lond), MA, FRCA, FRCP(C)
Professor Emeritus, Department of Anesthesia, Perioperative Medicine and Pain Management, Stanford University School of Medicine, Stanford, California, USA

LUIS GAITINI, MD
Associate Clinical Professor, Department of Anesthesiology, Bnai-Zion Medical Center, Haifa, Israel

NEIL A. HALPERN, MD, MCCM, FCCP, FACP
Service Chief, Critical Care Medicine, Director, Critical Care Center, Professor of Medicine in Clinical Anesthesiology, Professor of Clinical Medicine, Weill Cornell Medical College, Department of Anesthesiology and Critical Care, Memorial Sloan Kettering Cancer Center, New York, New York, USA

D. KIRK HAMILTON, BArch, MSOD, PhD
Professor Emeritus, Texas A&M University, College Station, Texas, USA

MAY HUA, MD, MS
Department of Anesthesiology, Columbia University, Department of Epidemiology, Mailman School of Public Health, New York, New York, USA

JOHN H. KERR, MA, DM (Oxon), FFARCS
Retired Consultant Anaesthetist, Nuffield Department of Anaesthetics, University of Oxford, Radcliffe Infirmary, Oxford, United Kingdom

MICHELLE E. KHO, PT, PhD
School of Rehabilitation Science, McMaster University, Institute for Applied Health Science, Physiotherapy Department, Research Institute of St. Joe's Hamilton, Hamilton, Ontario, Canada

JEANNE KISACKY, MArch, PhD
Independent Historian, Ithaca, New York, USA

MATTHEW F. MART, MD, MSc
Critical Illness, Brain Dysfunction, and Survivorship (CIBS) Center, Division of Allergy, Pulmonary, and Critical Care Medicine, Department of Medicine, Vanderbilt University Medical Center, Geriatric Research and Education Clinical Center (GRECC), Veterans Affairs Tennessee Valley Health System, Nashville, Tennessee, USA

IBRAHIM MATTAR, MD
Associate Clinical Professor, Department of Surgery, Bnai-Zion Medical Center, Haifa, Israel

KERRY A. MILNER, DNSc, APRN, FNP-BC, EBP-C
Professor, Sacred Heart University, Dr. Susan L. Davis, RN and Richard J. Henley College of Nursing, Fairfield, Connecticut, USA

RONALD G. PEARL, MD, PhD, FCCM
Dr. Richard K. and Erika N. Richards Professor, Department of Anesthesiology, Perioperative and Pain Medicine, Stanford University, Stanford University School of Medicine Palo Alto, California, USA

JANSIE PROZESKY, MB, ChB
Associate Professor of Anesthesiology and Perioperative Medicine, Department of Anesthesiology, Penn State College of Medicine, Penn State Milton S. Hershey Medical Center, Hershey, Pennsylvania, USA

MICHELLE RAUSEN, MS, RRT, RRT-NPS
Technical Director, Respiratory Therapy, Department of Anesthesiology and Critical Care, Critical Care Center, Memorial Sloan Kettering Cancer Center, New York, New York, USA

KIMBERLY F. RENGEL, MD
Critical Illness, Brain Dysfunction, and Survivorship (CIBS) Center, Department of Anesthesiology, Division of Anesthesia Critical Care Medicine, Vanderbilt University Medical Center, Nashville, Tennessee, USA

ELIZABETH SCRUTH, PhD, MPH, RN, CNS, CCRN-K, CCNS, FCCM, FCNS, CPHQ
Regional Director Clinical Quality Programs, Data Analytics and Tele Critical Care, NCAL Safety, Quality and Regulatory Services, Kaiser Foundation Hospital and Health Plan, Oakland, California, USA

ANDREA SIKORA, PharmD, MSCR, BCCCP, FCCM
Clinical Associate Professor, Department of Clinical and Administrative Pharmacy, University of Georgia College of Pharmacy, Department of Pharmacy, Augusta University Medical Center, Augusta, Georgia, USA

MOSTAFA SOMRI, MD
Associate Clinical Professor, Department of Anesthesiology, Bnai-Zion Medical Center, Haifa, Israel

SONIA VAIDA, MD
Professor of Anesthesiology and Perioperative Medicine, Department of Anesthesiology, Penn State College of Medicine, Penn State Milton S. Hershey Medical Center, Hershey, Pennsylvania, USA

JO ELLEN WILSON, MD, MPH
Critical Illness, Brain Dysfunction, and Survivorship (CIBS) Center, Geriatric Research and Education Clinical Center (GRECC), Veterans Affairs Tennessee Valley Health System, Department of Psychiatry and Behavioral Sciences, Vanderbilt University Medical Center, Nashville, Tennessee, USA

HANNAH WUNSCH, MD, MSc
Department of Critical Care Medicine, Sunnybrook Health Sciences Centre, Professor of Anesthesiology and Critical Care Medicine, Department of Anesthesiology and Pain Medicine and Interdepartmental Division of Critical Care Medicine, University of Toronto, Toronto, Ontario, Canada

FRANK ZILM, DArch
Founding Director, Institute for Health and Wellness Design, The University of Kansas, Lawrence, Kansas, USA

Contents

practice including the importance of light sedation and the avoidance of deliriogenic drugs such as benzodiazepines. Best practices are now strategically incorporated in targeted bundles of care like the ICU Liberation Campaign's ABCDEF Bundle.

Michelle E. Kho and Bronwen Connolly

Critically ill patients are at risk of post-intensive care syndrome, including physical, cognitive, and psychological sequelae. Physiotherapists are rehabilitation experts who focus on restoring strength, physical function, and exercise capacity. Critical care has evolved from a culture of deep sedation and bed rest to one of awakening and early mobility; physiotherapeutic interventions have developed to address patients' rehabilitation needs. Physiotherapists are assuming more prominent roles in clinical and research leadership, with opportunities for wider interdisciplinary collaboration. This paper reviews the evolution of critical care from a rehabilitation perspective, highlights relevant research milestones, and proposes future opportunities for improving survivorship outcomes.

Andrea Sikora

Critical care pharmacy has evolved rapidly over the last 50 years to keep pace with the rapid technological and knowledge advances that have characterized critical care medicine. The modern-day critical care pharmacist is a highly trained individual well suited for the interprofessional team-based care that critical illness necessitates. Critical care pharmacists improve patient-centered outcomes and reduce health care costs through three domains: direct patient care, indirect patient care, and professional service. Optimizing workload of critical care pharmacists, similar to the professions of medicine and nursing, is a key next step for using evidence-based medicine to improve patient-centered outcomes.

James Downar, May Hua, and Hannah Wunsch

In this article, the authors review the origins of palliative care within the critical care context and describe the evolution of symptom management, shared decision-making, and comfort-focused care in the ICU from the 1970s to the early 2000s. The authors also review the growth of interventional studies in the past 20 years and indicate areas for future study and quality improvement for end-of-life care among the critically ill.

Kerry A. Milner

This article gives a historical perspective of visitation in the intensive care unit (ICU) since the establishment of critical care units. Initially, visitors were not allowed because it was thought to be harmful to the patient. Despite the evidence, ICUs with open visitation have consistently been in the minority and the COVID-19 pandemic halted progress in this area. Virtual visitation was introduced during the pandemic to maintain family presence, but limited evidence suggests that this is not equivalent to in-person visitation. Going forward ICUs and health systems must consider family presence policies that allow for visitation under any circumstance.

CRITICAL CARE CLINICS

Preface

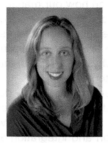

Hannah Wunsch, MD, MSc
Editor

Critical care has its roots in many different areas of medicine: infectious disease, surgery and anesthesia, neurology, cardiology, and nursing. However, one disease, polio, was an outsized driver of many of the key developments that led to this new field.

The first organ support, in the form of negative pressure ventilation, occurred in 1928. The development of the iron lung at Harvard's School of Public Health was spurred on by the need to save people paralyzed by polio who were unable to breathe. Next came positive pressure ventilation. This breakthrough in management occurred at the Blegdam Hospital in Copenhagen in 1952, proposed by a young anesthesiologist, Bjørn Ibsen. Again, the reason was respiratory failure due to polio. The modern concept of an intensive care unit (ICU), with both expertise and equipment to keep an array of critically ill patients alive, only came into existence in 1953 as Ibsen took his knowledge from polio patients and the operating room and applied them to any and all who were critically ill. Experience from the care of patients who had overdosed, the resuscitation of soldiers in hemorrhagic shock on battlefields, and complex post-surgical care were then all incorporated into these nascent ICUs.

Critical care is, therefore, a young specialty. The first ICUs in the United States and Canada (units capable of organ support and able to care for a range of patients) all began around 1958. A little less than seventy years later, there are still a few people alive who can remember those early years—the immense trial and error; the tinkering with machines; the excitement of saving individuals that they couldn't save before; and the morass of ethics created by dependence on machines for life. It is imperative that we capture those memories, so we can understand and learn from the mistakes that were made, and also feel pride in how far we have come. Drs Barrie Fairley and John Kerr were two of those early physicians in the first ICUs. Dr Fairley founded the first ICU in Toronto, Canada in 1958 and shares his memories of some of those earliest challenges. Dr Kerr worked in the respiratory unit in Oxford, UK and reflects on the changes in care and observation of patients.

However, it is also important that we look beyond those early years to understand the evolution of our specialty in the nearer past—as the care of the critically ill evolved beyond early struggles just to stabilize and ventilate patients, to include more

Crit Care Clin 39 (2023) xi–xii
https://doi.org/10.1016/j.ccc.2023.01.001
0749-0704/23/© 2023 Published by Elsevier Inc.

criticalcare.theclinics.com

sophisticated approaches to intubation and airway management, nuanced ventilator management, and approaches to sedation, with recognition of how these choices might impact short- and long-term outcomes.

Traditionally, much of the history of critical care has focused on how our management of specific illnesses has changed over time, particularly for key disease states such as sepsis, hemorrhagic shock, pneumonia, and the acute respiratory distress syndrome. But the history of critical care is as much about the evolution in thinking around the care team, the organization of care, and even the physical facilities, that all help to allow for the best delivery of sophisticated, coordinated care.

While critical care conjures up the image of a room with a patient surrounded by devices providing organ support and monitoring, it is also the individuals who matter, including the interdisciplinary team of pharmacists, physical therapists, palliative care physicians, and many others. The history of their evolution and integration as team members in the ICU for the care of the critically ill is essential to the story of the maturation of our specialty.

Seventy years ago, the majority of our patients would have entered the hospital and never left. Some would never have sought out hospital care, aware that little to nothing was on offer. In a short time, we have witnessed a sea change in who lives and who dies. Yet while ours is a specialty that comes with the privilege of experiencing the extraordinary moments of unexpected recovery and the joyful (and often tearful) reunion of loved ones, it still involves heart-wrenching grief in many moments of death. We are also only beginning to come to grips with the enormous disability and life-altering changes that often occur even with critical care that is well delivered, and despite the "success" of an individual able to leave the ICU.

The next seventy years will doubtless bring enormous new advances. However, we cannot ever forget that the ability to receive critical care is a privilege not extended to all across the globe. With climate change, large migration of populations, and vaccine hesitancy leading to potential resurgences of diseases such as polio, measles and diphtheria, our services will be needed more than ever, and our ability to provide such high-tech care to most will continue to be limited. Our greatest future challenge will be to provide equitable care in an increasingly inequitable world.

Hannah Wunsch, MD, MSc
Department of Critical Care Medicine, Sunnybrook Health Sciences Centre, 2075 Bayview Avenue, Room D1.08, Toronto, ON M4N 3M5, Canada

Department of Anesthesiology and
Pain Medicine
Interdepartmental Division of Critical Care Medicine
University of Toronto

E-mail address:
hannah.wunsch@sunnybrook.ca

Challenges of ICU Care in the Early Days

H. Barrie Fairley, MB, BS (Lond), MA, FRCA, FRCPC*

KEYWORDS

- Toronto General Hospital • Chronic obstructive pulmonary disease
- Intermittent positive pressure • Intensive therapy unit • PVC
- Acute respiratory distress syndrome • ICU

The first intensive care unit (ICU) in Toronto was opened at the Toronto General Hospital (TGH) as a "Respiratory Unit" in 1958. The early days of this unit have been described in various articles published at the time, such as a description in the *Canadian Medical Assn. Journal* of the establishment of the Unit itself, including the 4 *sine qua non*s for intensive care.[1] These were…a special location, a specialized team of nurses, a team of physicians in charge of the patient care, and intermittent positive pressure (IPP) as the mode of respiratory support. We further published a 38-page detailed account in the *Canadian Anaesthetists' Society Journal* outlining our thinking and activities arising from the care of our first 100 patients.[2] The following account will focus particularly on some of the significant issues that arose in the initial years between the opening of the Unit in 1958 and the arrival of clinically available blood gas measurement in the early 1960s.[a,b] It is of interest that what was one of the first coronary units was established independently at TGH about the same time.[3] We had yet to recognize the advantage of combining these and other critical care needs! Critical care as a discipline was not yet recognized in North America[c] but, eventually, individual special-purpose units that had been established in each locale as needed were combined under that label.

Department of Anesthesia, Perioperative Medicine and Pain Management, Stanford University, School of Medicine
* Corresponding author. c/o Dr. Hannah Wunsch, Department of Critical Care Medicine, Sunnybrook Hospital, 2075 Bayview Avenue, Room D1.08, Toronto, ON M4N 3M5.
E-mail address: bfairley@stanford.edu

[a] The author's colleagues, Drs Richard Chambers (Neurology), Colin Woolf (Pulmonology), and Hugh Barber (ENT) unfortunately are not alive to assist with memory recall.

[b] In preparing to write this account, the author has been unable to find surviving contemporaries elsewhere with whom to compare notes. These would have included, for instance, Pontoppidan, Bendixen, and Laver (at Harvard), Safar and Grenvik (Pittsburgh), Secher (Copenhagen), Crampton-Smith (Oxford), Norlander (Stockholm), and Holmdahl (Uppsala).

[c] The Society of Critical Medicine was founded in 1971.

Crit Care Clin 39 (2023) 427–435
https://doi.org/10.1016/j.ccc.2022.12.001
0749-0704/23/© 2022 Elsevier Inc. All rights reserved.

FIRST, A DESCRIPTION OF THE CIRCUMSTANCES THAT EXISTED IN THE LATE 1950S

Communication was difficult without the Internet, and with air travel and long-distance phone calls very expensive, there was a degree of isolation not experienced today. In major centers, the different specialties were setting up units to meet their own patients' needs, most notably for respiratory failure, coronary-related events, and post-cardiac surgery care. Open-heart surgery was in its infancy and trauma and stroke units, for example, came much later. The participants were publishing in their own specialty (as well as national, rather than international) journals, resulting in further isolation. We were relatively uninformed as to what was happening elsewhere.

As was typical in many hospitals in the 1950s, TGH did not have mechanical ventilators, piped wall gases or suction, continuous monitoring of electrocardiogram (ECG), intravascular pressure monitoring, or respiratory measurements. Prepackaged and disposable sterile plastic items did not yet exist. Intravenous (IV) infusions, including blood, were dispensed from glass bottles connected by rubber tubing to IV needles, and fluid and electrolyte balance was incompletely understood. Metal IV cannulas were also in use but required a "cut down" for their insertion. These were replaced initially with Rochester needles with attached plastic cannulas, until the latter's successors became widely available from multiple commercial sources. If oxygen was needed, a cylinder would be brought from storage by an "orderly." The field of respiratory therapy had not yet been created. There would be one-on-one nursing. However, until the Unit was established, when such dedicated nursing was required, the nurse would often be from an agency and have no prior experience of managing a patient requiring respiratory support.

The Toronto General Hospital Unit and Medical Staff

The Unit arose in the first place because Richard Chambers, a British neurologist on the TGH junior staff, had trained in London and experienced IPP ventilation of patients with respiratory paralysis. He found himself looking after a TGH patient with poliomyelitis in a tank respirator (iron lung). He was told there was a UK-trained anesthesiologist in charge of cardiac anesthesia (the author), and so approached me one afternoon while I was looking after a patient rewarming after hypothermia for open heart surgery, to enquire if I knew anything about the use of IPP ventilation for paralyzed patients. After visiting his patient, we then recruited Colin Woolf, a South Africa-trained pulmonologist in charge of our pulmonary function laboratory, and Hugh Barber, a Toronto-trained ear, nose and throat (ENT) surgeon who would oversee our tracheostomy arrangements, and so forth.

Physicians who did not work in the operating rooms were in general unfamiliar with airway maintenance and IPP ventilation. Indeed, some internists doubted that venous return and cardiac output could be maintained for long without the intermittent negative intrapleural pressure of spontaneous respiration. In creating the Unit, this was one of the issues to be clarified in order to obtain the Medical Board's approval for the care we proposed to provide. In that regard, when the initial proposal to establish a unit was made to the Medical Board by junior medical staff,[d] the decision was made to have them form a "Poliomyelitis Committee" but with a chair to be appointed from among the uninvolved senior staff of the Department of Internal Medicine. Therefore, at the

---

[d] The author was aged 31 years at the time, and a cardiac anesthesiologist whose sole prior experience of respiratory failure management (other than of curarized anesthetized patients in the operating room [OR]) was anesthesia for bronchoscopy of a few patients in tank respirators (iron lungs), and (in the United Kingdom) in the IPP ventilation of a few others with drug overdoses (Nembutal most commonly).

outset we were all—nurses, physicians, orderlies, hospital administration, outside referring physicians, ambulance companies—together in the learning mode as we established very elementary routines. It was like a specialized form of camping out!

The Respiratory Unit's Medical Team

Since the medical staff were funded from fee-for-service payments (and worked with indigent patients on a pro bono basis), availability of staff 24/7 could be a problem. The insurance companies did not recognize what we would now call "critical care" as a reimbursable item but the Anesthesia Department staff worked as a partnership, thereby permitting allocation of its members to patient care without considering the financial aspects and were generous in freeing the author to spend considerable unreimbursed time in the Unit.[e] Later, when a fellow, Murray Mendelson, and, years later, residents became involved, this started to ease. However, the lack of reimbursement certainly influenced decisions on the part of graduating residents. In locations where practice partnerships had yet to recognize the new responsibility, the lack of reimbursement discouraged anesthesiologists from moving in this direction.

From the start, it was obvious that decision-making regarding patient care could not be made based only on daily "rounds." Chambers and Woolf certainly paid unscheduled daily visits, but without residents or students, and at other times as required. One of them would be the primary physician for each patient but all 3 of us were always very familiar with all the patients. I was there more frequently, as much of the initial need was to resolve problems related to respiratory support. However, in the early days, I was still involved with providing cardiac anesthesia in the operating room as well. I made it a point when otherwise unoccupied to drop by the Unit and respond to queries from the nursing staff who were establishing their own routines and accumulating questions related to the ventilators and their use. The unit only involved 4 or 5 beds until we moved into the new Urquhart wing in late 1959.

INTERACTIONS WITH OTHER MEDICAL STAFF

This was interesting. There were 2 issues that stay in my memory. One was that we found it necessary, with the Medical Board's approval, to insist that only the medical staff of the Unit could write orders for patients admitted there. The interaction with our colleagues on the medical staff regarding handing over the care of their patients to our group ranged from enthusiastic to distrustful. Fortunately, the former predominated because it was quickly recognized that the new unit was a place where patients could receive unusually close attention from medical staff with the necessary insight. This was not the case elsewhere. For example, a colleague in the United Kingdom has since described his experience in the early 1960s on assuming his post as the first cardiac surgeon for a region of the country. When he wanted to set up a special "intensive therapy" unit (ITU) for the postoperative care of his patients, a senior internist on the staff told him that "he would rather his patients died in his ward with dignity, than they be subjected to the awful instruments of the anaesthetists (sic) in the ITU."

That said, regardless of the need for respiratory support, the TGH Unit offered a level of nursing care not available elsewhere in the hospital. A head nurse and a team of registered nurse (RNs) were allocated full-time to the Unit. Once trained, it was understood that only those with this special skill (and insight) would work there. These predecessors of today's ICU nurse became the essential core of any success that was achieved. As a

---

[e] Because I was usually the one to be called for respiratory support in emergency situations, including at night, I was given admitting privileges, which most anesthesiologists did not have.

result we would be approached, particularly by some surgeons, who requested admission of their more complicated cases. Unfortunately, lack of beds at that time often did not permit us to admit these patients in the absence of a specific respiratory problem.[f]

Equipment and Routines

Respiratory support
It happened that, at TGH, an anesthesiologist was one of the founders of the Unit and became an integral part of the patient care team. In those early days, as ICUs were being set up, the founders were usually not anesthesiologists. However, in those instances, the medical staff would call on their anesthesia colleagues to supervise the set-up and operation of the ventilators. Thus, the involvement of the specialty in this activity varied from broad inclusion in the patient's care in some teaching hospitals, such as TGH, to that of more role-limited "ventilator managers" elsewhere. It was to fill this latter role that respiratory therapy evolved.

Airway
From the start, tracheostomies were usually reserved for patients requiring mechanical ventilation for longer than a day or two. One problem was that the use of cuffed tubes was foreign to all the staff other than anesthesiologists. It was not intuitive to inflate the cuffs to just the point where there was no escape of inspired air but no prolonged excessive pressure on the tracheal mucosa. Simple now, but not then—and just one example of so many features that are completely routine today.

Selection of a ventilator
The only machines in the hospital at the outset that could produce a positive inspiratory pressure were primarily designed to deliver bronchodilator aerosols to patients with chronic obstructive pulmonary disease (COPD) receiving these "treatments" through a mouthpiece. Operated from an oxygen cylinder, they could be adjusted to continue each inflation until a preset pressure was reached and could be set to repeat this to provide successive respiratory cycles. The oxygen flow used for inflation could be set to entrain room air, and they would either be adjusted to operate at a specific frequency or, in the case of the treatments, to have each inspiration triggered by the patient creating a negative airway pressure at the start of each breath. We used these until we could obtain something better. In respiratory units in Europe that were set up to handle patients with respiratory paralysis, the ventilators designed for the purpose were set to deliver specific tidal volumes, some with a maximum pressure. Inevitable then was the resulting controversy in the following years as to the relative merits of pressure limited, volume-variable versus volume-limited, pressure-variable ventilation, with or without patient-triggering and, in due course, intermittent mandatory ventilation. The author's preference was very much for volume-limited ventilation, and the hospital administration was very cooperative in purchasing the necessary equipment, initially from European sources (the Engstrom, Blease and Morch ventilators) and, later, from the United States when these came on the market and as the need became more universally obvious. At the same time, we purchased other equipment common to centers dealing with respiratory paralysis—a rocking bed and cuirass respirators, for example, although the latter were almost never used and the rocking bed very rarely.

---

[f] Critical care units with different origins were being set up around the world. For example, in 1960 Peter Safar described one set up (but yet to be defined as such) as an expansion of a postoperative recovery room at Baltimore City Hospital.

Monitoring patient progress
Vital signs were recorded every half hour and tracheobronchial secretions suctioned. Special charts had to be designed to record not only the vital signs but also the quantity, color, and consistency of the secretions.

As the initial *raison d'être* of the unit was to maintain adequate ventilation for patients with normal lungs but respiratory paralysis (such as in patients with polio), the objective of the respiratory support was seen as maintaining a minute volume sufficient to achieve adequate CO_2 elimination. PCO_2 and PO_2 measurements were not yet available, and so it was assumed that, if an adequate minute volume was maintained,[9] adequate gas exchange would follow. If the patient showed clinical signs of hypoxia such as cyanosis, then the inspired oxygen could be increased. If the ventilator was not adjustable to provide specific tidal volumes, a Wright respirometer could be inserted in line to provide ongoing volume measurements when determining the appropriate peak inspiratory pressure setting.

How best to ventilate an abnormal lung?
Very quickly, the emphasis on respiratory paralysis was diluted by the arrival of a few of Dr Colin Woolf's patients with pulmonary disease, particularly COPD, with flare-ups of their chronic respiratory tract infections. This created a new focus and new challenges. As we acquired new ventilators, we were interested first in seeing how they delivered each inspiration and then deciding the variables to monitor. In the laboratory, we "ventilated" oil drums filled with water to the level at which a given inspired volume generated the peak pressure representing the compliance to be studied. From this model, for example, we could observe the pressure–volume and volume–time curves, in response to differing downstream pressures. Immediately, it became clear that some ventilators delivered a constant flow and a "square wave" profile, whereas others were more gradual in reaching peak flow and pressure. These simple studies stimulated questions as to the best ways to inflate not only the normal lung but also lungs with parenchymal disease. These studies also raised questions of which variables were most important to monitor. From the start, pressure and volume were obviously important. However, to an anesthesiologist with special training in anesthesia for thoracic surgery who had watched umpteen normal and diseased lungs in the open chest receive IPP ventilation, it was an intriguing question as to what else mattered. Even in the normal lung, there are regional differences in compliance and airway resistance, in part related to gravity, but also to posture and the presence or absence of abdominal distension. It becomes complicated when regional disease is also considered, and therefore, this became of considerable interest to many of us in the years that ensued. Two of my own interests in the early days that were later discarded were the possible value of being able to have an online calculation of work of breathing as a measure of the status of the ventilated lung-thorax, and the use of an esophageal balloon to permit measurement of lung as opposed to lung-thorax status. Neither caught on at the time, although we did get as far as having a company produce gastric tubes with attached balloons that had a pressure measuring line incorporated, and more recently, interest has returned regarding the potential use of esophageal manometry.

Weaning from the ventilator
Weaning patients involved considerable trial and error until the most useful indicators of likely success could be recognized. The availability of a patient-triggering setting on

---

[9] Determined by referring to the Radford nomogram that related normal tidal volume and frequency to body weight (and sex).

ventilators was of assistance in the transition from completely controlled to assisted ventilation. Moreover, eventually, measurements such as the vital capacity and blood gas measurements, coupled with the status of the underlying condition, were used to assist in when to start a trial of spontaneous respiration.

Management of secretions

There were no suction catheters designed for the purpose of suctioning through endotracheal tubes or tracheostomies, so we used red rubber urinary catheters that were cleaned and sterilized after each use. At each bedside, there was a container filled with an antiseptic solution, ready to receive these catheters after use. The initial ventilators were used to deliver an aerosol of sterile water on each inspiratory cycle but this was quite inadequate, and various in-line water containers were then used. It was not until later, in the 1960s, that for-the-purpose in-line humidifiers with heaters appeared on the market. In patients with normal lungs and respiratory paralysis, it was common to find that secretions would collect in dependent parts of the bronchial tree, and so the patient would be turned from side to side and chest physiotherapy administered twice daily.[h] If atelectasis occurred, this was initially managed by "artificial coughing." With the patient in the lateral position and the atelectatic side uppermost, a large positive pressure inspiration would be delivered, and the physiotherapist would then compress the chest to assist and produce an exaggerated, somewhat rapid expiration, followed by chest percussion then tracheo-bronchial "toilet."

Complications and Unanticipated Situations

Tracheal stenosis

Initially, our cuffed endotracheal and tracheostomy tubes were made of red rubber and reusable. As mentioned above, careful attention was paid to the degree to which the cuff was inflated. In due course, the red rubber tubes were replaced by disposable ones made of plastic (polyvinyl chloride [PVC]). As we moved on in the 1960s, our volume of patients was increasing and some developed subglottic edema following extubation, sometimes with stenosis and respiratory difficulty. In the more severe cases, a tracheostomy below the stenosis was necessary. The initial assumption was that this was secondary to excessive cuff pressure that had caused ischemia in the tracheal mucosa. Although this complication was becoming recognized in North America, it was not a feature in the United Kingdom or in Scandinavian countries, and it eventually turned out that the cause lay in the different manufacturing process of the tubes used on the 2 sides of the Atlantic. The US manufacturer was using organotin as a stabilizer in the PVC production process, and this tissue-toxic substance was leaching out and causing the damage.[4] The European companies' process did not use organotin.[i]

Pulmonary "consolidation"

It was not unusual that a patient would develop radiologic opacities in the lung fields. The cause was frequently clinically obvious bronchopneumonia but there were situations where this was not the case. The acute respiratory distress syndrome had yet to be described, and 2 possibilities were commonly entertained. One was the possibility that prolonged IPP might cause alveolar damage, particularly when high inflation pressures were used. Certainly, the occasional tension pneumothorax occurred for this

---

[h] Passive movement of paralyzed limbs was applied routinely during these physiotherapist visits.

[i] Before this was sorted out, the thoracic surgeons became skilled in excision of the stenotic area in the more severe cases and, on occasion, implanting prosthetic tubing.

reason.[j] The other possibility came to the fore when 1 or 2 patients with "consolidation" in the lungs went to autopsy. The histology was described as being very similar to that seen in experimental oxygen toxicity. This possibility was in due course supported by our finding that one of the most commonly used pressure-limited ventilators that was by then in use worldwide (The Bird, Mark 7) and that was claimed to deliver 40% oxygen by entraining room air into a venturi was, in fact, delivering a percentage that varied directly with the patient's airway pressure.[5] Thus, as increasing consolidation occurred and compliance decreased, requiring higher peak pressures, less air was entrained and the inspired oxygen level increased. That device disappeared from the market shortly thereafter.

Accidental airway disconnection

A major problem was the possibility of the ventilator becoming disconnected from the endotracheal or tracheotomy tube, with obviously disastrous consequence when it went unnoticed. This caused us to design a disconnect alarm based on a pressure switch connected by tubing to a t-piece at the airway.[6] This approach was so effective at reducing complications from ventilator disconnections that we required one of these to be connected in line any time a patient was receiving mechanical ventilation at TGH. These alarms were initially built in our laboratory for TGH use but, in due course, their successors became a feature incorporated in all new ventilators coming to the market.

Prolonging the disease course

We provided ongoing respiratory support beyond the point at which, in some instances, death would otherwise have occured. Therefore, we found ourselves dealing with situations that are all too familiar now but were new to us then. Moreover, decision-making that required accurate prognostication was hampered by our not having experienced many of the situations before. Of course, when the support provided time for recovery from the underlying disease—the object of the exercise—this was very gratifying. However, the alternatives were new to us. For example, if the disease in a patient with respiratory paralysis or crippling pulmonary pathologic condition was not going to resolve, the new technique of IPP support could prolong life, perhaps indefinitely. An early example of this was a young ambulatory adult with gross kyphoscoliosis-related pulmonary compromise, and pneumonia, who required mechanical ventilation. When discharged, it was entirely possible that this individual would experience a recurrence and return to the Unit. We worried that on that second admission he might not be able to be weaned from ventilation. We discussed whether subsequent intubation and ventilation should even be undertaken, and the opinion that prevailed was that it should. That situation did arise, and the individual remained hospitalized with mechanical ventilation for decades while working part-time in the hospital's secretarial pool. A quite different scenario was the new possibility of permitting a patient to live while experiencing previously unthought of discomfort because the disease process progressed sometimes far beyond the previously observed lethal stage. One such example was an alert patient with 2 disease processes requiring conflicting therapy: advanced myasthenia gravis requiring respiratory support that worsened when steroids were administered to treat pemphigus covering a large proportion of his body including face and eyelids, which required tarsorrhaphy. He experienced severe discomfort without ultimate benefit from the treatment.

---

[j] In later years, it was shown that, posthospitalization, some prolonged mechanical ventilation had not impaired lung function.

Coupled with our inexperience with dealing with this level of patient care was our lack of insight into how to interact not only with the patients but also with the relatives. Compared with today, little information was provided, particularly to family members. A variation on this theme was the fact that a patient who would otherwise have died, and on occasion was "brain dead," was being maintained only if we continued support. The question then was whether we should withdraw support and, if so, when and how best to interact with the family. Looking back during the decades, each of us dealt with this in their own way, particularly in terms of conversation with the patients' families and with the patient, if conscious. I can remember only a very few instances where we, as an interdisciplinary group, discussed the best way to proceed with a specific patient (but did not always agree as to whether and how to continue). We never engaged in regular prescheduled patient reviews, as would be the case today. These were always handled on an impromptu basis and frequently during chance presences together in the Unit.

Patient psyche
A few aspects of a situation that is now better understood emerged from the beginning. Patients with obviously severe medical conditions found themselves isolated in strange surroundings and, if receiving mechanical ventilation, frequently not able to communicate. It was easy for visiting personnel, medical or otherwise, who were unfamiliar with the situation to assume the patient could not hear. Therefore, conversations often did not get modified and could be upsetting to patients. This was particularly the case when the underlying condition caused facial paralysis or the patient was paralyzed but incompletely sedated.

Fully conscious patients not able to see a clock or the outdoors could feel trapped in a very threatening situation. I recall a new unit at the Mayo Clinic being constructed in a circular format, with individual glass-walled patient rooms around the circumference, and the nurses' station in the middle. Each room had a large window to the outside and a wall clock. The patient could see help was available even if his or her nurse was out of the room. The intention was to allay some of the fears mentioned above.

Referrals and transport
As the success of the Unit became known not only to the medical staff at TGH but also at other institutions in the region, patients with increasing respiratory difficulty would sometimes be sent by ambulance without respiratory support and unaccompanied by skilled staff. On a few occasions, this resulted in serious consequences. When a cardio-respiratory arrest occurred on the way to the hospital, and another in the corridor leading to the Unit, all TGH medical staff were advised not to accept a referral without prior confirmation from one of the Unit's medical staff. We arranged with the leading ambulance company in the area to equip an ambulance with a step-up transformer that would permit a portable ventilator and suction equipment to operate. The trip would initiate from TGH, picking up an anesthesiologist and equipment before proceeding to bring the patient to TGH with the necessary support.

Disappearing conditions and their treatment
Two examples of this come to mind. Our early publications describing the types of patients we had treated included those with "stove-in chest" and tetanus. The former was an unfortunately well-recognized injury in the years preceding mandatory seat belts that arose from head-on motor vehicle accidents. The driver would be thrown against the steering wheel while being squeezed between it and the seat back as the momentum moved the whole seat forward. In the worst cases, multiple parasternal rib fractures would result in a "flail chest" with the anterior chest wall being drawn

inward on each gasping inspiration. This mechanical difficulty would be coupled with pulmonary bruising and serious respiratory difficulty. In the case of tetanus, universal vaccination has removed tetanus as one of the causes for admission to the ICU but, before that, the standard treatment included paralysis with muscle relaxants and IPP ventilation. Among our first 100 cases, we reported 8 with stove-in chest, 7 of whom survived, and 1 with tetanus who did not.

The advent of blood gas measurements in the clinical arena

Once electrodes that could measure PCO_2 and then PO_2 were developed, these were combined with a pH electrode into a single unit to provide the significant data with which we are now so familiar. In the early 1960s, we obtained the equipment developed by the Instrumentation Laboratory Company (Bedford, MA) and made the measurements Challenges of ICU Care in the Unit. We found Poul Astrup's use of the "blood buffer base" to be very useful. Of course, while the CO_2 and pH values from the arterial blood were important, the newly available PaO_2 measurements were completely transformative in the focus of respiratory management and in expanding our knowledge of pulmonary gas exchange. As an understanding of the use of this information spread among the hospital's medical staff, the blood gas equipment was transferred to the hospital's Clinical Laboratory, and a new era of respiratory care and related research began.

If I knew then what I know now..........

REFERENCES

1. Barber HO, Chambers RA, Fairley HB, et al. A respiratory unit: the Toronto General Hospital unit for the treatment of severe respiratory insufficiency. Can Med Assoc J 1959;81:97–101.
2. Fairley HB, Chambers RA. The management of the patient with respiratory insufficiency. Can Anaesth Soc J 1960;7:447–90.
3. Brown KW, MacMillan RL, Forbath N, et al. Coronary unit: an intensive care centre for acute myocardial infarction. Lancet 1963;2:349–52.
4. Guess WL, Stetson JB. Tissue reactions to organotin-stabilized polyvinyl chloride (PVC) catheters. JAMA 1968;204:580–4.
5. Fairley HB, Britt BA. The adequacy of the air-mix control in ventilators operated from an oxygen source. Can Med Assoc J 1964;90:1394–6.
6. Lamont A, Fairley HB. A pressure-sensitive ventilator alarm. Anesthesiology 1965; 26:359–61.

Mechanical Ventilation
Negative to Positive and Back Again

Laurent J. Brochard, MD[a,b],*

KEYWORDS

- Positive-pressure ventilation • Negative-pressure ventilation
- Ventilation-induced lung injury • Acute respiratory distress syndrome
- Acute respiratory failure • Respiratory physiology • Heart–lung interaction

KEY POINTS

- Historically, the first forms of mechanical ventilation were essentially noninvasive and using negative pressure.
- During the last 30 years, noninvasive positive-pressure ventilation extended its indications, with a large use during the recent COVID-19 pandemic.
- Tidal volume adjustment was initially based on the need to prevent atelectasis in the operating room. It took more than 30 years to prove tidal volumes were often excessive in the intensive care unit.
- The history of positive end-expiratory pressure is as long as the history of care for the adult (acute) respiratory distress syndrome and is ongoing.

During the poliomyelitis epidemics, the "iron lung" was a form of noninvasive ventilation (NIV).[1,2] Despite saving many lives, the "iron lung" had its limitations: it was cumbersome, allowed a limited access to the patient and was poorly efficient in its ability to treat parenchymal lung disease or to clear secretions. The later use of invasive positive-pressure ventilation allowed a more effective delivery of mechanical assistance through the endotracheal tube providing direct access to the lower airway. Since its introduction in the 1950s, positive-pressure ventilation became the standard form of mechanical ventilation (MV), coupling the patient to a ventilator through an endotracheal tube or a tracheostomy cannula. Because of the invasiveness of positive-pressure ventilation and its complications, newer forms of NIV came back in the intensive care unit (ICU) after several decades and, today, both types of techniques, invasive and noninvasive, have their respective indications.

[a] Keenan Research Centre, St Michael's Hospital, Unity Health Toronto, 209 Victoria Street, Room 4-08, Toronto, Ontario M5B 1T8, Canada; [b] Interdepartmental Division of Critical Care Medicine, University of Toronto, Toronto, Canada
* Corresponding author. Li Ka Shing Knowledge Institute - Keenan Research Centre, 209 Victoria Street, 4th Floor, Room 408, Toronto, ON M5B 1T8.
E-mail address: Laurent.Brochard@unityhealth.to

Crit Care Clin 39 (2023) 437–449
https://doi.org/10.1016/j.ccc.2022.12.002
0749-0704/23/© 2022 Elsevier Inc. All rights reserved.

It is useful to go back to this history,[1] and in this article, we will go through several examples of similar changes and alternative visions for the delivery of MV,[2] which offer an interesting perspective on the way we modify our knowledge and beliefs over time.

HISTORY

Galen was a Greek philosopher, writer, and physician (129 – c. AD 216) with a bright but also limited theory about the function of the human body, who described human physiology as influenced by the four humors (black bile, yellow bile, blood, and phlegm), and this was accepted for ...approximately 1300 years. It needed some brave pioneers to challenge the dogma and start the history of modern anatomy and physiology. Dissection of animal and human bodies had a fundamental importance to try to understand how the organs functioned, and therefore, this new anatomical knowledge helped to reinvent physiology while challenging what was thought to be the truth. These pioneers included Andreas Vesalius (1514–1564) whose famous anatomy lessons showed that insufflating air with a pipe in the trachea could insufflate the lungs[3] (**Fig. 1**), and Miguel Servet (1511–1553) who reasoned out the role of circulation in the lung, observing that the blood became pink and aerated after passing through the lungs in the pulmonary circulation. Although Servet's views proved ultimately to be correct, this was published in a theology book, *Christianismi Restitutio*, in which he also challenged the dogma of the Trinity, which set both Catholics and Protestants against him. His writings were considered heretical at the time, and he was subsequently burned at the stake—along with most copies of his book— in 1553 in Geneva. The pulmonary circulation was more completely described a few years later (1578–1657) by William Harvey. The concept of artificial respiration needed to wait longer and was mostly developed for the treatment of nearly-drowned persons from the eighteenth century to the first quarter of the nineteenth century, and included some of the artificial internal ventilation techniques or principles of today. Interestingly, Leroy d'Étiolles published and presented an "alarming" dissertation in 1827, underlining the pleuro-pulmonary risks of endotracheal insufflation—as a visionary description of ventilator-induced lung injury—and recommended

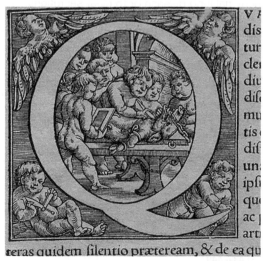

V ʃ
dis
tur
clei
dit
diſ
mu
tis
dif
un
ipſi
qu
ac
art

ʃeras quidem ſilentio præteream, & de ea qu

Fig. 1. The initial "Q" showing vivisection experiment and tracheostomy on a pig, by Vesalius.

external manual methods instead.[4] Positive-pressure techniques were abandoned in part because of these debates. In 1854, Eugene Woillez described the Spirophore, a forerunner of the future Iron Lung. This negative-pressure ventilator was hand powered by the use of bellows and adjusted to the body with a neck collar but there are no reports of its clinical use.

THE IRON LUNG

Other inventors used the principle of negative pressure around the body (Dr Alfred Jones who used a prototype in a patient) but it is only in 1928 that Dr Phillip Drinker (1894–1972) and Dr Louis Agassiz Shaw (1886–1940), faculty members at Harvard University, developed the first widely used negative pressure "respiration apparatus."[5] The bellows generated pressures down to −60 cmH20 with rates from 10 to 40 breaths per minute. The iron lung was later "improved" in a different version by Emerson in 1931, after a fight over patents that he eventually won.

These negative-pressure tanks, or "iron lungs," were used clinically for patients suffering from poliomyelitis with respiratory insufficiency, and several centers in the United States became well-equipped with these devices because of generous donations (they were expensive) during the first half of the twentieth century and into the 1950s. They were rarely used for patients without polio, were large and cumbersome for provision of nursing care, and offered no airway protection. During the same time period, positive-pressure ventilators were invented for patients in the operating room but were not in routine use, and were viewed as safe only for short-term care.

POSITIVE-PRESSURE VENTILATION

The demonstration that prolonged, positive-pressure ventilation was a safe and effective means of respiratory support came during a Copenhagen polio epidemic. A severe polio outbreak took place starting in July 1952, possibly because one year earlier an international conference on polio was held in this city (physicians and patients attended what would be called today a super spreader event). In the summer of 1952 in Copenhagen, dozens of patients were suffering from respiratory forms of polio with an extremely high mortality. The Blegdam Hospital, the infectious disease hospital, had only one iron lung and 6 cuirass respirators. Bjørn Ibsen, an anesthesiologist who had spent some training period in Boston where he had noted that a patient was easy to ventilate in the operating room with a tracheostomy, proposed to tracheostomize the patients and hand-ventilate them.[6] This was done with the help of hundreds of medical students at the bedside. Dramatically, the mortality dropped from 87% to ∼30% in the following weeks, and, after the publication of the results by Lassen[7] (the Chief physician at the Blegdam), positive-pressure ventilation subsequently became the norm for the management of respiratory failure, with dedicated personnel taking care of the patients on a 24 h/7 d basis. This defined what was soon going to be called an ICU. Soon after, the first electrodes used for blood gas measurements were developed and described by Severinghaus (CO_2) and Clark (O_2), and subsequently used to help in adjusting ventilation.[8] Claus Bang, a Danish physician, and Carl-Gunnar Engström, a Swedish anesthesiologist, developed some of the first efficient mechanical ventilators.[9] Positive-pressure ventilators were designed around the globe, such as the Morch Piston respirator in the United States, and the Draeger Spiromat in Europe. These were followed by more flexible ventilators such as the Bird Mark 7, with all of them delivering different forms of positive-pressure ventilation. The Servo 900 (Siemens-Elema, Solna, Sweden) invented in Sweden (by Bjorn Jonson a clinical physiologist and a team of an anesthesiologist, surgeon and engineer) was released in 1972 and was the first mechanical ventilator with a valve for adjusting a real positive end-expiratory pressure (PEEP) as we understand it today. The "scissor" servo valves controlling the flow allowed the introduction of new modes of ventilation such as pressure-controlled ventilation and pressure support ventilation (PSV).[10] Ventilators became progressively more compact, user-friendly, and electronically driven, and much less based on predominantly pneumatic systems. These devices used precision valves, such as electromagnetic servo-valves, and incorporated a host of modes of ventilation and advanced monitoring capabilities.[2]

VENTILATION DURING CARDIOPULMONARY RESUSCITATION

In his "memoire sur l'asphyxie" to the French Academy of Sciences, Leroy d'Etiolles described in 1826 the terrible effects on the lungs of forced insufflation directly into the trachea of rabbits, rapidly leading to their deaths with lesions looking like pulmonary hemorrhage, pneumothoraces, diaphragm distension, and circulatory collapse. His conclusions were a strong opposition to the use of bellows inserted in the trachea as an attempt to resuscitate human beings, and he gave a strong warning against what we would refer to today as high tidal volume ventilation.

For resuscitation, the next major date was 1960 when a description of the closed chest cardiac massage technique as a simple and revolutionary method to maintain circulation during a cardiac arrest was published.[11] Soon after, Peter Safar and coworkers demonstrated that positive-pressure ventilation was also required for adequate resuscitation, either in the form of mouth-to-mouth ventilation or with a self-inflating bag or a ventilator.[12] They showed that, in most cases, no air movement could be generated by chest compressions alone, despite actively compressing and decompressing the chest. They pointed first to the obstruction of the upper airways as one of the reasons for this absence of air displacement (putting "Airway" first in their "ABC" for resuscitation). However, this lack of ventilation also happened in intubated patients. It is only very recently (50 years later approximately) that intrathoracic airway closure was understood as a pathophysiological phenomenon contributing to this impediment to ventilation.[13]

NONINVASIVE VENTILATION COMING BACK IN THE INTENSIVE CARE UNIT

Novel NIV techniques started to be used in parallel at the end of the 1980s both for home ventilation in chronic patients who needed respiratory support, and for care of acute patients in ICUs.

Home Mechanical Ventilation for Chronic Respiratory Failure

Home MV had been traditionally delivered through tracheostomies, mostly in patients with severe chronic restrictive—and much less frequently obstructive respiratory disorders—with varying results in terms of long-term survival. At the end of the 1980s, concerns about the quality of life for these patients prompted the testing and use of noninvasive techniques, some of which had previously been considered only for polio patients with respiratory sequelae.[14–16] With the main objective of improving patients' quality of life for people who otherwise needed a tracheostomy for home ventilation, home NIV was progressively implemented. Later, manufacturers devoted considerable technological effort to develop specific home ventilators for "leaky" ventilation and to provide comfortable and adaptable interfaces. The recognition that major sleep disturbances could be caused by abnormal respiration has also contributed to the widespread use of different kinds of home ventilatory support.[17] NIV progressively became, therefore, the standard of care for home MV, especially for patients with restrictive lung diseases.

Acute Respiratory Failure

Soon after the introduction of endotracheal MV and positive-pressure ventilation in the ICU, complications of this technique were identified. These complications generated concerns about the "invasiveness" of MV and raised the possibility of avoiding this technique while still supporting the patient. Endotracheal intubation (ETI) and the tube itself were implicated in a large number of complications. Some were directly related to the intubation procedure, such as cardiac arrest at time of ETI, and laryngeal or tracheal injury leading to long-term sequelae.[18] Others were ascribable to the fact that the endotracheal tube bypasses the barrier of the upper airway, setting the stage for ventilator-associated pneumonia that carries its own risk of morbidity and mortality. MV also required sedation, which is itself a cause of a prolonged duration of MV. These major safety considerations prompted efforts to develop noninvasive methods for delivering positive-pressure ventilation.[19] Therefore, in parallel with the development of home NIV, clinicians started to demonstrate a major interest in this technique in the late 1980s and early 1990s as a way to avoid ETI in the acute care setting. This development took place at the time where a new mode of ventilation called PSV appeared on ICU ventilators.[20] This mode seemed to offer flexibility to adapt to spontaneously breathing patients. The possibility to deliver pressure with a decelerating flow profile in a reasonably well-synchronized manner was an interesting improvement, augmenting the acceptance of the technique.

In patients with acute respiratory failure, the main goal of NIV was to provide ventilatory assistance while lowering the risk of adverse events by reducing the need for invasive MV. Convincing evidence that NIV diminishes the risk of infectious complications has been obtained from randomized controlled trials and meta-analyses, and from large cohort studies and case-control studies, which showed substantial decreases in all categories of nosocomial infection.[21] NIV was associated with a reduction in the overall invasiveness of patient management: sedation was not given or at low levels, and there was less, or shorter, use of central venous lines, urinary catheters, and other invasive devices compared with patients receiving endotracheal MV. Another factor favoring the use of NIV has been the growing number of patients who are unwilling to accept ETI or who are considered poor candidates for endotracheal MV because of a fragile underlying health status.[22] By postponing ETI, NIV could also provide a window of opportunity for the physician, family, and patient to make informed decisions about the goals of therapy.

Exacerbations of Chronic Respiratory Failure

Numerous studies have now demonstrated the utility and benefits of the application of facemask NIV for exacerbations of chronic obstructive pulmonary disease (COPD). In the early 1990s, this was new, and both physiological studies and randomized clinical trials demonstrated that intubation could be avoided due to a reduction in a patient's effort to breathe and an improvement in alveolar ventilation allowing a reduction in the mortality related to exacerbations.[23,24] Technical improvements in the interface (oronasal mask, total facial mask, and later helmet) came (**Fig. 2**), as well as technical progress in the ventilators delivering NIV, either using dedicated NIV modes on ICU ventilators or using dedicated turbine-based portable ventilators for delivering the two levels of positive-pressure required.[25–27] Since 2007, the Global Initiative for Chronic Obstructive Lung Disease (https://goldcopd.org/) reinforced the importance of NIV when treating COPD exacerbations with a high level of evidence (Evidence A)

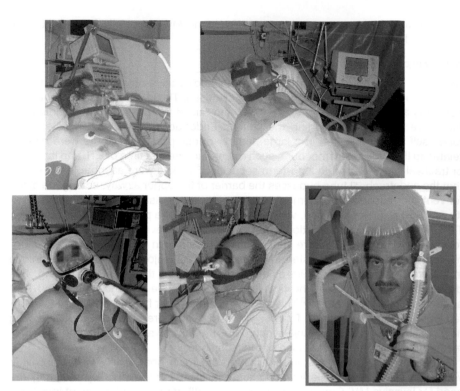

Fig. 2. Five different interfaces used for noninvasive ventilation: oronasal mask, oral full-face mask, another oral full-face mask, mouth-piece, and helmet for the latter. (*Courtesy of* Prof. Massimo Antonelli, shown on the picture using the helmet, Rome, Italy.)

based on its considerable rate of success (80%–85%) in this clinical situation. A Cochrane database review observed in 2017 that facemask NIV decreases mortality, reduces the need for intubation, has less treatment failure and faster clinical improvement, as well as reduces treatment complications and length of hospital stay compared with a classical treatment including oxygen, medications and ETI as clinically indicated.[28] An international consensus conference in 2017 recommended that facemask NIV-PSV should be considered as a first-line treatment in patients with COPD exacerbation and different national guidelines advocated this practice.[29] In an analysis of more than 7 million of admissions for COPD exacerbations in the United States from 1998 to 2008, of which 8.1% required respiratory support, an increase in the use of NIV could be demonstrated over time (1.0% increasing to 4.5% of admissions) with a 42% decline in invasive MV (from 6.0% down to 3.5% of admissions). Intubation and in-hospital mortality declined during this period and, by 2008, NIV was used more frequently than invasive MV as the first-line therapy for this indication.

Today, the epidemiology of chronic respiratory failure has changed. Many patients are admitted with "undifferentiated hypercapnic respiratory failure" in the emergency department or in ICU.[30,31] Obesity has become a major cause of acute hypercapnic episodes, sometimes due to pure obesity hypoventilation, sometimes mixed with cardiac failure, airway disease, or COPD.[32] Among these more mixed chronic respiratory failure groups, the available data suggest that NIV prevents subsequent deterioration and need for intubation at least as efficiently as for patients with pure COPD, although less evidence is available.

Hypoxemic Respiratory Failure and COVID-19

Advances in the technology also made possible the wider use of NIV, which started to be employed for other indications, such as hypoxemic respiratory failure. In acute hypoxemic respiratory failure, NIV had frequently moderate success rates and the risks of delaying intubation associated with prolonged NIV use have been debated.[33,34] There have been large fluctuations in the use of invasive MV for patients with hypoxemic respiratory failure during the coronavirus disease 2019 (COVID-19) pandemic. During the initial wave of patients with COVID-19-induced acute respiratory distress syndrome, very high rates of ETI were observed, and there were some strong signals indicating that the high-intubation rate observed initially could have resulted in an excessive numbers of patients receiving invasive MV, resulting in harm to patients.[35] The use of NIV was progressively favored, and later during the pandemic, numerous studies, including randomized clinical trials (RCTs), demonstrated that noninvasive techniques (including high-flow nasal cannula, NIV, continuous positive airway pressure [CPAP], and helmet NIV) could be used successfully to prevent ETI. These results recently described during the COVID-19 pandemic, confirm meta-analysis of previous studies in non-COVID patients that NIV techniques have now several possible indications to prevent intubation for patients with acute hypoxemic respiratory failure.[36]

Cardiogenic Pulmonary Edema

Positive pressure applied at the mouth was shown in the 1930s to improve patients' dyspnea in case of cardiogenic pulmonary edema.[37,38] In 1936, Poulton explained that "...acute pulmonary edema of circulatory origin was due to incoordination between the right and left ventricle such that the volume of blood delivered per minute into the pulmonary circulation is not completely passed on into the systemic circulation by the left ventricle creating congestion of the pulmonary circulation and local rise of blood pressure."[37] He showed that the use of "...the pulmonary plus pressure machine" applied with a face mask was beneficial for the symptomatic relief of the patient by "providing pressure in the air passages of the lungs, so as to oppose the increase of intrapulmonary blood pressure." The device was an "inverted" vacuum cleaner (properly cleaned before use to avoid delivering dust). He mentioned that the optimum pressure must be "determined experimentally, using the patient's feelings as a guide." They also described trying the machine out on some cases of bronchial asthma.

Evidence of therapeutic efficacy of positive pressure use during acute pulmonary edema was only formally shown in 1991 in a randomized trial of 39 patients assigned to conventional oxygen therapy or facemask CPAP of 10 cm H_2O.[39] The interventional group showed improvement of gas exchange, a decrease of respiratory rate, and a lower intubation rate. Subsequently, additional randomized trials comparing either CPAP or NIV to standard therapy found similar benefits.

A QUICK STORY OF POSITIVE END-EXPIRATORY PRESSURE FOR ADULT (ACUTE) RESPIRATORY DISTRESS SYNDROME

A major step in the evolution of MV was the use of PEEP. Although the application of PEEP was first described in the 1930s,[37,38] it came into common use for treating respiratory failure at the end of the 1960s, mainly encouraged by the identification of the adult (acute) respiratory distress syndrome (ARDS). Ashbaugh and colleagues described the ARDS in a seminal article published in the *Lancet* (the article had been rejected by 3 journals previously).[40] They mentioned that, to prevent an immediate death from hypoxemia, the use of PEEP provided an apparent benefit (more precisely, they used the "expiratory retard knob" that they discovered on the Engstrom ventilator). However, in the intervening 50 years, a clear consensus around how to manage PEEP in general, and for patients with ARDS specifically, has remained elusive despite a series of RCTs comparing high versus low PEEP.[41,42]

Traditionally, PEEP has been used to improve oxygenation in ARDS. PEEP was found to be "very helpful to prevent atelectasis and to combat hypoxemia" by Ashbaugh and colleagues.[40] Rapidly, however, it became unclear whether the goal should be to simply avoid lethal hypoxemia or to improve oxygenation as much as possible and decrease the inspired oxygen fraction. This latter idea was supported by the early notion that part of the lung injury observed in the cases of patients dying while on a ventilator was mostly the result of oxygen toxicity. Indeed, the "ventilator lung," as it has been referred to, looked very much like oxygen toxicity on autopsy studies.[43] In the following years, multiple oxygenation targets, based on a minimal FiO_2 or shunt values, have been proposed. Using high PEEP was also soon recognized to induce hemodynamic alterations.[44] Some authors considered that it was a necessary side effect, easily controlled by fluids and hemodynamic support, whereas others tried to find the best balance between gas exchange and effects on cardiac output. Falke and colleagues[45] first described the relationships between lung mechanics, lung volumes, gas exchange, and hemodynamics, and this concept was superbly articulated later by Suter and colleagues in 1972.[46] These authors showed that oxygen transport, the product of oxygen content and cardiac output, reached a maximum level—the so-called optimum—when increasing PEEP, before being reduced for higher PEEP values, alongside parallel changes in respiratory system compliance and despite a continuous improvement in PaO_2. Soon after, it was also demonstrated that a decrease in cardiac output induced by PEEP was, in itself, causing better oxygenation.[44] The idea behind PEEP titration was, therefore, to find the most efficient way to increase oxygen delivery to the tissue, as well as using the best surrogate to make it available and feasible at the bedside. The goal was the best oxygen transport, and compliance was then the best surrogate target for titration of PEEP but, unfortunately, there are multiple ways to titrate PEEP and to subsquently measure and interpret compliance.[47] In the studies looking at the effects of PEEP, these fundamental interactions of circulation, oxygenation, and oxygen transport have been progressively forgotten, in part, because of the abandonment of the pulmonary artery catheter in the ICU (which is another story).

Another mechanical approach for titrating PEEP has been the use of the pressure–volume curve to better understand changes in lung mechanics over a large lung volume and find the best pressure to "physically" reopen the lung.[48–50] This technique has also been the first mechanical descriptor for quantifying lung recruitment.[50,51] Reopening the lung seemed necessary for better gas exchange but also, perhaps, for helping to "cure the disease" by combating the consequences of repeated opening and closure. Subsequently, because the evidence of risks of distension-induced lung injury became more apparent from experimental studies, reaching the upper part of the curve where distension occurred was proposed as something to be avoided, providing an incentive to reduce tidal volume in clinical practice.[52] Many different strategies have since been proposed for titrating PEEP as a way to avoid recruitment/derecruitment but hypoxemia has remained the most frequent clinical target for PEEP titration because it was felt to be the simplest surrogate available at the bedside.[53] Moreover, treating hypoxemia was often perceived, erroneously to a large extent, as a cure for the disease. Although there are differences in the design and clinical results among the RCTs that compared low versus high PEEP,[54–56] none has demonstrated a reduction in mortality when testing PEEP alone. One possible reason may be a lack of individualization of the PEEP titration in these studies. Indeed, increasing PEEP has different effects depending on the potential for lung recruitability and studies demonstrate a large variability in lung recruitability among patients with ARDS.[57] Therefore, the benefit/risk balance could differ markedly between patients depending on their individual potential for recruitment.[58] We may not yet be at the end of the PEEP story for ARDS.

TIDAL VOLUME

In 1963, Bendixen and colleagues[59] published a very influential study addressing whether the pattern of ventilation, by itself, could influence oxygenation during anesthesia and surgery. In 18 patients, they could show how oxygenation was falling dramatically when applying shallow ventilation during anesthesia for the surgical procedure. Their results supported the hypothesis that progressive mechanical atelectasis leads to increased venous admixture to arterial blood by shunting in atelectatic areas. This was further illustrated by the reversibility of the fall in oxygen tension that followed hyperinflation. These convincing data were used to set the ventilator not only in the operating room but also rapidly in the ICU, especially because oxygenation was seen as the primary problem of patients with ARDS.[60] Therefore, for years, it has not been uncommon to use tidal volumes up to 20 mL/kg to ventilate patients with ARDS in an attempt to try to reach normal blood gases.

Experimental studies by Webb and Tierney in 1974[61] and later by Dreyfuss and Saumon and others in a series of illuminating experiments in the 1990s[62,63] demonstrated the direct injury generated to the lungs by excessive tidal volumes (back to Leroy d E'tiolles). Because of this strong experimental evidence and of physiological observations in patients, for the first time in 1993 a consensus conference chaired by AS Slutsky mentioned that "...alveolar overdistention could cause alveolar damage or air leaks (barotrauma) and maneuvers to prevent the development of excess alveolar (or transpulmonary) pressure should be instituted if necessary. While recognizing that the causes of ventilator-induced lung injury are multifactorial ...the consensus committee generally believed that end-inspiratory occlusion pressure (i.e., plateau pressure) was the best, clinically applicable estimate of average peak alveolar pressure...and many individuals on the consensus committee believed that high plateau pressures (>35 cm H^2O) may be more harmful in most patients than high values of FiO_2." The approach of favoring limited tidal volume to minimize pressures and accepting hypercapnia had already been proposed for patients with severe asthma by Darioli and Perret in 1984,[64] and in obstructive lung disease by Tuxen and Lane in 1987,[65] following the seminal study of Pepe and Marini on auto-PEEP.[66] Hickling had been the first to propose the concept of permissive hypercapnia in 1990 for ARDS.[67] However, it is only in 2000, that the reality of harm due to excessive tidal volume was strongly demonstrated by ARMA, a clinical trial from the ARDS Network.[68] A tidal volume of 6 mL/kg of predicted body weight has since largely been accepted to be used as a default value. Later, the demonstration that the driving pressure was the best simple available marker for the risk of ventilator-induced lung injury[69] raised new discussions about adapting the tidal volume to such a measurement instead of using one size for all.[70] Once again, the story has not reached a definitive conclusion.

SUMMARY

Looking back at the history of MV tells us two things: (1) we have made enormous progress during a relatively short amount of time since the birth of the modern management of acute respiratory failure and (2) things have so frequently changed in opposite directions that we need to continue to keep our minds open to new concepts and consider our current knowledge with some humility.

CLINICS CARE POINTS

- History tells us that our vision of pathophysiology continuously evolves, and this has important clinical implications.
- Our primary reasoning is based on physiological evidence but needs experimental and clinical confirmation.
- Some major adaptations of MV are justified by a less risky or harmful approach (fewer complications of intubation, lfewer hemodynamic effects, less injury due to ventilation) but require a careful thinking regarding the trade-offs and the consequences of new approaches.

CONFLICTS OF INTEREST

L.J. Brochard's laboratory received research grants from Medtronic, Draeger, Vitalaire and Stimit; equipment from Sentec, Fisher Paykel and Philips; lecture fees from Fisher Paykel.

REFERENCES

1. Slutsky A. History of mechanical ventilation: from Vesalius to ventilator-induced lung injury. Am J Respir Crit Care Med 2015;19:1106–15.
2. Kacmarek R. The mechanical ventilator: past, present, and future. Respir Care 2011;56:1170–80.
3. Vesalius A. De humani corporis fabrica. Basel, Switzerland: Johannes Oporinus; 1543.
4. d'Étiolles L. Second Mémoire sur l'Asphyxie. Académie des Sci 1828;8:97–135.
5. Drinker P, Shaw L. An apparatus for the prolonged administration of artificial respiration, I: a design for adults and children. J Clin Invest 1929;72:229–47.
6. Ibsen B. The anæsthetist's viewpoint on the treatment of respiratory complications in poliomyelitis during the epidemic in Copenhagen, 1952. Proc R Soc Med 1954;47:72–4.
7. Lassen H. A preliminary report on the 1952 epidemic of poliomyelitis in Copenhagen with special reference to the treatment of acute respiratory insufficiency. Lancet 1953;6749:37–41.
8. Severinghaus JW. The invention and development of blood gas analysis apparatus. Anesthesiology 2002;97:253–6.
9. Engström C-G. Treatment of severe cases of respiratory paralysis by the Engström universal respirator. Br Med J 1954;2:666–9.
10. Ingelstedt S, Jonson B, Nordström L, et al. A servocontrolled ventilator measuring expired minute volume, airway flow and pressure. Acta Anaesthesiol Scand Suppl 1972;47:7–27.
11. Kouwenhoven WB, Jude JR, Knickerbocker GG. Closed-chest cardiac massAGE. JAMA 1960;173:1064–7.
12. Safar P, Brown TC, Holtey WJ, et al. Ventilation and circulation with closed-chest cardiac massage in man. JAMA 1961;574:92–4.

13. Grieco DL, Brochard L, Drouet A, et al. Intrathoracic airway closure impacts CO2 signal and delivered ventilation during cardiopulmonary resuscitation. Am J Respir Crit Care Med 2019;199:728–37.
14. Leger P, Bedicam JM, Cornette A, et al. Nasal intermittent positive pressure ventilation. Long-term follow-up in patients with severe chronic respiratory insufficiency. Chest 1994;105:100–5.
15. Robert D, Willig TN, Leger P, et al. Long-term nasal ventilation in neuromuscular disorders: report of a consensus conference. Eur Respir J 1993;6:599–606.
16. Bach JR, Alba AS. Management of chronic alveolar hypoventilation by nasal ventilation. Chest 1990;97:52–7.
17. Sullivan C, Issa F, Berthon-Jones M, et al. Reversal of obstructive sleep apnoea by continuous positive airway pressure applied through the nares. Lancet 1981;1:862–5.
18. Brochard L. Noninvasive ventilation for acute respiratory failure. JAMA 2002;288: 932–5.
19. Brochard L, Mancebo J, Elliott MW. Noninvasive ventilation for acute respiratory failure. Eur Respir J 2002;19:712–21.
20. Brochard L, Pluskwa F, Lemaire F. Improved efficacy of spontaneous breathing with inspiratory pressure support. Am Rev Respir Dis 1987;136:411–5.
21. Girou E, Brun-Buisson C, Taille S, et al. Secular trends in nosocomial infections and mortality associated with noninvasive ventilation in patients with exacerbation of COPD and pulmonary edema. JAMA 2003;290:2985–91.
22. Azoulay E, Demoule A, Jaber S, et al. Palliative noninvasive ventilation in patients with acute respiratory failure. Intensive Care Med 2011;37:1250–7.
23. Brochard L, Isabey D, Piquet J, et al. Reversal of acute exacerbations of chronic obstructive lung disease by inspiratory assistance with a face mask. N Engl J Med 1990;323:1523–30.
24. Brochard L, Mancebo J, Wysocki M, et al. Noninvasive ventilation for acute exacerbations of chronic obstructive pulmonary disease. N Engl J Med 1995;333:817–22.
25. Carteaux G, Lyazidi A, Cordoba-Izquierdo A, et al. Patient-ventilator asynchrony during noninvasive ventilation: a bench and clinical study. Chest 2012;142: 367–76.
26. Vignaux L, Tassaux D, Carteaux G, et al. Performance of noninvasive ventilation algorithms on ICU ventilators during pressure support: a clinical study. Intensive Care Med 2010;36:2053–9.
27. Fraticelli AT, Lellouche F, L'Her E, et al. Physiological effects of different interfaces during noninvasive ventilation for acute respiratory failure. Crit Care Med 2009; 37:939–45.
28. Osadnik C, Tee V, Carson-Chahhoud K, et al. Non-invasive ventilation for the management of acute hypercapnic respiratory failure due to exacerbation of chronic obstructive pulmonary disease. Cochrane Database Syst Rev 2017;7: CD004104.
29. Rochwerg B, Brochard L, Elliott MW, et al. Official ERS/ATS clinical practice guidelines: noninvasive ventilation for acute respiratory failure. Eur Respir J 2017;50(2):1602426.
30. Cavalot G, Dounaevskaia V, Vieira F, et al. One-year readmission following undifferentiated acute hypercapnic respiratory failure. COPD 2021;18:602–11.
31. Chung Y, Garden FL, Marks GB, et al. Population prevalence of hypercapnic respiratory failure from any cause. Am J Respir Crit Care Med 2022;205:966–7.
32. Carrillo A, Ferrer M, Gonzalez-Diaz G, et al. Noninvasive ventilation in acute hypercapnic respiratory failure caused by obesity hypoventilation syndrome and chronic obstructive pulmonary disease. Am J Respir Crit Care Med 2012;186:1279–85.

33. Bellani G, Laffey JG, Pham T, et al. Noninvasive ventilation of patients with acute respiratory distress syndrome. Insights from the LUNG SAFE study. Am J Respir Crit Care Med 2017;195:67–77.
34. Carteaux G, Millan-Guilarte T, De Prost N, et al. Failure of noninvasive ventilation for de novo acute hypoxemic respiratory failure: role of tidal volume. Crit Care Med 2016;44:282–90.
35. Doidge JCGD, Ferrando-Vivas P, Mouncey PR, et al. Trends in intensive care for patients with COVID-19 in England, Wales, And Northern Ireland. Am J Respir Crit Care Med 2021;203:565–74.
36. Ferreyro BL, Angriman F, Munshi L, et al. Association of noninvasive oxygenation strategies with all-cause mortality in adults with acute hypoxemic respiratory failure: a systematic review and meta-analysis. JAMA 2020;324:57–67.
37. Poulton E, Oxon D. Left-sided heart failure with pulmonary edema: its treatment with the "pulmonary plus pressure machine. Lancet 1936;228:981–3.
38. Barach AL, Fenn WO, Ferris EB, et al. The physiology of pressure breathing; a brief review of its present status. J Aviat Med 1947;18(1):73–87.
39. Bersten A, Holt A, Vedig A, et al. Treatment of severe cardiogenic pulmonary edema with continuous positive airway pressure delivered by face mask. N Engl J Med 1991;325:1825–30.
40. Ashbaugh DG, Bigelow DB, Petty TL, et al. Acute respiratory distress in adults. Lancet 1967;2:319–23.
41. Millington SJ, Cardinal P, Brochard L. Setting and titrating positive end-expiratory pressure. Chest 2022;161:1566–75.
42. Dianti J, Tisminetzky M, Ferreyro BL, et al. Association of positive end-expiratory pressure and lung recruitment selection strategies with mortality in acute respiratory distress syndrome: a systematic review and network meta-analysis. Am J Respir Crit Care Med 2022;205:1300–10.
43. Nash G, Blennerhassett JB, Pontoppidan H. Pulmonary lesions associated with oxygen therapy and artifical ventilation. N Engl J Med 1967;276:368–74.
44. Dantzker DR, Lynch JP, Weg JG. Depression of cardiac output is a mechanism of shunt reduction in the therapy of acute respiratory failure. Chest 1980;77:636–42.
45. Falke KJ, Pontoppidan H, Kumar A, et al. Ventilation with end-expiratory pressure in acute lung disease. J Clin Invest 1972;51:2315–23.
46. Suter PM, Fairley B, Isenberg MD. Optimum end-expiratory airway pressure in patients with acute pulmonary failure. N Engl J Med 1975;292:284–9.
47. Hickling KG. Best compliance during a decremental, but not incremental, positive end-expiratory pressure trial is related to open-lung positive end-expiratory pressure: a mathematical model of acute respiratory distress syndrome lungs. Am J Respir Crit Care Med 2001;163:69–78.
48. Jonson B, Richard JC, Straus C, et al. Pressure-volume curves and compliance in acute lung injury: evidence of recruitment above the lower inflection point. Am J Respir Crit Care Med 1999;159:1172–8.
49. Amato MB, Barbas CS, Medeiros DM, et al. Effect of a protective-ventilation strategy on mortality in the acute respiratory distress syndrome. N Engl J Med 1998;338:347–54.
50. Ranieri VM, Eissa NT, Corbeil C, et al. Effects of positive end-expiratory pressure on alveolar recruitment and gas exchange in patients with the adult respiratory distress syndrome. Am Rev Respir Dis 1991;144:544–51.
51. Maggiore SM, Jonson B, Richard JC, et al. Alveolar derecruitment at decremental positive end-expiratory pressure levels in acute lung injury: comparison with the lower inflection point, oxygenation, and compliance. Am J Respir Crit Care Med 2001;164:795–801.

52. Roupie E, Dambrosio M, Servillo G, et al. Titration of tidal volume and induced hypercapnia in acute respiratory distress syndrome. Am J Respir Crit Care Med 1995;152:121–8.

53. Bellani G, Laffey JG, Pham T, et al. Epidemiology, patterns of care, and mortality for patients with acute respiratory distress syndrome in intensive care units in 50 countries. JAMA 2016;315:788–800.

54. Briel M, Meade M, Mercat A, et al. Higher vs lower positive end-expiratory pressure in patients with acute lung injury and acute respiratory distress syndrome: systematic review and meta-analysis. JAMA 2010;303:865–73.

55. Brower RG, Lanken PN, MacIntyre N, et al. Higher versus lower positive end-expiratory pressures in patients with the acute respiratory distress syndrome. N Engl J Med 2004;351:327–36.

56. Mercat A, Richard JC, Vielle B, et al. Positive end-expiratory pressure setting in adults with acute lung injury and acute respiratory distress syndrome: a randomized controlled trial. JAMA 2008;299:646–55.

57. Gattinoni L, Caironi P, Cressoni M, et al. Lung recruitment in patients with the acute respiratory distress syndrome. N Engl J Med 2006;354:1775–86.

58. Chen L, Del Sorbo L, Grieco DL, et al. Potential for lung recruitment estimated by the recruitment-to-inflation ratio in acute respiratory distress syndrome. A clinical trial. Am J Respir Crit Care Med 2020;201:178–87.

59. Bendixen HH, Hedley-Whyte J, Laver MB. Impaired oxygenation in surgical patients during general anesthesia with controlled ventilation. A concept of atelectasis. N Engl J Med 1963;269:991–6.

60. Lellouche F, Delorme M, Brochard L. Impact of respiratory rate and dead space in the current era of lung protective mechanical ventilation. Chest 2020;158:45–7.

61. Webb H, Tierney D. Experimental pulmonary edema due to intermittent positive pressure ventilation with high inflation pressures. Protection by positive end-expiratory pressure. Am Rev Respir Dis 1974;110:556–65.

62. Dreyfuss D, Saumon G. Ventilator-induced lung injury: lessons from experimental studies. Am J Respir Crit Care Med 1998;157:294–323.

63. Slutsky A, Ranieri V. Ventilator-induced lung injury. N Engl J Med 2013;369:2126–36.

64. Darioli R, Perret C. Mechanical controlled hypoventilation in status asthmaticus. Am Rev Respir Dis 1984;129:385–7.

65. Tuxen DV, Lane S. The effects of ventilatory pattern on hyperinflation, airway pressures, and circulation in mechanical ventilation of patients with severe air-flow obstruction. Am Rev Respir Dis 1987;136:872–9.

66. Pepe PE, Marini JJ. Occult positive end-expiratory pressure in mechanically ventilated patients with airflow obstruction: the auto-PEEP effect. Am Rev Respir Dis 1982;126:166–70.

67. Hickling KG, Henderson SJ, Jackson R. Low mortality associated with low volume pressure limited ventilation with permissive hypercapnia in severe adult respiratory distress syndrome. Intensive Care Med 1990;16:372–7.

68. Acute Respiratory Distress Syndrome N, Brower RG, Matthay MA, et al. Ventilation with lower tidal volumes as compared with traditional tidal volumes for acute lung injury and the acute respiratory distress syndrome. N Engl J Med 2000;342:1301–8.

69. Amato MB, Meade MO, Slutsky AS, et al. Driving pressure and survival in the acute respiratory distress syndrome. N Engl J Med 2015;372:747–55.

70. Goligher EC, Costa ELV, Yarnell CJ, et al. Effect of lowering vt on mortality in acute respiratory distress syndrome varies with respiratory system elastance. Am J Respir Crit Care Med 2021;203:1378–85.

Airway Management During the Last 100 Years

Sonia Vaida, MD[a,*], Luis Gaitini, MD[b], Mostafa Somri, MD[b], Ibrahim Matter, MD[c], Jansie Prozesky, MB, ChB[a]

KEYWORDS

- Airway management • History • Endotracheal tube • Fiberoptic scope intubation
- Supraglottic airway devices • Laryngeal mask airway • Laryngeal tube

KEY POINTS

- Airway management is an essential skill for anesthesiologists and critical care and emergency medicine practitioners.
- The past 100 years are marked by the development of modern-day laryngoscopy, fiberoptic laryngoscopy, supraglottic airway devices, algorithms for difficult airway and video-laryngoscopy.
- Technical and nontechnical skills developed during the past 100 years have revolutionized airway management.

Expertise in airway management is an essential skill for anesthesiologists and critical care and emergency medicine physicians. One of the earliest airway management techniques was the tracheotomy procedure documented on ancient Egyptian tablets, dating back to the first dynasty around 3060 BCE.[1] Thankfully, many other devices and techniques have evolved since then to ensure secure and safe oxygenation and ventilation. Specifically, in the last 100 years, a plethora of innovative technical advancements have revolutionized airway management altogether.

DIRECT LARYNGOSCOPY

Despite many advancements in airway management, direct laryngoscopy first performed in 1895[2] is still the most commonly used technique to visualize the larynx in order to enable endotracheal tube (ETT) insertion. The laryngoscope blades used today were developed in the 1940s and, remarkably, continue to serve as standard devices for intubation. The Miller straight blade was described in 1941 by Dr Robert

[a] Department of Anesthesiology, Penn State College of Medicine, Penn State Milton S. Hershey Medical Center, 500 University Drive, Hershey, PA 17033, USA; [b] Department of Anesthesiology, Bnai-Zion Medical Center, 31048, 47 Golomb Street, Haifa, Israel; [c] Department of Surgery, Bnai-Zion Medical Center, 31048, 47 Golomb Street, Haifa, Israel
* Corresponding author.
E-mail address: svaida@pennstatehealth.psu.edu

Crit Care Clin 39 (2023) 451–464
https://doi.org/10.1016/j.ccc.2022.12.003
0749-0704/23/© 2023 Elsevier Inc. All rights reserved.

Miller[3] while the curved MacIntosh laryngoscope that came after has arguably become the most commonly used around the world[4] **(Fig. 1)**.

The inventor of the blade, Sir Robert Reynolds Macintosh, was born in New Zealand in 1897. After spending his childhood in Argentina and New Zealand, he enlisted in the Royal Scots Fusiliers during World War I. After the war, he enrolled in medical school in England and later became the first Professor of Anesthesia in Europe, at Oxford University. In honor of his extraordinary achievements in medicine, he was knighted in 1955.[5] Sir MacIntosh (or Mac, as he was known by his friends) died in Oxford in 1989 at the age of 91.[6] Without any doubt, his famous letter "A new laryngoscope" published in the "New Innovations" session of the *Lancet* in 1943 has forever changed the way we approach airway management. Dr MacIntosh described as the approach to intubation with his new laryngoscope: "When the short-curved blade is in position the tip will fit into the angle made by the epiglottis with the base of the tongue," going on to add that, "using the laryngoscope I can expose the larynx more easily and at a lighter plane of anesthesia."[7]

Multiple studies comparing straight and curved blades for laryngoscopic view, ease of intubation, time to achieve an effective airway, upper airway trauma, and so forth reported mixed results regarding the superiority of one type over the other. The straight "Miller" laryngoscope blade described by Robert Miller is still popular for intubation in infants because it is better suited to the upper airway anatomy in these patients. In adults, laryngoscopy with Miller-type straight blades seems to be associated with more pronounced sympathetic-mediated increases in blood pressure and heart rate, which can be problematic in patients with underlying cardiac diseases.[8]

In an attempt to optimize visualization of the larynx and intubation conditions in general, throughout the years, more than 50 modifications with particular characteristics have been made to both the original Macintosh and Miller blades.[9]

As clearly delineated by Unzueta and colleagues,[10] "the laryngoscope designed by Macintosh is probably the most successful and lasting instrument in the history of anesthesia; it has survived plastic translation and the adoption of fiber light."

FIBEROPTIC BRONCHOSCOPY

Gustav Killian from Freiberg, Germany is considered the father of modern bronchoscopy. In 1897, he used a technique, which he named "directe bronkoscopie" to examine the trachea and main bronchi of a volunteer and also to remove airway foreign bodies.[11]

In 1904, the American otolaryngologist Chevalier Jackson, considered the father of American bronchoesophagoscopy, developed a forerunner of the modern

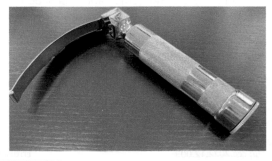

Fig. 1. Mcintosh laryngoscope.

bronchoscope consisting of a rigid U-shaped ocular device with a light source and suction tube.[12]

A versatile, flexible bronchoscope with a diameter of less than 6 mm, containing 15,000 glass fibers was developed in 1962 by a Japanese thoracic surgeon, Shigeto Ikeda, and presented in 1968 in Copenhagen.[13] After further changes, including the addition of a "working channel" that provides a tube separate from the glass fibers, the first flexible bronchoscope was launched in 1968. This was followed in 1970 by the first Olympus model, with improved imaging and easier handling.

Fiberoptic scope intubation (FSI) with a flexible fiberoptic bronchoscope has become the gold standard for awake intubation in a spontaneously breathing patient with difficult airway (**Fig. 2**). It allows intubation to be performed before general anesthesia is induced, thereby avoiding the risk of losing upper airway patency or a failed intubation with a life-threatening cannot intubate/cannot oxygenate situation. FSI may be indicated in patients with a history of difficult intubation and various anatomic features indicative of difficult laryngoscopy, such as limited mouth opening, reduced thyromental distance, limited neck mobility, inability to protrude the mandible, poor oropharyngeal view, and obesity. It may also be indicated in patients with known or suspected cervical spine instability; anatomical malformations of the mandible or larynx; congenital deformities of the head and neck; and a history of head, neck, and spine trauma.[14,15]

The modern flexible fiberoptic scope consists of an insertion cord with a video chip at the distal part of the cord. The insertion cord is attached to a handle equipped with a lever that allows the operator to move the tip up and down so that the flexible cord can adapt to the anatomical structures of the upper airway. The optical basis of the fiberscope is the lens, the image transmission bundle, and the eyepiece. The working channel can be used for suctioning secretions or blood, drug administration (such as local anesthetics), oxygen delivery, or as a vehicle for different instruments (such as biopsy forceps). Several adjunct tools can be used to help the operator center the orotracheal tube and displace the tongue during oral FSI. Most widely used are the Ovassapian fiberoptic intubating airway (Teleflex Medical Research, Triangle Park, NC) Williams Airway Intubator (SunMed Medical Systems LLC, Grand Rapids, MI) and the Berman Oropharyngeal Airway Teleflex Medical Research, Triangle Park, NC).[16] FSI in an awake or sedated patient requires adequate topical anesthesia of the upper airway, patient cooperation, and advanced operator skills. Therefore, it should only be performed by experienced, fully trained clinicians who are aware of

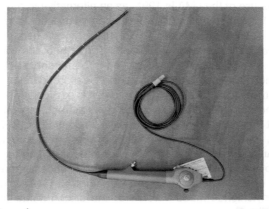

Fig. 2. Fiberoptic bronchoscope.

the need of following the basic principles of FSI to ensure adequate oxygenation and ventilation.

Awake FSI is now the technique of choice for management of the anticipated difficult airway as recommended by all national societies for airway management around the world.

SUPRAGLOTTIC AIRWAY DEVICES
Laryngeal Mask Airway

Airway management practices dramatically improved in the 1980s with the addition of supraglottic airway devices (SADs) to the airway armamentarium. SADs are noninvasive airway devices inserted blindly, sealing the oropharynx and capable of delivering oxygen or anesthetic gases above the level of the glottis.

Dr Archie Ian Jeremy Brain, the inventor of the famous Laryngeal Mask Airway (LMA), is a British Anesthesiologist born in Kobe, Japan, on July 2, 1942. He began developing the LMA in 1981 as an alternative to the facemask while working as a lecturer in anesthesia at the Royal London Hospital. It consisted of an inflatable mask placed in the hypopharyngeal space to seal the glottic opening and connected to a ventilation tube. The LMA patent was approved in 1982. The first homemade prototype built from a Goldman Dental Mask was used in a young patient undergoing inguinal hernia repair at the William Harvey Hospital in Ashford, United Kingdom.[17]

The first article on "The Laryngeal Mask Airway- A new concept in airway management" was published in 1983 in the British Journal of Anaesthesia, reporting the results of a pilot study of 23 patients who received LMAs. Dr Brain described the LMA as "an alternative to either the endotracheal tube (ETT) or the face-mask with either spontaneous or positive-pressure ventilation."[18] That year, the LMA prototype was used for the first time to rescue the airway in a morbidly obese patient after a failed intubation.

Dr Brain continued to improve the design of the LMA with tens of homemade prototypes, evolving to the factory-made prototype in 1987. By that time, the LMA had been trialed in more than 7000 patients.[19] It became commercially and clinically available in the United Kingdom in 1988. The same year, Alexander and colleagues, in a letter titled "Use your Brain," reported the successful use of the LMA in more than 150 patients including cases of known difficult airway. It quickly became obvious that the LMA has multiple advantages over facemask ventilation (eg, hands free ventilation) and ETT (noninvasive, easy insertion, short learning curve, lfewer hemodynamic changes at insertion and removal).[20] In the United States, the Food and Drug Administration (FDA) approved the use of the LMA in 1991, as an alternative to the facemask only.[17]

Critics of the LMA worried about possible airway obstruction caused by downfolding of the epiglottis. To address that, 2 epiglottis retention bars were added to the initial design of the ventilation aperture (**Fig. 3**). Throughout the years, a wide range of sizes and LMA variants have also been added to better serve different clinical situations. LMA flexible introduced in 1992 has a wire-reinforced longer tube attached to the cuff to reduce the risk of kinking, and therefore, it is particularly suited for head and neck surgery.[21] The intubating LMA (also known as Fastrach), specifically designed to serve as a conduit for endotracheal intubation, was released in 1997. It has a curved, rigid airway tube, with the 2 epiglottis retention bars replaced by one epiglottic elevating flap.[22] An ETT can be inserted through the intubating LMA both blindly or by an assistance of the fiberoptic scope with very high success rates, including in patients with known or suspected difficult airway[23] (**Fig. 4**). LMA Unique, a single use, disposable polyvinylchloride-made version of the silicon-made classic LMA, was released in 1998 (**Fig. 5**).

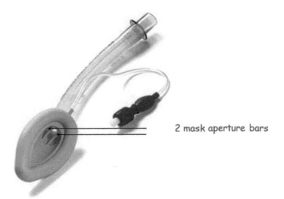

2 mask aperture bars

Fig. 3. Classic LMA with epiglottis retention bars.

The classic LMA's main shortcomings are as follows: low oropharyngeal pressure seal and lack of protection from aspiration with regurgitant stomach contents. Low oropharyngeal seal pressure can cause both ventilation gas loss and gastric insufflation mainly in situations where the airway pressure exceeds the seal pressure. To address this, in 2001, Dr Brain designed the LMA Proseal, a multi-use silicone-made LMA variant with an added esophageal drain tube to improve protection against aspiration by isolating the esophagus from the respiratory tract, and a dorsal cuff to improve the oropharyngeal seal pressure (**Fig. 6**). As compared with the classic LMA, LMA Proseal provided a better seal and effectively facilitated gastric tube placement; however, its insertion was more difficult, causing more frequent epiglottic downfolding.[24] Following that, there were further refinements as the LMA Supreme was introduced in 2007 as a single use, improved version of the LMA Proseal. A rigid curved shaft replaced the flexible shaft of the Proseal for an easier insertion. LMA Supreme has a decreased transverse diameter of the upper part of the mask facilitating insertion in patients with smaller mouth opening. In addition to a bite block, a reinforced tip and molded distal cuff were added to avoid folding over of the tip during the insertion of the device (**Fig. 7**).

The SADs with added design features intended to reduce the risk of pulmonary aspiration of gastric contents are referred to as "second-generation" SADs. LMA Protector

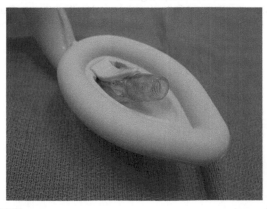

Fig. 4. Intubating LMA.

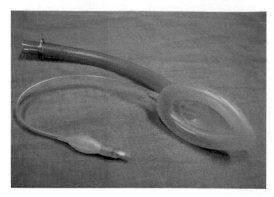

Fig. 5. LMA unique.

released in 2016, is a silicon-made, single-use, advanced second-generation device, incorporating features of previously described LMAs. It has dual gastric drainage channels, an integrated cuff pressure indicator and a larger airway tube to serve as a conduit for endotracheal intubation. LMA gastro, released in 2017, is also a second-generation SAD designed with 2 channels, 1 for ventilation and another 16-mm internal diameter channel dedicated for upper gastrointestinal access. Endoscopic procedures, including endoscopic retrograde cholangiopancreatography are reported to be successfully performed through the dedicated endoscopic channel.[25]

Thousands of articles and hundreds of millions of safe administrations later, LMA and LMA variants have become the most commonly used airway devices for routine cases requiring general anesthesia. However, although the LMA and its variants are the most frequently used SADs, they are not always successful. Other SADs types with different features and designs may provide oxygenation and ventilation in circumstances where the LMAs fail.

Combitube

The Esophageal Tracheal Combitube known as the "Combitube," was designed by Dr Michael Frass in cooperation with Reinhard Frenzer and Dr Jonas Zahler, in Vienna, Austria, in 1983. It became commercially available in 1988. It is a double-lumen, double-cuff airway device for emergency intubation (**Fig. 8**). It allows ventilation independent of its position, in either the esophagus or the trachea. However, blind insertion results in successful esophageal insertion in nearly all patients. Due to concerns of oropharyngeal and esophageal trauma associated with insertion and prolonged use,

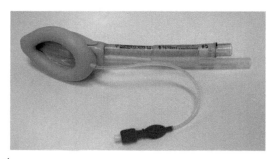

Fig. 6. LMA proseal.

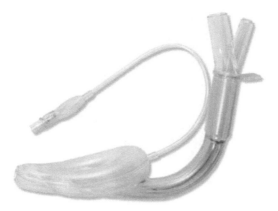

Fig. 7. LMA supreme.

the role of the Combitube in airway management has been significantly reduced in recent years. To address some of these concerns, the EasyTube was developed and approved in the European Union in 2003 and by the FDA 2005. Specifically, it was designed in an attempt to improve the performance of the Combitube and reduce incidences of traumatic complications (**Fig. 9**). Its pharyngeal lumen has a single supraglottic ventilation outlet ending below the oropharyngeal balloon as opposed to Combitube that has 8 perforations between the cuffs and tracheoesophageal lumen. It has a smaller outer diameter, and compared with the Combitube, the Easy-Tube is easier and quicker to insert.[26]

Laryngeal Tube (King Laryngeal Tube)

The Laryngeal Tube (LT) was designed by Volker Bertram in Sulz, Germany, and introduced to the European Union in 2002. King Systems company (now Ambu, Noblesville, IN, USA)) introduced the LT in USA in 2004, under the name of "King LT." The original LT consisted of a single lumen SAD closed at the distal end, 2 inflatable interconnected cuffs inflated by a single pilot tube and a ventilation orifice between the cuffs. Later, an additional channel for gastric tube placement was added posterior

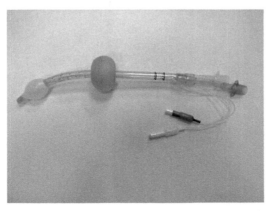

Fig. 8. Combitube.

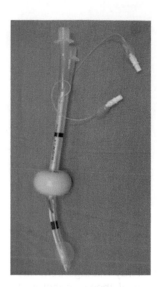

Fig. 9. EasyTube.

to the ventilation lumen and the device named LT Suction (LTS). Multiple LT variants have been developed throughout the years to optimize its performance. In 2004, the LTS II was replaced by LTS II with a modified distal cuff shape for a better fit to the esophageal inlet. The LTS-D is a single-use polyvinyl chloride device marketed in Europe in 2005 and in the United States in 2006. It was further modified in 2014, by creating a steeper curvature of the ventilation tube and multiple ventilation orifices in addition to the original large ventilation aperture in order to prevent occlusion of the main airway inlet (**Fig. 10**). The intubating LT tube suction–disposable (iLTS-D) was later developed with the additional capability to serve as conduit for blind of fiberoptic-guided intubation.

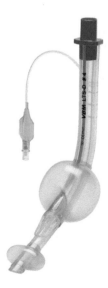

Fig. 10. Laryngeal tube.

Due to its slim design and easy insertion, the LT variants have gained much in popularity for emergency airway management as primary or rescue airway device, including in the prehospital area.[27] Exchanging a LT for an ETT is often needed for prolonged ventilation and can be done by various techniques ranging from direct laryngoscopy to advanced techniques requiring fiberoptic-guided assistance. Prolonged overinflation of the cuffs can lead to traumatic upper airway complications. Therefore, cuff inflation, using a manometer, and frequent monitoring of the intracuff pressure are highly recommended.

i-Gel

The i-gel is an anatomically designed SAD with a noninflatable cuff made of soft material resembling a gel, and a gastric tube, marketed in 2007. It was invented by Dr Muhammed Nasir a United Kingdom anaesthetist, originally from Pakistan (**Fig. 11**). One of the most remarkable features of the i-Gel is the low incidence of postoperative pharyngolaryngeal complications due to its soft cuff.

Throughout the years, following the success of the original LMA, a variety of SADs have been developed and marketed with different degrees of commercial success. There is no ideal SAD, and the decision to choose one SAD over another should be based on factors such as clinical situation, patient characteristics, availability, proficiency, and costs. However, second-generation SADs should be used whenever possible because they have distinct advantages over first-generation SADs. In the future, we will most likely witness the development of more sophisticated SADs to further enhance their safety profile.

ALGORITHMS FOR DIFFICULT AIRWAY

A significant step toward increased airway management safety was achieved by promoting advanced planning for a difficult airway. In 1985, Mallampati and colleagues[28,29] introduced a famous screening tool to predict a difficult airway, based on the visibility of the oropharyngeal structures. The authors described "a relatively simple grading system which involves preoperative ability to visualize the faucial pillars, soft palate and base of uvula," grading 3 classes of oropharyngeal view. Later, in 1987, Samson and Young added a fourth class. Even though the accuracy of the original and modified Mallampati score was questioned by many, it remains one of the most important tools for assessing the upper airway.

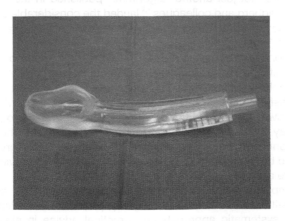

Fig. 11. i-Gel.

The American Society of Anesthesiologists (ASA) published the first "Practice Guidelines for the Management of the Difficult Airway," in 1993, after recognizing the complexity of airway management, morbidity caused by difficult or failed intubation, and the increased medical malpractice claims against anesthesiologists. These guidelines were developed by an ASA-appointed task force of 10 members. The task force based the guidelines on existing peer reviewed literature and expert opinion and created predefined stepwise algorithms.[30] As stated by the authors, "the purpose of these guidelines is to facilitate the management of difficult airway and to reduce the likelihood of adverse outcomes."[31] Key points emphasized in these algorithms are recommendations for awake intubation in patients with recognized difficult airway, and planned alternate strategies based on existing resources and skills. Graphic representations of the information presented in flowcharts were added to aid clinicians in the decision-making process.

An updated version of the first algorithms was published in 2003, incorporating the LMA and LMA variants for emergency and nonemergency airway management, both as rescue ventilator devices and as conduits for endotracheal intubation.[32] Ten years later, in 2013, a revised and updated version of the algorithms was released to address the continued changes and technological improvements in airway management. In this version, videolaryngoscopy has been added for cases where difficulty was encountered with direct laryngoscopy.[33] In addition to the LMA, other SADs such as the LT have been added in this version to be used in cases of difficult ventilation, or as conduits for endotracheal intubation.

The recently published guidelines in 2022, replacing the 2013 version, were developed by an international task force of 15 anesthesiologists from the United States, India, Ireland, Italy, and Switzerland, and 2 methodologists.[34] These guidelines emphasize the importance of supplemental oxygen administration throughout the critical steps of airway management and attention to "passage of time, the number of attempts, and oxygen saturation." For the first time, these guidelines also include a pediatric airway algorithm.

Over time, other national anesthesia societies have developed their own difficult airway guidelines. Notably, the 2015 guidelines for the management of unanticipated difficult intubation, published by the Difficult Airway Society (DAS) in the United Kingdom, has become very popular as a reference. DAS has also created subspecialty specific guidelines for pediatric, obstetric, and critically ill patients. In an editorial titled "Difficult Airway Society 2015 guidelines for the management of unanticipated difficult intubation in adults: not just another algorithm," published in the *British Journal of Anaesthesia*, Dr Hagberg and colleagues[35] lauded the considerable emphasis placed by these guidelines on "preparedness and accountability of the practitioner by optimizing conditions."

The "Vortex" concept was developed by Dr Chrimes as a visual cognitive aid to help implement difficult airway-management algorithms. It was created to specifically address the complexity of the decision-making process when optimizing care under such highly stressful situations.[36] The Vortex graphical provides a visual representation of looking down into a funnel that symbolizes the rapid and progressive deterioration of an airway crisis toward the "blue zone," which represents the life-threatening situation of a "cannot intubate/cannot oxygenate scenario." The "green zone" of the Vortex is reached by reestablishing airway patency, which then provides the opportunity to reorganize and plan the next steps.

Successful implementation of algorithms requires frequent simulation-based training with institutionally available airway equipment. The evidence shows that adherence to a systematic approach and practical advice in managing the very complex situation of a difficult airway results in an improved outcome. However, although algorithms are very important strategic tools for managing expected and un-expected difficult airways, they are very complex, and so far, there is no evidence of improved outcomes using one algorithm over another.[37]

VIDEOLARYNGOSCOPY

The beginning of the twenty-first century has brought major advances in airway video technology and fiberoptics resulting in the development of video-assisted laryngos-copy. Videolaryngoscopes (VLs) are equipped with a small video camera, a fiberoptic bundle or a system of prisms attached distally at the end of the blade, allowing indirect visualization of an enlarged image of airway structures on a monitor screen.[38] VLs have gained rapid popularity as both rescue and primary airway devices due to an improved visualization of the vocal cords and shorter learning curve. Several VLs with different designs are available such as the following:

- Optical laryngoscopes (eg, Bullard laryngoscope, Circon ACMI, USA).
- VL with a guide channel and a preloaded ETT (eg, Airtraq Avant (ATQ; Prodol Meditec, Vizcaya, Spain, Pentax Airway Scope, Hoya Corporation, Tokyo, Japan).
- VL with a hyperangulated blade (eg, Glidescope) **(Fig. 12)**.
- VL with standard McIntosh blade (eg, Storz C-Mac Storz, Tuttlingen, Germany, McGrath MACMedtronic, Minneapolis, MN, USA).

Even though "optical stylets" have been available since 1979, Dr John A Pacey, a Canadian vascular and general Surgeon, the inventor of Glidescope, is regarded by many as the father of modern videolaryngoscopy.[39] The first reported elective use of the Glidescope was in 2003, by Agro and colleagues,[40] in a case series of 15 pa-tients with cervical spine immobilization. The same year Copper reported the success-ful use of the Glidescope in a patient with a history of failed intubation who refused an awake fiberoptic intubation.[41]

A wide range of VLs with different designs is available today. Significant research resulting in numerous publications focuses on comparing various VLs against each other, as well as to direct laryngoscopes, in patients with known or unknown difficult airways. Reported outcome measures used for comparison are as follows: improved visualization of the glottis, first attempt intubation success rate, time for intubation, he-modynamic changes during intubation, force used during laryngoscopy, and so forth.

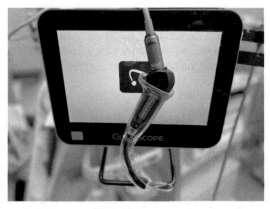

Fig. 12. Glidescope.

Videolaryngoscopy clearly offers the advantage of improved glottic visualization and a higher first-attempt endotracheal intubation success rate in both predicted and unexpected difficult airways. Its use also is associated with a high success rate of rescue intubation.[42,43] However, because video laryngoscopy has gained in popularity, there have been increasing numbers of publications reporting upper airway trauma caused by different types of video laryngoscopes.

Despite the remarkable improvement in managing the difficult airway, videolaryngoscopy may fail in patients with limited mouth opening, upper airway bleeding, oropharyngeal tumor, and so forth, and therefore, practitioners should always have a backup plan to rescue the airway within the structure of a difficult airway algorithm.

Many different types of VLs have been compared. With help clinicians can choose the optimal device for their practice. Considering that no VL is 100% efficient in all clinical circumstances, the decision to choose a specific type of VL should by based on multiple local factors including user preference, costs, and training availability.

The latest technological addition, the Glidescope Core, offers simultaneous dual vision with a Glidescope and a bronchoscope connected to a large monitor touch screen.

As hard as it is to predict future developments, with constant technological advances and innovations, we are confident that the future will bring more exciting devices and cognitive tools to improve the safety of airway management.

CLINICS CARE POINTS

- Difficulty securing the airway is a common clinical problem encountered by anesthesiologists, critical care and emergency medicine physicians.
- The development of advanced technology over the past 100 years has revolutionized airway management and significantly increased patient safety.
- Adherence to a systematic approach offered by difficult airway algorithms leads to improved outcome.

REFERENCES

1. Pahor AL. Ear, nose and throat in ancient Egypt. J Laryngol Otol 1992;106: 863–73.
2. Burkle CM, Zepeda FA, Bacon DR, et al. A historical perspective on use of the laryngoscope as a tool in anesthesiology. Anesthesiology 2004;100:1003–6.
3. Miller RA. A new laryngoscope. Anesthesiology 1941;2:317–20. 17.
4. Scott J, Baker PA. How did the Macintosh laryngoscope become so popular? Pediatr Anesth 2009;19(Suppl. 1):24–9.
5. Croft TM. Professor sir robert macintosh, 1897- 1989. Resuscitation 2002;54: 111–3.
6. Roberts FW. Obituary. Robert Reynolds macintosh. Anaesth Intensive Care 1990; 18:132.
7. Macintosh RR. A new laryngoscope. Lancet 1943;1:205.
8. Nishiyama T, Higashizawa T, Bito H, et al. Which laryngoscope is the most stressful in laryngoscopy; Macintosh, Miller, or McCoy? Masui 1997;46:1519–24.
9. Doherty JS, Froom SR, Gildersleve CD. Pediatric laryngoscopes and intubation aids old and new. Paediatr Anaesth 2009;19(Suppl 1):30–7.

10. Unzueta MC, Casas JI, Merten A. Macintosh's laryngoscope. Anesthesiology 2005;102:242.
11. Zöllner F. Gustav Killian, father of bronchoscopy. Arch Otolaryngol 1965;82: 656–9.
12. Boyd AD. Chevalier Jackson: the father of American bronchoesophagoscopy. Ann Thorac Surg 1994;57:502–5.
13. Panchabhai TS, Mehta AC. Historical perspectives of bronchoscopy. Connecting Dots Ann Am Thorac Soc 2015;12:631–41.
14. Frerk C, Mitchell VS, McNarry AF, et al. Difficult Airway Society intubation guidelines working group. Difficult Airway Society 2015 guidelines for management of unanticipated difficult intubation in adults. Br J Anaesth 2015;115:827–48.
15. Apfelbaum JL, Hagberg CA, Connis RT, et al. American society of anesthesiologists practice guidelines for management of the difficult airway. Anesthesiology 2022;136:31–81.
16. Greenland KB, Irwin MG. The Williams Airway Intubator, the Ovassapian Airway and the Berman Airway as upper airway conduits for fibreoptic bronchoscopy in patients with difficult airways. Curr Opin Anaesthesiol 2004;17:505–10.
17. van Zundert TCRV, Brimacombe JR, Ferson DZ, et al. Archie Brain: celebrating 30 years pf development in laryngeal mask airway. Anaesthesia 2012;67: 1375–85.
18. Brain AI. The laryngeal mask–a new concept in airway management. Br J Anaesth 1983;55:801–5.
19. Hernandez MR, Klock PA Jr, Ovassapian A. Evolution of the extraglottic airway: a review of its history, applications, and practical tips for success. Anesth Analg 2012;114:349–68.
20. Alexander CA, Leach AB, Thompson AR, et al. Use your Brain. Anaesthesia 1988; 43:893–4.
21. van Zundert TC, Cattano D. The LMA-Flexible: time to celebrate a unique extraglottic airway device. Minerva Anestesiol 2017;83:895–8.
22. Gerstein NS, Braude DA, Hung O, et al. The Fastrach intubating laryngeal mask airway: an overview and update. Can J Anaesth 2010;57:588–601.
23. Ferson DZ, Rosenblatt WH, Johansen MJ, et al. Use of the intubating LMA-Fastrach in 254 patients with difficult-to-manage airways. Anesthesiology 2001; 95:1175–8.
24. Brimacombe J, Keller C. The proseal laryngeal mask airway. Anesthesiology 2000;93:104–9.
25. Hagan KB, Carlson R, Arnold B, et al. Safety of the LMA®Gastro™ for endoscopic retrograde cholangiopancreatography. Anesth Analg 2020;131:1566–72.
26. Gaitini LA, Yanovsky B, Somri M, et al. Prospective randomized comparison of the EasyTube and the esophageal-tracheal Combitube airway devices during general anesthesia with mechanical ventilation. J Clin Anesth 2011;23:475–8.
27. Driver BE, Scharber SK, Horton GB, et al. Emergency department management of out-of-hospital laryngeal tubes. Ann Emerg Med 2019;74:403–9.
28. Mallampati SR, Gatt SP, Gugino LD, et al. A clinical sign to predict difficult tracheal intubation: a prospective study. Can Anaesth Soc J 1985;32:429–34.
29. Samsoon G, Young J. Difficult tracheal intubation: a retrospective study. Anaesthesia 1987;42:487–90.
30. Rosenblatt WH, Yanez D. A decision tree approach to airway management pathways in the 2022 difficult airway. Algorithm Am Soc Anesthesiologists Anesth Analg 2022;134:910–5.

31. Practice guidelines for management of the difficult airway. A report by the American society of anesthesiologists task force on management of the difficult airway. Anesthesiology 1993;78:597–602.
32. Practice guidelines for management of the difficult airway. An updated report by the American society of anesthesiologists task force on management of the difficult airway. Anesthesiology 2003;98:1269–77.
33. Practice guidelines for management of the difficult airway an updated report by the American society of anesthesiologists task force on management of the difficult airway. Anesthesiology 2013;118:251–70.
34. Apfelbaum JL, Hagberg CA, Caplan RA, et al. American society of anesthesiologists task force on management of the difficult airway. Practice guidelines for management of the difficult airway: an updated report by the American society of anesthesiologists task force on management of the difficult airway. Anesthesiology 2022;136:31–81.
35. Hagberg CA, Gabel JC, Connis RT. Difficult Airway Society 2015 guidelines for the management of unanticipated difficult intubation in adults: not just another algorithm. Br J Anaesth 2015;115:812–4.
36. Chrimes N. The Vortex: a universal 'high-acuity implementation tool' for emergency airway management. Br J Anaesth 2016;117(suppl 1):i20–7.
37. Artime CA, Hagberg CA. Is there a gold standard for management of the difficult airway? Anesthesiol Clin 2015 Jun;33(2):233–40.
38. Pott LM, Murray WB. Review of video laryngoscopy and rigid fiberoptic laryngoscopy. Curr Opin Anaesthesiol 2008;21(6):750–8.
39. McNarry AF, Patel A. The evolution of airway management – new concepts and conflicts with traditional practice. Br J Anaesth 2017;119(S1):i154–66.
40. Agrò F, Barzoi G, Montecchia F. Tracheal intubation using a Macintosh laryngoscope or a GlideScope in 15 patients with cervical spine immobilization. Br J Anaesth 2003;90:705–6.
41. Cooper RM. Use of a new videolaryngoscope (GlideScope) in the management of a difficult airway. Can J Anaesth 2003;50:611–3.
42. de Carvalho CC, da Silva DM, Lemos VM, et al. Videolaryngoscopy vs. direct Macintosh laryngoscopy in tracheal intubation in adults: a ranking systematic review and network meta-analysis. Anaesthesia 2022;77:326.
43. Pieters BMA, Maas EHA, Knape JTA, et al. Videolaryngoscopy vs. direct laryngoscopy use by experienced anaesthetists in patients with known difficult airways: a systematic review and meta-analysis. Anaesthesia 2017;72:1532–41.

Thinking Clearly
The History of Brain Dysfunction in Critical Illness

Kimberly F. Rengel, MD[a,b,*], Matthew F. Mart, MD, MSc[a,c,d],
Jo Ellen Wilson, MD, MPH[a,d,e], E. Wesley Ely, MD, MPH[a,c,d]

KEYWORDS

- Critical illness • Level of consciousness • Delirium • Cognition • ABCDEF Bundle

KEY POINTS

- Brain dysfunction in the intensive care unit (ICU), which manifests as delirium and coma, is an underrecognized form of organ failure that has only been fully appreciated in the history of critical care medicine in the last 2 decades.
- Delirium in the ICU is the strongest independent predictor of ongoing brain dysfunction after the ICU in the form of long-term cognitive impairment among survivors.
- Preventing short and long-term cognitive deficits due to critical illness is centered upon non-pharmacologic approaches including light sedation, delirium screening, avoiding benzodiazepines, early rehabilitation, and engaging family—all part of the ICU Liberation Campaign's ABCDEF Bundle.

INTRODUCTION

Brain dysfunction in critical illness ranges from delirium and coma to long-term cognitive dysfunction. These conditions, and the history that brought them to our attention, are multi-faceted and intricately intertwined with the history of mechanical ventilation, sedation, mobility, and the management of organ failure during critical illness. Over the

We do not plan to order reprints.
[a] Critical Illness, Brain Dysfunction, and Survivorship (CIBS) Center, Vanderbilt University Medical Center, 2525 West End Avenue, Suite 450, 4th Floor, Nashville, TN 37203, USA; [b] Department of Anesthesiology, Division of Anesthesia Critical Care Medicine, Vanderbilt University Medical Center, 1211 21st Avenue South, MAB 422, Nashville, TN 37213, USA; [c] Division of Allergy, Pulmonary, and Critical Care Medicine, Department of Medicine, Vanderbilt University Medical Center, 1161 21st Avenue South, Nashville, TN 37232, USA; [d] Geriatric Research, Education, and Clinical Center (GRECC), Tennessee Valley Veterans Affairs Health System, VA Tennessee Valley Healthcare system, 1310 24th Avenue South, Nashville, TN 37212, USA; [e] Department of Psychiatry and Behavioral Sciences, Vanderbilt University Medical Center, Vanderbilt Psychiatric Hospital, 1601 23rd Avenue South, Nashville, TN 37212, USA
* Corresponding author. 1211, 21st Avenue South, 422 Medical Arts Building, Nashville, TN 37212-1120.
E-mail address: kimberly.rengel@vumc.org

Crit Care Clin 39 (2023) 465–477
https://doi.org/10.1016/j.ccc.2023.01.004
0749-0704/23/© 2023 Elsevier Inc. All rights reserved.

past 30 years, we have become increasingly adept at ensuring our patients survive their critical illness with mortality rates decreasing across multiple common admission diagnoses including chronic obstructive pulmonary disease (COPD) exacerbation, ruptured aortic aneurysm, congestive heart failure, and subarachnoid hemorrhage.[1] At the same time, we see a second trend of increasing discharge to post-acute care facilities with fewer patients able to return home,[1] indicating that despite surviving their presenting problem, patients are discharged with an ongoing burden of problems requiring professional care. These trends sparked two important questions: why are patients not recovering back to their normal and, more importantly, is the care we provide contributing to this problem? In this review, we present a brief description of the journey to answer these questions, the landmark discoveries that impact the field, and the advances we have made in minimizing long-term cognitive injury to patients during and after critical illness. Finally, we briefly explore the effects of the recent coronavirus disease-2019 (COVID-19) pandemic that upended critical care medicine and health systems at large and led to a breakdown in many of the advances we have made in the past 25 years. We will soon face the opportunity to explore the ramifications of both the care we provided and the yet-unknown effects of long COVID.

The Advent of Critical Care Organ Support and Its Complications

The origins of the practice of critical care medicine and, subsequently cognitive dysfunction, are rooted in the 1952 Danish polio epidemic where anesthesiologist and innovator Dr Bjorn Ibsen first used positive pressure ventilation through a tracheostomy to support a young patient in Denmark.[2,3] Application of this technology grew rapidly in the coming years along with a growing understanding of lung injury and the early definition of acute respiratory distress syndrome (ARDS) in 1967.[4] These landmark developments and insights, along with parallel work on the care of postoperative patients and resuscitation of shock, led to the formal development of dedicated hospital units that could manage complex life support devices across multiple patients and gave rise to the specialty of critical care medicine. Understandably, early intensive care physicians focused primarily on the devastating injury occurring in the lung and other organs, such as the liver and kidneys, where the function could be readily measured. Brain dysfunction was not at the forefront of consideration.

Over the ensuing years, new strategies of mechanical ventilation emerged to better treat advanced lung injury including positive end-expiratory pressure and inverse ratio ventilation.[5] Although these developments in mechanical ventilation drastically improved our ability to oxygenate damaged lungs and improve survival, many ventilator settings were uncomfortable to patients and poorly tolerated. Drawing from the operating room environment, the use of deep sedation and paralytic agents became increasingly common in the newly formed intensive care unit (ICUs). Thus began an era of heavy sedation with high-dose benzodiazepine, opioid, and paralytic infusions as the standard of care. Intensivists recount memories of units filled with room after room of quiet, unmoving patients "resting" on the ventilator and healing their lungs. Underneath the surface of that seemingly peaceful drug-induced coma, however, an equally devastating storm was brewing in the brain and the body that would leave patients fighting an entirely new battle as they recovered from their critical illness. Patients who were awake and displaying manifestations of acute brain dysfunction, including disorientation, agitation, confusion, and hallucinations, were given the diagnosis of "ICU psychosis," a condition viewed as a temporary but expected finding in critical illness that was more of an inconvenience to providers than a serious problem for patients.[6]

Gradually toward the end of the twentieth century, skepticism and concern grew regarding the practice of deep sedation. Intensivists increasingly recognized the growing problem of the brain and physical dysfunction in patients' lives as they recovered from a critical illness. In a poignant editorial for the journal Chest in 1998, Dr Thomas Petty expressed his frustration with the state of critical care medicine and concern about the implications of the practices of the time, stating, "what I see these days are paralyzed, sedated patients, lying without motion, appearing to be dead, except for the monitors that tell me otherwise. Why this syndrome of sedation and paralysis has emerged baffles me, because this was not the case in the past."[7] He recounts that early in the history of critical care medicine and mechanical ventilation, only modest amounts of analgesia and sedation were used so that patients would be awake and alert and "sustain a zest for living, which is a requirement for survival."[7] He goes on to discuss the multitude of complications resulting from deep sedation and immobility including "critical care neuropathy, pulmonary emboli from immobilization, and sepsis from bacterial invasion of the atrophic gastrointestinal (GI) tract, but also clouded sensorium that often results in what has been termed as intensive care delirium. I am afraid that the conspiracy between the requirements of high acuity care and available pharmacologic therapy has led to the present situation."[7] These cautionary observations were an early call to attention about the outright potential dangers of the care we provide that we would spend the next 2 decades unraveling.

Delirium: A Hidden Menace

At the time of Dr Petty's observations, the medical community's awareness of acute brain dysfunction, or delirium, in critical illness was still in its nascency. Pioneering work from Drs Engel and Romano in 1959 sought to draw attention to 2 salient features of delirium that most physicians tended to overlook: (1) delirium has an organic etiology and (2) is not a primary neurologic problem, but rather a state of "cerebral insufficiency" in the same way other end-organ dysfunctions occur such as renal insufficiency, pulmonary insufficiency, or cardiac insufficiency.[8] Recognition of delirium in daily clinical practice increased throughout the 1980s as a condition that frequently plagued older adults, contributed to adverse outcomes, and was often preventable.[9,10] Postulating that "ICU psychosis" may actually be delirium, providers urgently needed a tool to diagnose and measure the prevalence of delirium in intubated ICU patients. Thus, the Confusion Assessment Method for the ICU (CAM-ICU)[11] and the Intensive Care Delirium Screening Checklist[12] were created in 2001 to fill this need. The CAM-ICU and ICDSC were validated against the formal DSM criteria and found to be highly sensitive and specific.[11,12] These instruments allow for the rapid and accurate assessment of both verbal and nonverbal (intubated) patients by any trained care provider for the presence of the hallmark features of delirium: acute presentation, fluctuating mental status, inattention, altered consciousness, and disorganized thinking.[13] Armed with validated tools to actually measure delirium in the ICU, multiple studies screened hundreds of ICU patients and found staggering estimates of delirium; as many as 60% to 80% of patients across medical, surgical, and trauma ICUs were found to have delirium during their critical illness.[11,14] In addition to discovering the high prevalence of ICU delirium, investigators found that patients who developed delirium had worse outcomes than those patients who did not develop delirium, even after accounting for confounders such as severity of illness.[15,16] During acute hospitalization, delirium is an independent predictor of increased time on mechanical ventilation, longer ICU stays, longer time in the hospital, and increased health care costs.[15–18] Further, patients with delirium experienced higher mortality in the ICU and during the hospital stay.[16,19] These data provided the framework for our growing understanding of brain dysfunction in the ICU: delirium is not an innocent yet inevitable bystander of critical illness. It is a complex disease process and an independent predictor of poor outcomes in the ICU.

Long-Term Cognitive Impairment and the Link to Delirium

Concurrent with the growing recognition of the impact delirium in a vast number of critically ill patients, intensivists also noticed that survivors of critical illness were experiencing lasting difficulties with cognition, an unexpected finding for a population that initially presented with respiratory failure or sepsis. In a small cohort of ARDS survivors who completed a battery of neuropsychological tests 1 year after discharge from their illness, 30% showed global cognitive dysfunction and 78% showed impairment in at least one domain of memory, attention, concentration, or processing speed.[20] Over the next two decades, investigators worldwide found similar results; ICU survivors were experiencing persistent cognitive dysfunction for months to years after discharge[21,22] with some failing to recover up to 8 years later.[23–25] A longitudinal study of older adults without preexisting dementia showed that participants hospitalized with critical illness had significantly lower scores on cognitive testing compared with those who did not experience critical illness.[26] Even mild deficits can be disruptive and, in some cases, survivors with no prior cognitive issues showed cognitive function at the level of patients with traumatic brain injuries or Alzheimer's disease at 12 months after discharge from the ICU (**Fig. 1**).[27] Later imaging studies would confirm that patients with cognitive dysfunction had physical changes to the brain including gross atrophy and disruption of white matter.[28,29]

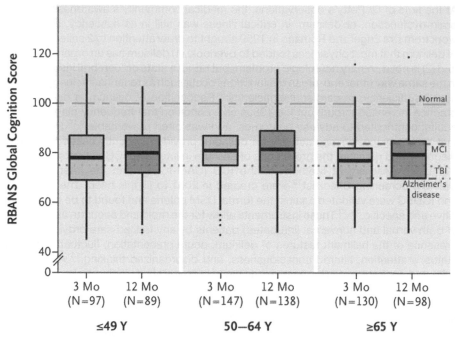

Fig. 1. The box-and-whisker plots show the age-adjusted global cognition scores on the Repeatable Battery for the Assessment of Neuropsychological Status (RBANS) according to age in survivors of critical illness. The age-adjusted population mean is 100 for healthy adults, and the green band indicates the standard deviation (15). As shown, survivors have significantly lower global cognition scores upon testing with values comparable to those of patients with mild cognitive impairment (MCI), moderate traumatic brain injury (TBI), and mild Alzheimer's disease based on other cohort studies. (*From* Pandharipande PP, Girard TD, Jackson JC, et al. Long-Term Cognitive Impairment after Critical Illness. New England Journal of Medicine. 2013;369(14):1306-1316; with permission.)

Increasing awareness of post-ICU cognitive dysfunction prompted a search to identify risk factors and prevention strategies to mitigate its impact. Many studies found overlap in the baseline risk factors for delirium and cognitive dysfunction (ie, increasing age and comorbidity burden).[27,30,31] Seminal work published in the early 2000s found that both the presence and increasing duration of delirium was one of the strongest risk factors for subsequent cognitive dysfunction in ICU survivors.[27,30,31] This further highlighted the importance of recognizing delirium in the ICU as a form of organ dysfunction with both short and long-term implications.

The lasting effects of critical illness and cognitive dysfunction were discovered to permeate multiple and far-reaching aspects of survivors' lives. They developed disabilities in functional activities like managing medications, tracking finances, and arranging transportation to medical appointments.[32] They experienced new depression and posttraumatic stress disorder, were unable to return to work, and reported overall low quality of life.[25,32,33] The Society of Critical Care Medicine convened a key stakeholders conference in 2010 to raise awareness about the long-term consequences of critical illness for patients and their families, introducing the term Post Intensive Care Syndrome (PICS) to encompass the physical, cognitive, and mental health challenges many patients were facing.[34]

Managing Brain Dysfunction in the Intensive Care Unit: From Sedation to Exercise

In a new movement to understand the factors driving brain dysfunction in the ICU, a surprising but compelling body of evidence found that benzodiazepine administration increased the risk of developing delirium.[14,35–37] This disrupted a widely accepted sedation practice and prompted a change in 2002 guidelines on sedation management from promoting the use of longer-acting benzodiazepines (ie, lorazepam and midazolam)[38] to recommending *against* benzodiazepine use in 2013.[39] Sedation practices further came into question with the evolving knowledge that prolonged sedation via continuous infusion was associated with longer duration of mechanical ventilation and length of stay in the ICU, increasing risk of iatrogenic harm.[40–43] These guideline changes moved us toward the current era in critical care medicine where we recognize the real risks of brain dysfunction in the ICU and the iatrogenic injury that can occur to our patients during their critical illness. The increasing recognition of delirium and long-term cognitive impairment has prompted continuous evaluation and updates to the evidence-based Society of Critical Care Medicine Clinical Practice Guidelines for the Prevention and Management of Pain, Agitation/Sedation, Delirium, Immobility, and Sleep Disruption (PADIS Guidelines—last updated in 2018) and the formation of a national quality improvement initiative, the ICU Liberation Collaborative. The Collaborative is tasked with promoting the implementation of the guidelines and helping critical care programs worldwide operationalize evidence-based practices into their everyday workflow to improve outcomes for patients. We will now briefly review some of the landmark studies showing how the strategies outlined in the ICU Liberation Bundle reduce delirium and subsequent cognitive impairment.

Managing Delirium and Preventing Cognitive Impairment with Intensive Care Unit Liberation

The ICU Liberation Bundle, also known as the "ABCDEF Bundle," is the keystone strategy to implement the recommendations of the PADIS guidelines and reduce the impact of delirium, long-term cognitive impairment, mental health disparities, and disability after critical illness.[44] The bundle itself represents a collation of hundreds of studies conducted with the goal of improving outcomes for ICU patients into six key components considered essential for reducing iatrogenesis **(Table 1)**.[45] Rather than

Table 1	
Key components of the ABCDEF bundle	
A	Assess and manage pain
B	Both spontaneous awaking and breathing trials
C	Choice of sedation
D	Delirium: assess, prevent, and manage
E	Early mobility and exercise
F	Family engagement and empowerment

being an afterthought during the care of critically ill patients, the goal of the ICU Liberation Bundle is to initiate key components shown to improve outcomes, such as routine delirium screening and early mobility, as a part of routine ICU care, beginning at the time of admission.

The first component of the bundle is "A" for "Assess, Treat, and Manage Pain." Studies confirm that ICU patients experience pain both at rest and during procedures and providers are prone to mistaking sedation as adequate treatment of pain.[46,47] Perioperative delirium studies show increased delirium in patients whose pain is inadequately controlled,[48] however a recent large cohort study in a mixed medical-surgical ICU from the Netherlands found that administration of opioids increased the odds of transitioning to delirium in a dose-dependent fashion.[49] It is likely that delirium can be impacted by both overuse, and underuse, of opiates in managing pain. Nevertheless, providers agree that assessing for and managing pain should be a priority in ICU patients as the implementation of pain assessments has been shown to decrease ICU mortality and length of stay, and duration of mechanical ventilation.[50] The second component of the bundle is "B" for daily performance of "Both Awakening and Breathing Trials." Hypothesizing that prolonged periods of sedation were likely detrimental to patients, investigators sought to test the safety and efficacy of unified weaning protocols from sedation and mechanical ventilation. An early study of standardized daily sedative interruption showed a drastic reduction in the duration of mechanical ventilation and ICU stay.[51] Subsequent work by Girard and colleagues[52] paired this interruption of sedation or a "Spontaneous Awakening Trial" (SAT) with a daily "Spontaneous Breathing Trial" (SBT) and showed a significant reduction in duration of mechanical ventilation, earlier discharge from the ICU and hospital, and a *reduction in mortality up to 1 year after critical illness* in the intervention group (**Fig. 2**). In addition, paired SATs and SBTs clearly reduce ICU delirium.[53]

"C" represents "Choice of Sedation and Analgesia," based on the discovery that avoiding long-acting benzodiazepines is associated with less delirium, which is a clear deviation from prior practice patterns. In addition, we have learned that deeper planes of sedation are associated with an increased risk of death, delirium, and time to extubation, favoring targeting lighter levels of sedation for any patient requiring sedative medication (**Fig. 3**).[54-56] "D" for "Delirium: Assess, Prevent, & Manage" serves as a reminder that the development of tools that could identify delirium in the ICU, such as CAM-ICU or ICDSC, was essential to developing practices to target brain dysfunction. Without the consistent implementation of a delirium screening tool, many providers miss the presence of delirium and the opportunity to implement management strategies including identifying and correcting factors contributing to delirium (ie, medications, electrolyte imbalances, and sleep disturbances).

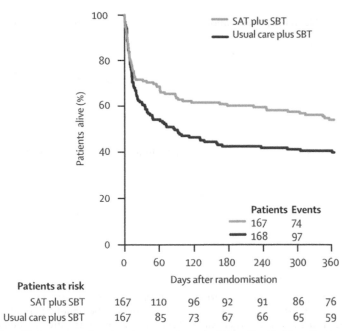

Fig. 2. Kaplan–Meier curve showing improved survival in critically ill patients undergoing paired spontaneous awakening and breathing trials, which form a key component of the ABCDEF bundle and help reduce delirium. (Reprinted with permission from Elsevier. The Lancet, 2008; 371(9607):126-134.)

The "E" component of the ABCDEF bundle advocates for the use of "Early Mobility and Exercise". Studies of early mobility and rehabilitation were developed to counteract muscle loss, acquired weakness, and physical impairment and led to improved functional independence at discharge.[57,58] Notably, two studies by Schaller and Schweickert showed that early rehabilitation clearly reduced the duration of delirium, providing one of the few *active* interventions shown to reduce the duration of delirium.[57,58] The final and most recent addition to the bundle is the "F" component for "Family Engagement and Empowerment." Family presence can help tremendously with patient re-orientation and comfort during critical illness. Further, families are at high risk for mental health problems triggered by the psychological stress of a loved one's critical illness.[59] Though the ideal model for family engagement has yet to be established, there is evidence that both patients[60] and families[61] have better mental health outcomes when families are directly involved in care.

Although each individual component of the ABCDEF bundle was developed from high-quality evidence and represents the historical arc of scientific evidence over the last several decades in critical care medicine, the bundle in aggregate offers extremely positive results in improving patient outcomes. Two large studies of more than 6000 and 15,000 patients across multiple hospitals showed that increasing compliance with the bundle led to decreased ICU mortality, less use of physical restraints, decreased duration of mechanical ventilation, increase in delirium- and coma-free days, decreased risk of readmission to the ICU, and increased discharge to home.[62,63] The demonstrated benefit of bundling each of these components highlights the importance of multi-faceted interventions that target numerous causes of brain dysfunction in the ICU. For the ABCDEF bundle, the whole is greater than the sum of its parts.

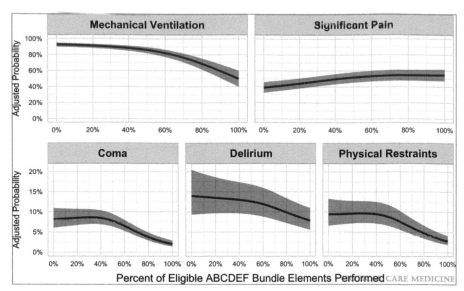

Fig. 3. Increased proportional performance of the ABCDEF bundle reduces the risk of delirium, coma, and other outcomes the next day, showing the benefit of multifaceted, holistic bundles of care in preventing brain dysfunction and other negative sequelae of critical illness. (*From* Pun BT, Balas MC, Barnes-Daly MA, et al. Caring for Critically Ill Patients with the ABCDEF Bundle: Results of the ICU Liberation Collaborative in Over 15,000 Adults. Crit Care Med. 2019;47(1):3-14; with permission.)

The Challenges of the Coronavirus Disease-2019 Pandemic

The emergence of the severe acute respiratory syndrome coronavirus 2 (SARS-CoV-2) pathogen in early 2020 and its associated manifestation in the coronavirus disease 2019 or COVID-19 strained critical care resources worldwide. Critical care clinicians were suddenly faced with an overwhelming number of patients receiving non-invasive respiratory support or mechanical ventilation. Because of the profound hypoxemia and respiratory distress experienced by many patients with ARDS due to COVID-19, increasing amounts of sedation were given to patients to assist with ventilator synchrony. Patients also suffered from severe multi-organ failure, setting up the perfect storm for increased brain dysfunction at the same time the world was facing one of the largest threats to public health in decades. In an international study of over 2000 patients admitted to ICUs with severe COVID-19, up to 80% of patients developed delirium and/or coma during the 21-day study period.[64] In comparison, a study of the ABCDEF bundle in 15,000 patients across the United States before the COVID-19 pandemic found that patients experienced delirium on 29% of ICU days.[63] Notably, patients in the COVID-19 study received significantly more benzodiazepines compared with previous cohorts. Lastly, patients in the COVID-19 study only received some components of the ABCDEF bundle on 25% of eligible days at most. The progress that had been made in implementing strategies to reduce brain dysfunction and delirium had been rolled back under the strain of the pandemic. There were numerous reasons for these practice changes: patient volume, drug shortages, prolonged periods of mechanical ventilation, and concerns about aerosolization of virus in less sedated patients. The implications of COVID-19 and the increased public health burden of delirium remain to be evaluated in large prospective cohort studies; yet, based on prior research, we anticipate that a substantial number of survivors will be burdened with long-term cognitive impairment and disability for years to come.

The Future of Brain Dysfunction in Critical Illness

Our understanding of cognition and the brain during critical illness has evolved substantially in the last several decades, revolutionizing how we practice and understand the trajectories of recovery our patient's experience. There remain several unsolved problems - the lack of effective pharmaceutical interventions for acute delirium, management strategies in ICU survivors for long-term cognitive impairment, and fundamental questions regarding the driving pathologies that lead to brain dysfunction during critical illness. Importantly, however, delirium and coma are no longer considered benign byproducts of the ICU environment but instead are more aptly understood as an important form of organ failure to prevent and manage prospectively. Physicians and scientists worldwide have grown to appreciate the enormity of "brain failure" in the ICU and are working toward improving care from inside the ICU to outside the walls of the hospital. The COVID-19 pandemic created a substantial hurdle in the work toward improving cognitive function during and after critical illness. It is vital that clinicians and ICU environments return to strong evidence-based practices in caring for our most vulnerable patients. Managing pain, early liberation from mechanical ventilation, choosing appropriate light sedation, screening for delirium, engaging patients in early rehabilitation, and conducting patient- and family-centered care are the keys to reducing the global burden of delirium and cognitive impairment in the ICU. The arc of history in critical care medicine is one toward both a better physiologic understanding of critical illness and one of more humanistic care, and we must plot our course with that end in mind.

CLINICS CARE POINTS

- Delirium in the ICU is extremely prevalent and providers must routinely use validated screening tools to identify all cases and implement management strategies.
- Routine use of benzodiazepines and deep sedation is discouraged when possible due to the long-term detrimental effects on cognition.
- Implementation of the multi-component ABCDEF bundle is highly effective at reducing delirium and improving outcomes.

FUNDING/SUPPORT

This work was supported by the Department of Veterans Affairs Tennessee Valley Health Care System, Geriatric Research Education and Clinical Center (GRECC), United States, the National Institutes of Health, United States under awards (R01AG027472 and R01AG058639), and the Vanderbilt Faculty Research Scholars Program. This material is based upon work supported by the U.S. Department of Veterans Affairs, United States (VA) Office of Aviation Analysis, United States, VA National Quality Scholars Program, and with resources and use of facilities at VA Tennessee Valley Healthcare System in Nashville, Tennessee.

ROLE OF THE FUNDER/SPONSOR

The funding sources had no role in the design and conduct of the study; collection, management, analysis, and interpretation of the data; preparation, review, or approval of the article; and decision to submit the article for publication. The contents of this paper are solely the responsibility of the authors and do not necessarily represent those of the Department of Veterans Affairs, the National Institutes of Health, or Vanderbilt University Medical Center.

REFERENCES

1. Zimmerman JE, Kramer AA, Knaus WA. Changes in hospital mortality for United States intensive care unit admissions from 1988 to 2012. Crit Care 2013;17(2):R81.
2. Ibsen B. The anaesthetist's viewpoint on the treatment of respiratory complications in poliomyelitis during the epidemic in Copenhagen, 1952. Proc R Soc Med 1954;47(1):72–4.
3. Lassen HC. A preliminary report on the 1952 epidemic of poliomyelitis in Copenhagen with special reference to the treatment of acute respiratory insufficiency. Lancet 1953;1(6749):37–41.
4. Ashbaugh DG, Bigelow DB, Petty TL, et al. Acute respiratory distress in adults. Lancet 1967;2(7511):319–+.
5. Levine BE. Fifty years of research in ARDS. ARDS: how it all began. Am J Respir Crit Care Med 2017;196(10):1247–8.
6. Justic M. Does "ICU psychosis" really exist? Crit Care Nurse 2000;20(3):28–37, quiz 38-29.
7. Petty TL. Suspended life or extending death? Chest 1998;114(2):360–1.
8. Engel GL, Romano J. Delirium, a syndrome of cerebral insufficiency. J Chronic Dis 1959;9(3):260–77.
9. Francis J, Kapoor WN. Delirium in hospitalized elderly. J Gen Intern Med 1990; 5(1):65–79.
10. Inouye SK. The dilemma of delirium: clinical and research controversies regarding diagnosis and evaluation of delirium in hospitalized elderly medical patients. Am J Med 1994;97(3):278–88.
11. Ely EW, Inouye SK, Bernard GR, et al. Delirium in mechanically ventilated patients - validity and reliability of the Confusion Assessment Method for the intensive care unit (CAM-ICU). JAMA, J Am Med Assoc 2001;286(21):2703–10.
12. Bergeron N, Dubois MJ, Dumont M, et al. Intensive care delirium screening checklist: evaluation of a new screening tool. Intensive Care Med 2001;27(5): 859–64.
13. Diagnostic and statistical manual of mental disorders : DSM-5. Arlington, VA: American Psychiatric Association; 2013.
14. Pandharipande P, Cotton BA, Shintani A, et al. Prevalence and risk factors for development of delirium in surgical and trauma intensive care unit patients. J Trauma 2008;65(1):34–41.
15. Ely EW, Gautam S, Margolin R, et al. The impact of delirium in the intensive care unit on hospital length of stay. Intensive Care Med 2001;27(12):1892–900.
16. Ely EW, Shintani A, Truman B, et al. Delirium as a predictor of mortality in mechanically ventilated patients in the intensive care unit. JAMA, J Am Med Assoc 2004; 291(14):1753–62.
17. Milbrandt EB, Deppen S, Harrison PL, et al. Costs associated with delirium in mechanically ventilated patients. Crit Care Med 2004;32(4):955–62.
18. Vasilevskis EE, Chandrasekhar R, Holtze CH, et al. The cost of ICU delirium and coma in the intensive care unit patient. Med Care 2018;56(10):890–7.
19. Ouimet S, Kavanagh BP, Gottfried SB, et al. Incidence, risk factors and consequences of ICU delirium. Intensive Care Med 2007;33(1):66–73.

20. Hopkins RO, Weaver LK, Pope D, et al. Neuropsychological sequelae and impaired health status in survivors of severe acute respiratory distress syndrome. Am J Respir Crit Care Med 1999;160(1):50–6.

21. Jackson JC, Hart RP, Gordon SM, et al. Six-month neuropsychological outcome of medical intensive care unit patients. Crit Care Med 2003;31(4):1226–34.

22. Sukantarat KT, Burgess PW, Williamson RC, et al. Prolonged cognitive dysfunction in survivors of critical illness. Anaesthesia 2005;60(9):847–53.

23. Iwashyna TJ, Ely EW, Smith DM, et al. Long-term cognitive impairment and functional disability among survivors of severe sepsis. JAMA, J Am Med Assoc 2010; 304(16):1787–94.

24. Hopkins MW, Libon DJ. Neuropsychological functioning of dementia patients with psychosis. Arch Clin Neuropsychol 2005;20(6):771–83.

25. Rothenhausler HB, Ehrentraut S, Stoll C, et al. The relationship between cognitive performance and employment and health status in long-term survivors of the acute respiratory distress syndrome: results of an exploratory study. Gen Hosp Psychiatry 2001;23(2):90–6.

26. Ehlenbach WJ, Hough CL, Crane PK, et al. Association between acute care and critical illness hospitalization and cognitive function in older adults. JAMA, J Am Med Assoc 2010;303(8):763–70.

27. Pandharipande PP, Girard TD, Jackson JC, et al. Long-term cognitive impairment after critical illness. N Engl J Med 2013;369(14):1306–16.

28. Gunther ML, Morandi A, Krauskopf E, et al. The association between brain volumes, delirium duration, and cognitive outcomes in intensive care unit survivors: the VISIONS cohort magnetic resonance imaging study. Crit Care Med 2012; 40(7):2022–32.

29. Morandi A, Rogers BP, Gunther ML, et al. The relationship between delirium duration, white matter integrity, and cognitive impairment in intensive care unit survivors as determined by diffusion tensor imaging: the VISIONS prospective cohort magnetic resonance imaging study. Crit Care Med 2012;40(7):2182–9.

30. Girard TD, Jackson JC, Pandharipande PP, et al. Delirium as a predictor of long-term cognitive impairment in survivors of critical illness. Crit Care Med 2010; 38(7):1513–20.

31. Wolters AE, Slooter AJ, van der Kooi AW, et al. Cognitive impairment after intensive care unit admission: a systematic review. Intensive Care Med 2013;39(3): 376–86.

32. Jackson JC, Pandharipande PP, Girard TD, et al. Depression, post-traumatic stress disorder, and functional disability in survivors of critical illness in the BRAIN-ICU study: a longitudinal cohort study. Lancet Respir Med 2014;2(5): 369–79.

33. Norman BC, Jackson JC, Graves JA, et al. Employment outcomes after critical illness: an analysis of the bringing to light the risk factors and incidence of neuropsychological dysfunction in ICU survivors cohort. Crit Care Med 2016;44(11): 2003–9.

34. Needham DM, Davidson J, Cohen H, et al. Improving long-term outcomes after discharge from intensive care unit: report from a stakeholders' conference. Crit Care Med 2012;40(2):502–9.

35. Pandharipande P, Shintani A, Peterson J, et al. Lorazepam is an independent risk factor for transitioning to delirium in intensive care unit patients. Anesthesiology 2006;104(1):21–6.

36. Seymour CW, Pandharipande PP, Koestner T, et al. Diurnal sedative changes during intensive care: impact on liberation from mechanical ventilation and delirium. Crit Care Med 2012;40(10):2788–96.

37. Riker RR, Shehabi Y, Bokesch PM, et al. Dexmedetomidine vs midazolam for sedation of critically ill patients A randomized trial. JAMA, J Am Med Assoc 2009;301(5):489–99.

38. Jacobi J, Fraser GL, Coursin DB, et al. Clinical practice guidelines for the sustained use of sedatives and analgesics in the critically ill adult. Crit Care Med 2002;30(1):119–41.

39. Barr J, Fraser GL, Puntillo K, et al. Clinical practice guidelines for the management of pain, agitation, and delirium in adult patients in the intensive care unit. Crit Care Med 2013;41(1):263–306.

40. Cook DJ, Walter SD, Cook RJ, et al. Incidence of and risk factors for ventilator-associated pneumonia in critically ill patients. Ann Intern Med 1998;129(6):433–40.

41. Kollef MH, Levy NT, Ahrens TS, et al. The use of continuous i.v. sedation is associated with prolongation of mechanical ventilation. Chest 1998;114(2):541–8.

42. Payen JF, Chanques G, Mantz J, et al. Current practices in sedation and analgesia for mechanically ventilated critically ill patients: a prospective multicenter patient-based study. Anesthesiology 2007;106(4):687–95, quiz 891-682.

43. Pinhu L, Whitehead T, Evans T, et al. Ventilator-associated lung injury. Lancet 2003;361(9354):332–40.

44. Marra A, Ely EW, Pandharipande PP, et al. The ABCDEF bundle in critical care. Crit Care Clin 2017;33(2):225–43.

45. Ely EW. The ABCDEF bundle: science and philosophy of how ICU liberation serves patients and families. Crit Care Med 2017;45(2):321–30.

46. Chanques G, Sebbane M, Barbotte E, et al. A prospective study of pain at rest: incidence and characteristics of an unrecognized symptom in surgical and trauma versus medical intensive care unit patients. Anesthesiology 2007; 107(5):858–60.

47. Puntillo KA, Max A, Timsit JF, et al. Determinants of procedural pain intensity in the intensive care unit. The Europain(R) study. Am J Respir Crit Care Med 2014;189(1):39–47.

48. Morrison RS, Magaziner J, Gilbert M, et al. Relationship between pain and opioid analgesics on the development of delirium following hip fracture. J Gerontol A Biol Sci Med Sci 2003;58(1):76–81.

49. Duprey MS, Dijkstra-Kersten SMA, Zaal IJ, et al. Opioid use increases the risk of delirium in critically ill adults independently of pain. Am J Respir Crit Care Med 2021;204(5):566–72.

50. Payen JF, Bosson JL, Chanques G, et al. Pain assessment is associated with decreased duration of mechanical ventilation in the intensive care unit: a post Hoc analysis of the DOLOREA study. Anesthesiology 2009;111(6):1308–16.

51. Kress JP, Pohlman AS, O'Connor MF, et al. Daily interruption of sedative infusions in critically ill patients undergoing mechanical ventilation. N Engl J Med 2000; 342(20):1471–7.

52. Girard TD, Kress JP, Fuchs BD, et al. Efficacy and safety of a paired sedation and ventilator weaning protocol for mechanically ventilated patients in intensive care (Awakening and Breathing Controlled trial): a randomised controlled trial. Lancet 2008;371(9607):126–34.

53. Khan BA, Fadel WF, Tricker JL, et al. Effectiveness of implementing a wake up and breathe program on sedation and delirium in the ICU. Crit Care Med 2014; 42(12):e791–5.
54. Shehabi Y, Bellomo R, Kadiman S, et al. Sedation intensity in the first 48 hours of mechanical ventilation and 180-day mortality: a multinational prospective longitudinal cohort study. Crit Care Med 2018;46(6):850–9.
55. Shehabi Y, Bellomo R, Reade MC, et al. Early intensive care sedation predicts long-term mortality in ventilated critically ill patients. Am J Respir Crit Care Med 2012;186(8):724–31.
56. Stephens RJ, Dettmer MR, Roberts BW, et al. Practice patterns and outcomes associated with early sedation depth in mechanically ventilated patients: a systematic review and meta-analysis. Crit Care Med 2018;46(3):471–9.
57. Schweickert WD, Pohlman MC, Pohlman AS, et al. Early physical and occupational therapy in mechanically ventilated, critically ill patients: a randomised controlled trial. Lancet 2009;373(9678):1874–82.
58. Schaller SJ, Anstey M, Blobner M, et al. Early, goal-directed mobilisation in the surgical intensive care unit: a randomised controlled trial. Lancet 2016; 388(10052):1377–88.
59. Cameron JI, Chu LM, Matte A, et al. One-year outcomes in caregivers of critically ill patients. N Engl J Med 2016;374(19):1831–41.
60. Black P, Boore JR, Parahoo K. The effect of nurse-facilitated family participation in the psychological care of the critically ill patient. J Adv Nurs 2011;67(5): 1091–101.
61. Anderson WG, Arnold RM, Angus DC, et al. Passive decision-making preference is associated with anxiety and depression in relatives of patients in the intensive care unit. J Crit Care 2009;24(2):249–54.
62. Barnes-Daly MA, Phillips G, Ely EW. Improving hospital survival and reducing brain dysfunction at seven California community hospitals: implementing PAD guidelines via the ABCDEF bundle in 6,064 patients. Crit Care Med 2017;45(2): 171–8.
63. Pun BT, Balas MC, Barnes-Daly MA, et al. Caring for critically ill patients with the ABCDEF bundle: results of the ICU liberation collaborative in over 15,000 adults. Crit Care Med 2019;47(1):3–14.
64. Pun BT, Badenes R, Heras La Calle G, et al. Prevalence and risk factors for delirium in critically ill patients with COVID-19 (COVID-D): a multicentre cohort study. Lancet Respir Med 2021;9(3):239–50.

From Strict Bedrest to Early Mobilization
A History of Physiotherapy in the Intensive Care Unit

Michelle E. Kho, PT, PhD[a,b,*], Bronwen Connolly, MSc, PhD, MCSP[c]

KEYWORDS

- Physiotherapy • Physical therapy • Rehabilitation • Mechanical ventilation
- Intensive care units • Post-intensive care syndrome • Early mobility • Clinical trials

KEY POINTS

- Survivors of critical illness are at risk for post-intensive care sequelae including physical and cognitive impairments, mood disorders, fatigue, and frailty.
- Critical care is evolving from a culture of deep sedation and bed rest to one of the proactive strategies to improve long-term outcomes.
- Landmark clinical trials of early mobilization interventions in the late 2000s catalyzed increased awareness of the need for proven physiotherapeutic rehabilitation approaches to mitigate post-intensive care sequelae.
- Physiotherapists are experts in developing targeted, individualized management plans to address physical impairments in critically ill patients, throughout the recovery pathway.
- The evolution of physiotherapy clinician-scientists and their greater engagement and leadership in critical care research, including a specific focus on early mobilization and physical rehabilitation, will continue to change the field.

History is important because it teaches us about the past. And by learning about the past, you come to understand the present, so that you may make educated decisions about the future.

—Richelle Mead[1]

[a] School of Rehabilitation Science, McMaster University, Institute for Applied Health Science, Room 403, 1400 Main Street West, Hamilton, Ontario L8S 1C7, Canada; [b] Physiotherapy Department, Research Institute of St. Joe's Hamilton, 50 Charlton Avenue East, Hamilton, Ontario L8N 4A6, Canada; [c] Wellcome-Wolfson Institute for Experimental Medicine, Queen's University Belfast, 97 Lisburn Road, Belfast BT9 7BL, United Kingdom
* Corresponding author. School of Rehabilitation Science, McMaster University, Institute for Applied Health Science, Room 403, 1400 Main Street West, Hamilton, Ontario L8S 1C7, Canada
E-mail address: khome@mcmaster.ca

Crit Care Clin 39 (2023) 479–502
https://doi.org/10.1016/j.ccc.2023.01.003
0749-0704/23/© 2023 Elsevier Inc. All rights reserved.

criticalcare.theclinics.com

INTRODUCTION

Critical care medicine was founded upon principles of interdisciplinary teamwork. Notably, some of the first interdisciplinary interactions occurred between epidemiologists and anesthesiologists in Denmark to study strategies to improve outcomes of people with poliomyelitis and respiratory failure in the early 1950s.[2] Since those early days, physiotherapy as a profession has matured, academically, clinically, and in response to developments in research. In this article, we consider this professional evolution within the specialty of critical care, specifically focused on the context of early mobilization (EM). We examine two perspectives, the clinical and research remits. We explore advancements in these remits that have shaped physiotherapy within the interdisciplinary intensive care unit (ICU) team, moving from past, present, and looking ahead to the future.

CONCEPTS AND DEFINITIONS

Within this article, we will use the term "physiotherapy" and "physical therapy" interchangeably. Both terms refer to regulated health professions involving formalized training qualifications available at undergraduate and postgraduate levels. Traditionally, physiotherapy for critically ill patients within the ICU encompasses the management of both acute and chronic respiratory conditions, as well as the mitigation and treatment of physical deconditioning associated with prolonged immobility, invasive mechanical ventilation, and the deleterious effects of pharmacotherapy including sedation and neuromuscular blocking agents.[3] Within the context of this article, the emphasis will be on physical rehabilitation, although we also recognize the role of physiotherapists in airway clearance and ventilation management in some jurisdictions.

Our use of the concept "early mobility," and related terms, reflects the broad use in the literature. Although there is no universal agreement regarding the exact definition of EM,[4] in clinical practice, EM is typically characterized by a hierarchical progression of increasingly functional activities. In-bed activities such as positioning, assessment, and maintenance of joint range of motion, and bed mobility exercise, progress to out-of-bed activities such as sitting over the edge of the bed, transfers (eg, sit-to-stand or bed-to-chair, standing), and finally ambulation (eg, marching on the spot, gait training, and mobility away from the bed-space). Selection of EM activity depends on the clinical stability and level of active engagement of the patient, and recording of activities often uses established activity codes such as the ICU Mobility Scale.[5] At times, EM activities may be combined with activities of daily living (eg, washing, dressing, and bathing), in coordination with occupational therapy colleagues.

Brief History of Physiotherapy and Critical Care

The academic status and profile of physiotherapy as a profession has developed over the years, emerging around the early 1920s, with origins in therapeutic massage gymnastics, and with strong ties to medicine and nursing. A key driver in shaping modern physiotherapy was as a response to address the rehabilitation of physical impairments in individuals secondary to events such as World War I, and the polio epidemics of the first half of the twentieth century. In the late 1940s physiotherapists were enlisted in acute care to help care for patients with poliomyelitis requiring rehabilitation. Early guidance to physiotherapists included, "*The actual physical therapy measures should be carefully explained. This calls for a consideration of policies on muscle testing, muscle reeducation, preparation of the patient on admission, and for discharge, and limitations on patient activity.... At various times during an epidemic there probably will be medically conducted research with special equipment, medications, or statistical surveys. The therapist must cooperate to the fullest extent, and by doing so will find herself (sic) stimulated and be eager to further her knowledge of the disease."*[6]

Clinical education requirements were formalized in the first half of the twentieth century, but at different times in different countries. In the United States, the first Bachelor of Science program for physical therapists was launched in 1927,[7] in Canada, the first physiotherapists graduated with a combined physiotherapy and occupational therapy diploma in 1929,[8] the first physiotherapy degree was offered in Australia in 1950,[9] and in the United Kingdom, the first undergraduate physiotherapy course appeared later, in 1976.[10] Recent times has seen a move towards entry-level practice requiring Masters or Professional Doctorate (eg, DPT) qualification pathways.

The modern specialty of critical care was born during the polio epidemic in the early 1950s, with the demonstration by Dr Bjørn Ibsen of Denmark regarding the utility of positive pressure ventilation outside the operating room.[2] Early ICUs were documented in Canada, the United States, and by the late 1950s and early 1960s.[11] The Society of Critical Care Medicine was established in 1971, and the first world congress of critical care occurred in 1977.[11] Important growth of the critical care field occurred between 1980 and 1989, including the first textbook and establishment of critical care as a specialization.[11] The formation of the Canadian Critical Care Trials Group (CCCTG) in 1989[12] and its first major research output in the New England Journal of Medicine in 1994[13] helped inspire the development of trial groups worldwide. Since 2000, advances in the field of critical care, such as decreased mortality in acute respiratory distress syndrome (ARDS) patients through improved mechanical ventilation strategies,[14] prompted a shift in focus to consideration of life after the ICU, and led to seminal research of long-term outcomes in ARDS survivors.[15] **Fig. 1** outlines selected milestones in critical care. In the subsequent sections, we discuss the clinical and research landscapes of critical care and physical therapy—past, present, and future.

THE CLINICAL LANDSCAPE

In this section, we characterize how clinical physiotherapy practice has progressed in critical care, relevant guidance that has driven developments, and suggested areas of future advances (**Fig. 2**).

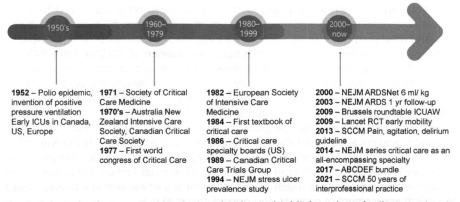

Fig. 1. Selected milestones in critical care. This figure highlights selected milestones in critical care over the last 70 years. ARDS, acute respiratory distress syndrome; ICUAW, ICU-acquired weakness; NEJM, *New England Journal of Medicine*; RCT, randomized clinical trial; SCCM, Society of Critical Care Medicine; US, United States.

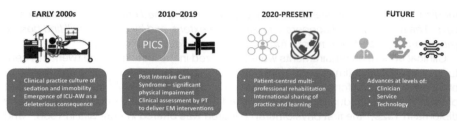

Fig. 2. Schematic representation of developments through the clinical landscape.

PAST
Early 2000s

Reports by Richard Asher, more than 70 years ago, highlighted the negative sequelae across multiple systems of the body associated with consigning acutely ill patients to bed rest.[16] Yet, prolonged immobilization and deep sedation have been characteristic features of critical care medicine for many decades. Traditionally, it had been considered that immobility (achieved through sedation) could preserve metabolic resources for systemic healing and recovery.[17] It was not until the early part of this century that a shift in culture began to appear in the management of critically ill patients in the ICU. One example is the incorporation of daily sedation interruptions (DSI) to potentially improve outcomes such as duration of mechanical ventilation and length of ICU stay.[18] Although subsequent meta-analyses of studies have shown inconsistent findings as a result of DSI,[19,20] the resultant prompt for clinicians to challenge longstanding empirical clinical practices triggered a cascade of further re-evaluation of care practices across multiple domains of patient care.

Alongside changes in the approach to sedation, there was growing recognition of intensive care unit-acquired weakness (ICUAW) as a common and detrimental clinical feature associated with a critical illness.[21] ICUAW is diagnosed clinically, most commonly with the Medical Research Sum-score (MRCSS), a volitional measure that requires the patient to generate muscle force against resistance provided by an examiner. The MRCSS was originally developed to assess critically ill patients with Guillain Barre syndrome,[22] and assesses 6 muscle groups bilaterally (upper extremity: shoulder abduction, elbow flexion, wrist extension; Lower extremity: hip flexion, knee extension, ankle dorsiflexion), rating each muscle group on a scale of 0 to 5 (no contraction, tolerates full resistance), and summing the scores for a minimum score of 0, and maximum score of 60. ICUAW was ascribed to patients scoring <48/60.[23]

Prospective studies showed the estimated prevalence of ICUAW from 24% to 65%.[23–26] Many patients experienced prolonged weaning from mechanical ventilation, which led to delayed rehabilitation, increased hospital length of stay, and mortality in both the ICU and hospital.[23–29] Increasing focus on understanding the biologic, pathophysiologic, and mechanistic nature of ICUAW followed throughout the decade, accompanied by clinical practice position pieces, the 2009 Brussels Roundtable Meeting,[21] and guidelines published by professional bodies such as the European Society of Intensive Care Medicine/European Respiratory Society,[3] and in later years, the American Thoracic Society.[30] With regard to physical rehabilitation, these guidelines recommended a graded approach to EM interventions of escalating intensity based on clinical assessment of patients and consideration of risk.

Incorporation of EM into clinical practice at this time was supported by emerging reports of its feasibility and safety.[31,32] Bailey and colleagues[31] prospectively recorded activity events and adverse events in patients with acute respiratory failure requiring mechanical ventilation > 4 days, including those with endotracheal tubes in situ. Activities that occurred included sitting over the edge of the bed (16%), sitting out in a chair (31%), and ambulation (63%), with a <1% rate of activity-related adverse events reported. Similar data were shown in a separate prospective quasi-randomized study.[32]

Furthermore, in the UK in 2009, the first national guidelines focusing on the rehabilitation of critically ill patients were published.[33] These guidelines advocated a multi-professional rehabilitation approach across the recovery continuum; for patients in the acute stage of critical illness during ICU admission, this involved an early clinical assessment to determine the risk of physical and nonphysical morbidity, associated rehabilitation requirements, and rehabilitation goal-setting.

Collectively, this decade was witness to the building of momentum of a culture toward embracing mobility as an increasingly important element in the management of patients, and the multiprofessional teamwork needed for its implementation.[33]

2010 to 2019

The landmark event in this decade influencing clinical practice in the field was the consensus roundtable and publication of the term "post-intensive care syndrome" (PICS) to encompass the impairments experienced by critically ill patients, across physical, mental, and cognitive domains, with additional recognition of the impact on families and caregivers.[34] To underpin the PICS concept, there was prolific publication of observational data longitudinally characterizing these impairments. Notably, with regard to the physical domain,[35–38] significant declines in muscle strength, physical function, and exercise capacity were observed in patients, but also in other physical aspects such as swallowing function.[39] For example, in a cohort of 193 survivors of ARDS, 86% experienced a decline in at least 1 physical measure (death, muscle strength [MRCSS], physical function, exercise capacity) at 5-year follow-up with older age, illness severity, and chronic comorbidity influential factors in the decline in physical performance.[36] In another, relatively young, cohort of ARDS survivors, again at 5 years, these patients showed an average walking distance of 76% that of age- and sex-matched predicted comparators (436 m), and physical health-related quality of life fell below average scores (score 41, compared with norm score of 50).[38]

To strengthen the case for early physical rehabilitation as a strategy to mitigate against these impairments, the financial cost savings associated with its implementation were shown, as well as the cost-to-outcome benefit in terms of the modest investment required to potentially improve patient outcomes.[40]

Clinical practice was also supported through further rigorous work detailing the safety of conducting EM interventions when appropriate clinical assessment had been undertaken. Hodgson and colleagues[41] reported the findings of expert multidisciplinary consensus recommendations on the safety criteria for active mobilization of mechanically ventilated critically ill adults. This report used a traffic-light system to indicate the risk associated with active mobilization, with a corresponding approach to the level of activity that could therefore be undertaken. The guidelines incorporated assessments across multiple systems (eg, cardiovascular, respiratory, neurological); clinical parameters according to each system were categorized as to whether they indicated a low risk of an adverse event occurring with mobilization (green = proceed with mobilization according to local policies and procedures), a potential risk/consequence of an adverse event, albeit these may be outweighed by any potential benefits (amber = clarify precautions or contraindications before mobilization and proceed with caution), or a significant potential risk or adverse consequence (red = do not proceed with active mobilization unless authorized by the senior ICU medical, nursing, and physiotherapy staff). From a clinical perspective, this simple-to-follow guidance offered practical support to clinicians in developing and implementing EM programs, in particular those settings where teams may have limited experience, skills, and resources. Furthermore, a large-scale systematic review synthesized safety data regarding patient mobilization rehabilitation in the ICU from 48 studies (7546 patients).[42] Potential safety events totaled 583 out of 22,351 treatment sessions (2.6%), and < 1% of reported interventions incurred a safety event with clinical consequences.

Other drivers of influence over clinical practice included the ABCDEF care bundle, where E reflects early mobilization and exercise.[43] Integrating EM into a composite package of care has increased its profile among clinicians who may have previously paid less attention, and also encouraged the multiprofessional team to collaboratively overcome barriers to implementation. Adoption of care bundles, where components are evidence-based and/or empirically considered valuable to patient management, facilitates the embedding of practices into the daily routine. New clinical practice guidelines recommending EM as a first-line nonpharmacological treatment of delirium,[26] and recommendations for early mobility activities started in the ICU[44] also increased the profile of EM activities.

Present (2020 to Current)

Undoubtedly the COVID-19 pandemic has dominated the shape of critical care rehabilitation over the last 2 to 3 years, both in relation to the clinical workforce (eg, significant additional pressures on ICUs, redeployment of noncritical care staff, development of makeshift critical care areas in alternative hospital settings) and patient demographics (eg, increased illness acuity of the unknown profile, trajectory, and prognosis). The emphasis of clinical care reverted to acute "medical" management to manage the severity of respiratory physiology that was evident in patients. Rehabilitation opportunities became limited. However, the global impact of the pandemic generated an international collaborative response from the clinical physiotherapy community,[45,46] as well as an explosion in the use of focused social media to promote collaboration, experiential learning, information provision, and sharing of practice. Examples such as the #RehabLegend initiative (via Twitter) was already in existence but became a platform for clinicians worldwide to offer peer support in a rapid, inclusive, and responsive manner, providing valuable contact between colleagues.

Separate to the pandemic, the wider clinical community has continued to explore and understand PICS in greater detail, expanding our previous knowledge by understanding the complex depth and breadth of impairments experienced by patients.[47] Examples of further domains requiring rehabilitation attention include sleep disorders, fatigue, occupational limitations (return to work),[48] chronic pain, and frailty.[49] The continued growth of interest in post-critical illness recovery and rehabilitation services highlights the need for a truly multiprofessional and multidisciplinary approach to following up with these patients and intervening accordingly.[50]

FUTURE

So where does the future lie for physiotherapy practice in the ICU? Areas for consideration include at the clinician, service, and technology levels.

- *Clinician*: Clinical physiotherapy teams will need to develop local approaches to ensure the rapid and efficient implementation of evidence to guide the delivery of EM interventions; this is likely to center on identifying patients who benefit most from interventions. EM interventions will continue to evolve as just one component of the multidomain rehabilitation required by critically ill patients. This will necessitate adaptive and flexible models of therapy delivery, integration with multiprofessional colleagues, and identifying areas of commonality in therapy delivery to maximize resources while retaining the delivery of interventions of unique physiotherapeutic value, and requiring bespoke physiotherapy skills. Rehabilitation, including EM and other physical rehabilitation interventions, will increase patient-centeredness to build a personalized rehabilitation approach.

- *Service*: At a service level, a detailed workforce review provides the opportunity for evaluating the profile of teams for skill-mix, experience, resources, relevant performance metrics, and innovative approaches to using support staff to complement qualified clinicians. Addressing these aspects can help to ensure the robustness and "fitness for purpose" of clinical teams for optimizing patient services.[51] Development of rehabilitation-focused competency frameworks may be valuable for building consistent and standardized quality of service. Such competency frameworks have been developed for critical care physiotherapy,[52,53] but with relatively little emphasis on mobilization; less than 5% of items deemed essential for competency reflected EM treatments (eg, competency with mobilization of nonventilated patients, competency of mobilization of ventilated patients, and delivery of bed exercise), with one other item addressing the performance of musculoskeletal and/or functional assessments. Furthermore, given the holistic approach to the delivery of rehabilitation to critically ill patients, competency frameworks may be beneficial across the multiprofessional team. Service managers should also be encouraged to explore opportunities around the use of "big data" to harness the value of routinely collected clinical data to inform service provision, team staffing profiles, and business cases.

- *Technology*: Advances in technology will undoubtedly shape future physiotherapy practice, especially in the context of EM interventions. Increasingly sophisticated assistive devices can provide practical support to rehabilitation practice and facilitate patient participation. Colleagues collaborating with clinical, engineering, computer, and robotics/automated intelligence experts are already exploring use of robotics in addition to in-person delivery of therapy. It is likely that carryover will be seen from enhanced technology supporting other domains of rehabilitation that may then improve physical interventions. For example, it is important to be able to effectively communicate with these patients to safely and accurately deliver interventions and maximize engagement from patients. New communication applications can support patients with impaired vocalization.

The Research Landscape: From Muscle Weakness to Post-Intensive Care Unit Sequelae

In this section, we summarize the evolution of evidence and inquiry for physiotherapy interventions in the ICU. We identify milestones of original research (including those led by physical therapists), knowledge synthesis, and propose areas for further inquiry. **Table 1** juxtaposes the clinical and research landscapes.

Past

Early 2000s: focus on muscle weakness and early randomized clinical trials
We highlight two landmark studies in this era. Herridge and colleagues[15,38] identified 1- and 5-year long-term sequelae in ARDS survivors, published in the New England Journal of Medicine. These articles raised awareness of post-ICU sequelae and paved

Table 1
Clinical and research landscape

	Past		Present	Future
	Pre-2010	2010 to 2019	2020 to Now	
Clinical Landscape				
Clinical events	Bedrest,[17] deep sedation; Brussels Round Table Conference—ICU-acquired weakness[21]; ERS and ESICM,[3] NICE guidelines[33]; Feasibility of early activity[31,32]	Post-intensive care syndrome[34]; SCCM guidelines[26,44]; Safety of rehabilitation activities[41,42]; Financial impact of early mobility[40]; ABCDEF bundle[43]; Frailty[49,61]	Post-intensive care syndrome-extended[47]; COVID-19[46]; Patient engagement; ECLS; Social media and sharing international practice	Clinical Service models; Technology
Original Research - Outcomes	ICU-acquired weakness[23]; Long-term follow-up of ARDS Survivors[15]	Rapid skeletal muscle atrophy in patients receiving mechanical ventilation[62]; Cognitive and functional outcomes[63,64]	COVID-19	
Research Landscape				
Research Synthesis - Interventions	Narrative reviews[55-60]	Systematic reviews,[65-67] scoping reviews,[68] and overview of reviews[69]	Bibliometric analysis; Network meta-analysis[70]	Integrated mixed-methods syntheses
RCT intervention focus	Early mobility; In-bed cycling	Neuromuscular electrical stimulation; In-bed cycling and adjuncts; Early in-bed cycling	Early mobility extended to other areas of critical care; Progressive mobility	Multidisciplinary rehabilitation
Published RCTs	Early mobility[54]; Mobility team[32] (quasi-randomized); In-bed cycling[71]; Neuromuscular electrical stimulation[72]	Goal-directed mobility (surgical)[73]; Mobility "dose"[74]; Exercise intervention from ICU to community[75]; Multicenter pilot studies[76,77]	International multicenter trials in progress	
Methodological advancements	Focus on muscle strength	Use of ICF framework[78]; Outcome measure psychometrics[79,80]; Core outcome sets[81]	Factorial trials[82]	Platform trials; Research process

the way for subsequent multicenter outcome studies. The second landmark study, led by Schweickert and colleagues,[54] was a multicenter RCT of early occupational and physical therapy started within the first 72 h of intubation versus the usual timing of therapy and was published in The Lancet. Narrative reviews identified treatments to proactively address immobility and muscle weakness, with interventions started in the ICU.[55-60]

RCTs focused on interventions started in the ICU, with some interventions occurring while patients received life support therapies such as mechanical ventilation or vaso-active agents. These approaches challenged commonly held beliefs that patients in the ICU were "too sick" for activity. One of the earliest clinical RCTs led by a physical therapist from Canada examined incentive spirometry and usual physiotherapy, which involved early mobility, versus usual PT alone.[83] Another RCT led by a physical therapist and team from Belgium evaluated in-bed cycling and routine PT versus routine PT alone, started after ICU day 14 in 90 patients, noting a clinically and statistically important improvement in 6-min walk test at hospital discharge (in-bed cycling median [interquartile range] = 196 [126 to 329] vs control 143 [37 to 226] m; 29 [19 to 43] vs 25 [8 to 36]% predicted, $p < 0.05$).[71]

Other studies evaluated neuromuscular electrical stimulation (NMES), an intervention that applies surface electrodes to muscles, initiating visible muscle contractions using a small device that sends a small electrical current to activate the muscle.[84] NMES focused on preserving muscle strength, is noninvasive, and can activate muscles without volitional control, thus it was very attractive to the ICU setting because it could be used with patients who were sedated or unable to follow commands. NMES is an intervention used by physical therapists with other patient populations, such as people with chronic obstructive pulmonary disease, to improve muscle strength.[85] An early RCT with 49 critically ill patients, noted better preservation of quadriceps muscle cross-sectional area measured by ultrasound at ICU day 10 in those receiving NMES within 2 days of ICU admission versus the control group.[72] A subsequent systematic review and meta-analysis of 6 RCTs from 2003 to 2018 enrolling 718 patients identified no difference in muscle strength at ICU discharge, duration of mechanical ventilation, ICU length of stay or mortality; however, included trials were heterogeneous.[86] Important considerations for implementation of NMES exist. Segers and colleagues[87] documented challenges consistently achieving muscle contractions. NMES requires continuous supervision and titration to ensure ongoing muscle contractions during ICU sessions which lasted from 30 to 60 min daily (excluding preparation and cleanup). Considerations for which ICU health care personnel administer this intervention are required, which could come at the opportunity cost of conducting other functional activities.

This period heralded the start of "early mobility" activities in the ICU. A quasi-randomized study evaluated whether a standard early mobility protocol increased the proportion of patients receiving physical therapy compared with usual care in 330 medical ICU patients with acute respiratory failure.[32] The premise of this study was elegant and simple—can an automatic physician order triggering the involvement of a mobility team including a nurse, nurse assistant, and physical therapist, increase the number of patients receiving at least one physical therapy session? Results were highly encouraging. More patients managed using the protocol received at least one physical therapy session than those not managed using the protocol (80% vs 47%, $p \leq 0.001$), with physical therapy commencing more frequently during ICU stay (91% vs 13%, $p \leq 0.001$). In addition, compared with usual care, protocol patients were out of bed earlier (5 vs 11 days, $p \leq .001$), had reduced ICU and hospital length of stay (5.5 vs 6.9 days, $p = 0.025$, and 11.2 vs 14.5 days, $p = 0.006$, respectively), and similar low complication rates with no adverse events during protocol-based mobility sessions. Together, with the landmark RCT of early physical and occupational therapy,[54] interest in physical therapy and engagement of physical therapists in the ICU increased substantially. **Table 2** summarizes selected clinical trials by population, intervention, comparison, and primary outcome.

2010 to 2019: early mobility, safety, and feasibility

Many activities in this decade advanced the field. ICU survivorship assumed a more prominent role with the publication of nomenclature for PICS, as described earlier.[34] This publication, with international multidisciplinary input, raised awareness about outcomes beyond muscle strength for clinical trials. In addition to PICS, the World Health Organization International Classification of Function, Disability, and Health provided a framework for ICU outcomes, considering a continuum from body structure and body function, to activities, and participation.[78,93] This era also saw an expansion of physiotherapist-led clinical research programs, including preparatory work culminating in randomized clinical trials,[75–77] and publications led by trainees from the next generation of research physiotherapists in graduate programs.[66,94,95]

The first systematic reviews of interventions started in the ICU identified few RCTs, mostly relying on observational studies.[65–67,96] Typical interventions assessed included NMES, "EM," "general physiotherapy," limb strengthening, active mobilization, and exercise training. However, reviewers identified important weaknesses in intervention descriptions. The systematic reviews also documented variable outcome measures across studies, with measurements occurring primarily at short-term timepoints (eg, ICU discharge, hospital discharge), and few studies reporting longer-term follow-up. Overall, the systematic reviews determined physical interventions initiated in the ICU were safe, with small effects favoring the intervention groups for muscle strength, function, ICU and hospital length of stay, and health-related quality of life.[65–67,96] However, new original research published during this decade began to question the efficacy of physical interventions started in the ICU.

As the field matured, investigators received national research funding to study ICU physical rehabilitation interventions in larger multicenter trials.[74,89] These novel RCTs explored different ways of implementing ICU physical rehabilitation. But study interventions and results for primary outcomes varied, introducing confusion to the field. Several larger studies of physical rehabilitation published during this decade reported variable results for their primary outcomes (see **Table 2**).[73–75,89,90] However, similar to the systematic reviews, these trials studied different interventions, for different duration, and measured different outcomes, a nuance that may have been underappreciated by the wider ICU community. For example, outcomes were heterogeneous in terms of both type and measurement time points (see **Table 2**). This heterogeneity of the primary outcome and results, and differences in secondary outcomes, made things unclear for the ICU community. A systematic review evaluating mortality outcomes raised concerns for possible harms with active mobilization activities in the ICU.[66] However, the small number of studies assessed, the small number of enrolled patients, as well as the overall low event rate (active mobility 12.3% (34/275) vs standard care 11.6% (32/276)) limits the certainty of currently available evidence.[97]

Other methodological advancements included the publication of quality improvement studies, and case series of the safety and feasibility of novel physical rehabilitation interventions in the ICU.[68] Building on clinical data, a systematic review documented a low adverse safety event rate (2.6%) in physical rehabilitation activities.[42] A scoping review identified reporting important gaps in key intervention attributes among ICU rehabilitation studies, notably protocol adherence and protocol

Table 2
Selected clinical rehabilitation trials

Author	Study Design	Population	Intervention	Comparison	Primary Outcome Results (Intervention vs Comparison)	
			Pre-2009			
Schweickert et al,[54] 2009	RCT; 2 centers, 1 country (United States)	Medical patients mechanically ventilated <72 h (N = 104)	Order for early exercise and mobilization during daily interruption of sedation beginning on day of enrolment (n = 49)	Daily interruption of sedation and therapy as ordered by primary care team (n = 55)	*Return to independent functional status* a hospital discharge (29 [59%] vs 19 [35%]; odd ratio [95% CI] 2.7 [1.2 to 6.1]) (blinded)	↘
Morris et al,[32] 2008	Quasi-randomized study; 1 center (United States)	Medical patients with acute respiratory failure requiring mechanical ventilation (N = 330)	Automatic order for ICU mobility team (critical care nurse, nursing assistant, physical therapist) (n = 165)	Patient-specific order for physical therapy (n = 165)	*% patients receiving physical therapy* of patients surviving to hospital discharge (80% vs 47%; p ≤ 0.001) (blinding not relevant for this objective outcome)	↘
Burtin et al,[71] 2009	RCT; 1 center (Belgium)	Medical or surgical patients with expected prolonged ICU stay (N = 90)	20 min of in-bed cycling and daily active respiratory physiotherapy and daily active motion of upper and lower limbs (n = 45)	Respiratory physiotherapy and daily active motion of upper and lower limbs (n = 45)	*6-min walk distance* at hospital discharge median (interquartile range)[88] (196 [126 to 329] vs 143 [37 to 226] m; 29 [19 to 43] vs 25 [8 to 36]% predicted, p < 0.05) (blinding unclear)	↘

(continued on next page)

Table 2
(continued)

Author	Study Design	Population	Intervention	Comparison	Primary Outcome Results (Intervention vs Comparison)	
			Pre-2009			
Gerovasilli et al,[72] 2009	RCT; 1 center (Greece)	Multidisciplinary ICU (*N* = 49)	60 min of neuromuscular electrical stimulation on quadriceps and peroneus longus × 7 days starting ICU day 2 (*n* = 24)	Not reported (*n* = 25)	Change in *quadriceps muscle cross-sectional diameter* at 7 to 8 days after randomization measured by ultrasound; R and L rectus femoris and vastus intermedius; both decreased significantly less for absolute difference (13 evaluated in each group; blinded)	✓
2010 to 2019						
Denehy et al,[75] 2013	RCT; 1 center (Australia)	Medical or surgical patients (*N* = 150 enrolled out of planned 200)	Intensive exercises in the ICU, ward, and as outpatients (*n* = 74)	Usual care (*n* = 76)	*6-min walk distance* at 6 months (402.4 [166.6] vs 394.2 [156.2] m; −4.9 [−68.0 to 58.3] 0.879) (blinded)	✗
Moss et al,[74] 2015	RCT; 5 centers (United States)	Patients requiring mechanical ventilation for at least 4 days (*N* = 120)	Intensive PT up to 28 days (7 days per week as an inpatient; 3 days per week at home or outpatient); 30 min in ICU; up to 60 min in on-ward and other settings) (*n* = 59)	Standard of care (3 days per week as an inpatient; no home or outpatient therapy) (*n* = 61)	*Continuous scale physical functional performance test short form* at 1 month (19.0 [3.7] vs 20.9 [4.1]; *p* = 0.73) (blinded)	✗

Study	Design/Setting	Population	Intervention	Control	Outcome	
Morris et al,[89] 2016	RCT; 1 center (United States)	Medical patients with acute respiratory failure requiring mechanical ventilation (N = 300)	Standardized rehabilitation therapy protocol including passive range of motion, physical therapy, and progressive resistance exercises by a rehabilitation team from enrolment to hospital discharge 7 days per week (n = 150)	Physical therapy (unprotocolized) Monday to Friday (n = 150)	*Hospital length of stay* (median 10 [6 to 17] vs 10 [7 to 16]; median difference [95% CI] 0 [−1.5 to 3] days, $p = 0.41$) (blinding not relevant for this objective outcome)	✗
Schaller et al,[73] 2016	RCT; five centers and three countries (Austria, Germany, United States)	Surgical patients mechanically ventilated <48 h (N = 200)	Early goal-directed mobilization facilitated by interprofessional closed-loop communication (n = 104)	Standard treatment (n = 96)	Mean (SD) SICU optimal mobilization score achieved during SICU stay (2.2 [1.0] vs [1.5 0.8]; mean difference [95% CI] 0.7 [0.4 to 1.0, $p < 0.0001$]) (blinded)	↘
Wright et al,[90] 2017	RCT; four centers, one country (United Kingdom)	Medical and surgical patients mechanically ventilated (invasive or noninvasive) >48 h (N = 308)	90 min of physical rehabilitation per day (Monday to Friday), split between at least 2 sessions (n = 150)	Standard care—30 min of physical rehabilitation per day (Monday to Friday) (n = 158)	*Physical Component Summary measure of Short Form 36 (Version 2) Quality of Life questionnaire* at 6 months (37[12.2] vs 37 [11.3]; the adjusted difference in means [95% CI] −1.1 [−7.1 to 5.0]) (blinded)	✗

(continued on next page)

Table 2
(continued)

Author	Study Design	Population	Intervention	Comparison	Primary Outcome Results (Intervention vs Comparison)	
2020 to present						
			Pre-2009			
Berney et al,[91] 2021	RCT; four centers, two countries (Australia, United States)	Mechanically ventilated patients with sepsis (N = 162)	Up to 60 min of functional electrical stimulation-assisted in-bed leg cycling (applied to 1 leg) and usual care rehabilitation ≥ 5 days per week (n = 80)	Usual care rehabilitation (n = 82)	*2 Primary outcomes (blinded):* 1. *Muscle strength at hospital discharge measured by hand-held dynamometry* Adjusted mean difference (95% CI) 3.3 (−5.0 to 12.1 Nm; p = 0.460) 2. *Cognitive impairment at 6 months (one test >2 SD below population norms or 2 tests > 1.5 SD population norms)* (41% [9/22] vs 40% [6/15]; odds ratio [95% CI] 1.1 [0.30 to 3.8; p = 0.929]; [22/46 and 15/46 of planned 92])	x
Waldauf et al,[92] 2021	RCT; 1 center (Czech Republic)	Multidisciplinary ICU; mechanically ventilated patients <72 h and predicted to need ICU > 1 week (N = 150)	Progressive tailored 90-min mobility program including functional electrical stimulation in-bed leg cycling initiated 1 day post-randomization up to 28 days (n = 75)	Standard physiotherapy 2 times per day, 6 days per week (nonprotocolized, initiated at request of treating physician) (n = 75)	*Physical Component Summary measure of Short Form 36 (Version 1) Quality of Life questionnaire at 6 months median (IQR)* (50 [21 to 69] vs 49 [26 to 77]; p = 0.261) (blinded)	x

fidelity.[68] Clinical trialists started publishing trial protocols[82,98] highlighting ongoing studies, and conducted pilot and feasibility studies in preparation for future large multicentre trials.[76,77,99] Finally, given the increase in the number of clinical studies across many disciplines, several groups developed core outcome sets to improve the standardization across studies,[81,100] including those extending to sub-specialty populations such as extra-corporeal membrane oxygenation.[101]

Present

2020 to now: coronavirus disease-2019

Systematic reviews have identified over 60 RCTs focused on physical rehabilitation in the ICU.[102] Multiple systematic reviews identified that in RCT intervention groups, there were no differences in mortality[102,103] or muscle strength,[102] but lower ICU length of stay,[102,103] small improvements in physical function at hospital discharge,[102] and no adverse safety events.[103] Inconsistency in pooled results for hospital length of stay occurred across reviews.[102,103] Authors identified ongoing gaps in primary study reporting, and opportunities to improve documentation of protocol adherence and intervention dose. Amidst the pandemic, two RCTs of in-bed cycling and electrical stimulation were published (see **Table 2**).[91,92] At the time of writing, results are pending for at least 2 international multicenter trials.[76,104]

The COVID-19 pandemic had devastating effects on ICUs worldwide. First, the overwhelming influx of patients into ICUs required immediate prioritization of clinical care of patients, with many research studies halted,[105] and ICUs focused on research identifying treatments for COVID-19. International ICU physiotherapists quickly mobilized to provide clinical guidance for the acute management of patients with COVID-19.[46] Ongoing ICU rehabilitation research studies were also interrupted,[104] and guidance to resume non-COVID ICU research emerged.[106] Processes of ICU care for COVID-19 patients reverted back to earlier paradigms, including deep sedation, neuromuscular blockade, and prolonged immobility.[107–109] Proning, both with and without invasive mechanical ventilation was common in patients with COVID-19.[109] All of these factors raise concerns for severe long-term post-ICU outcomes in COVID-19 survivors, and highlight the need to identify additional impairments caused by COVID-19. A core set of COVID-19 outcomes was recently published,[110] and information about Long COVID and outcomes post-COVID is of global concern.[111,112] Rehabilitation interventions within and beyond ICU will be required for COVID-19 survivors.

Future

In anticipation of more survivors of ICU, we urgently need innovative research to improve the outcomes of critically ill patients. Innovation may occur in research designs, research processes, or research personnel.

Innovation in research designs includes consideration of novel approaches such as platform trials and embedded studies within health care systems. A platform trial design provides the scaffolding to study multiple interventions for a disease or problem, rather than a single intervention.[113] Studies embedded in health care systems could allow the development of patient cohorts from ICU admission to hospital discharge, and also include post-hospital rehabilitation to home, facilitated by long-term longitudinal follow-up using health administrative databases.

Innovation in research processes includes careful and proactive study of research conduct from inception to completion. Rehabilitation interventions are complex,[114] and require ongoing monitoring to ensure the intervention is implemented as intended. Universal strategies to monitor protocol fidelity and adherence, improve enrolment, and optimize participant retention to minimize missing outcome data are needed.

Explicit description of rehabilitation interventions using an approach like the Rehabilitation Treatment Specification System[115] would help advance a multidisciplinary understanding of the "active ingredients" of treatments. Ideally, all research studies include an embedded process evaluation to improve the design and conduct of future research.[114]

Finally, we need innovations to build research personnel. Women, visible minorities, and nonphysicians are all underrepresented in critical care research.[116] Research by individuals in allied health and nursing represented only 10% of conference presentations at national or international meetings between 2010 and 2016.[116] **Fig. 3** is a schematic of the roles, training, and infrastructure required to develop research personnel. Students need exposure to research careers and practical opportunities to conduct clinical research. One model exposes students to the role of a clinician-scientist through a novel clinical placement of 50% clinical training and 50% embedded in a research team led by a physiotherapist as part of the entry-level university curriculum.[117] Clinicians need opportunities to contribute to research and learn about research career opportunities such as research physiotherapist or trial managers. One novel training opportunity by Sepsis Canada offers research methods modules and interactive sessions for clinicians.[118] Positions for clinician-scientists in health systems, and partnerships between universities and health systems will advance the field. Contemporary examples of clinical research leadership positions held by physiotherapists will help expand representation in the complex trials needed to improve patient outcomes.

DISCUSSION

In this article, we reflected on the clinical and research aspects of critical care and physiotherapy. As the critical care field evolved from a culture of bed rest, deep

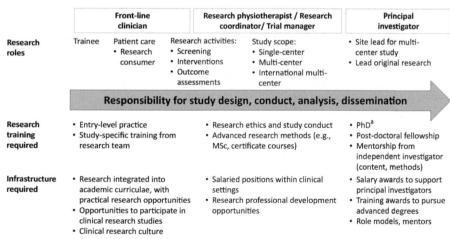

		Front-line clinician	Research physiotherapist / Research coordinator/ Trial manager		Principal investigator
Research roles	Trainee	Patient care • Research consumer	Research activities: • Screening • Interventions • Outcome assessments	Study scope: • Single-center • Multi-center • International multi-center	• Site lead for multi-center study • Lead original research

Responsibility for study design, conduct, analysis, dissemination

Research training required	• Entry-level practice • Study-specific training from research team	• Research ethics and study conduct • Advanced research methods (e.g., MSc, certificate courses)	• PhD[a] • Post-doctoral fellowship • Mentorship from independent investigator (content, methods)
Infrastructure required	• Research integrated into academic curriculae, with practical research opportunities • Opportunities to participate in clinical research studies • Clinical research culture	• Salaried positions within clinical settings • Research professional development opportunities	• Salary awards to support principal investigators • Training awards to pursue advanced degrees • Role models, mentors

Fig. 3. Schematic of roles, training, and infrastructure required to develop research personnel. This figure summarizes a continuum of research roles, training, and infrastructure required to increase capacity of research personnel. The far left of the continuum represents trainees, and the far right represents independent investigators. The arrow represents increasing responsibility for design, conduct, and oversight of research. [a]PhD training is typically required to lead larger-scale research studies. For healthcare professionals without a PhD or research training to lead research activities, we recommend seeking a research mentor with content and methodological expertise.

sedation, treatments to improve ICU outcomes also evolved from those solely focused on muscles to complex physical interventions. These complex interventions could impact many outcomes including physical function, cognition, mood, and the development of frailty. Thus, expanding the multidisciplinary team and patient and caregiver input to design new interventions is critical. As we plan future interventions, we need to consider implementability and generalizability across different settings, including academic and community settings, and different income settings and health care systems.

As critical care matures, we also anticipate a shift in terminology, progressing from early mobility to rehabilitation. "Early mobility" reflects an initial focus on muscle weakness, whereas "rehabilitation" reflects an anticipation of the future needs of ICU survivors and recognition of the need to start interventions in the ICU to address long-term outcomes.[93] For physiotherapists, we encourage our colleagues to seek broader exposure to developments in research methodology and critical care to inform clinical practice and research. The most clinically relevant interventions will represent the convergence of developments in clinical critical care and research methodology.

SUMMARY

Over the last century, the profession of physiotherapy has evolved tremendously. In this article, we have highlighted the journey of physiotherapists and their contributions to improving the outcomes of critical illness survivors. We witnessed a transition from bed rest to early mobility, and now to rehabilitation. And a focus from muscle weakness to returning to life participation. Clinical and research leadership are now key features of the profession, with an emphasis on interdisciplinary and interprofessional collaboration within the specialty.

CLINICS CARE POINTS

- Critical care clinicians should consider the depth, breadth, and complex inter-relationships of post-critical illness impairments that patients experience, during critical illness and recovery
- Physiotherapists can focus on bespoke restorative interventions to target muscle weaknesses, deficits in physical function, and limitations in exercise capacity
- Physiotherapists should undertake assessments of patients to determine clinical safety and appropriateness for delivering early mobilization and physical rehabilitation interventions
- Research has supported developments in clinical practice, and the future direction for the profession in the specialty of critical care should be greater convergence between research and clinical contexts

DISCLOSURE

M.E. Kho is funded by a Canada Research Chair in Critical Care Rehabilitation and Knowledge Translation. She currently holds grants from the Canadian Institutes of Health Research, the Canada Foundation for Innovation, and the Ontario Research Fund. She leads CYCLE, an international, multicenter randomized clinical trial of early in-bed cycling. Restorative Therapies (Baltimore, MD, United States) loaned Dr Kho 3 RT300 in-bed cycle ergometers to conduct her research. B. Connolly currently receives project grant funding from the National Institute for Health and Care Research (United Kingdom).

REFERENCES

1. Mead R., Bloodlines, 2011, Penguin Group, New York, NY.
2. Hilberman M. The evolution of intensive care units. Crit Care Med 1975;3(4): 159–65.
3. Gosselink R, Bott J, Johnson M, et al. Physiotherapy for adult patients with critical illness: recommendations of the European respiratory society and European society of intensive care medicine task force on physiotherapy for critically ill patients. Intensive Care Med 2008;34(7):1188–99.
4. Clarissa C, Salisbury L, Rodgers S, et al. Early mobilisation in mechanically ventilated patients: a systematic integrative review of definitions and activities. J Intensive Care 2019;7:3.
5. Hodgson C, Needham D, Haines K, et al. Feasibility and inter-rater reliability of the ICU mobility scale. Heart Lung 2014;43(1):19–24.
6. Graves DA. Emergency poliomyelitis policies: hints to the therapists. Phys Ther 1949;29(7):291–4.
7. Association APT. 100 milestones of physical therapy. 2022. Available at: https://centennial.apta.org/home/timeline/#story-852. Accessed August 14, 2022.
8. Toronto Uo. About the department of physical therapy. Available at: https://www.physicaltherapy.utoronto.ca/about/. Accessed August 14, 2022.
9. Association AP. The Australian physiotherapy association. Available at: https://australian.physio/aboutus/our-history. Accessed August 14, 2022.
10. Physiotherapy CSo. CSP history. Available at: https://www.csp.org.uk/about-csp/who-we-are/csp-history. Accessed August 14, 2022.
11. Grenvik A, Pinsky MR. Evolution of the intensive care unit as a clinical center and critical care medicine as a discipline. Crit Care Clin 2009;25(1):239–50, x.
12. Cook D, Todd T. The Canadian Critical Care Trials Group: a collaborative educational organization for the advancement of adult clinical ICU research. Intensive Care World 1997;14:68–70.
13. Cook DJ, Fuller HD, Guyatt GH, et al. Risk factors for gastrointestinal bleeding in critically ill patients. N Engl J Med 1994;330(6):377–81.
14. Ventilation with lower tidal volumes as compared with traditional tidal volumes for acute lung injury and the acute respiratory distress syndrome. N Engl J Med 2000;342(18):1301–8.
15. Herridge MS, Cheung AM, Tansey CM, et al. One-year outcomes in survivors of the acute respiratory distress syndrome. N Engl J Med 20 2003;348(8):683–93.
16. Asher RA. The dangers of going to bed. Br Med J 1947;2(4536):967.
17. Brower RG. Consequences of bed rest. Crit Care Med 2009;37(10 Suppl): S422–8.
18. Kress JP, Pohlman AS, O'Connor MF, et al. Daily interruption of sedative infusions in critically ill patients undergoing mechanical ventilation. N Engl J Med 2000;342(20):1471–7.
19. Chen T-J, Chung Y-W, Chen P-Y, et al. Effects of daily sedation interruption in intensive care unit patients undergoing mechanical ventilation: a meta-analysis of randomized controlled trials. Int J Nurs Pract 2022;28(2):e12948.
20. Burry L, Rose L, McCullagh IJ, et al. Daily sedation interruption versus no daily sedation interruption for critically ill adult patients requiring invasive mechanical ventilation. Cochrane Database Syst Rev 2014;7. https://doi.org/10.1002/14651858.CD009176.pub2.
21. Griffiths RD, Hall JB. Intensive care unit-acquired weakness. Crit Care Med 2010;38(3):779–87.

22. Kleyweg RP, van der Meche FG, Schmitz PI. Interobserver agreement in the assessment of muscle strength and functional abilities in Guillain-Barre syndrome. Muscle Nerve 1991;14(11):1103–9.

23. De Jonghe B, Sharshar T, Lefaucheur JP, et al. Paresis acquired in the intensive care unit: a prospective multicenter study. JAMA 2002;288(22):2859–67.

24. Sharshar T, Bastuji-Garin S, Stevens RD, et al. Presence and severity of intensive care unit-acquired paresis at time of awakening are associated with increased intensive care unit and hospital mortality. Crit Care Med 2009; 37(12):3047–53.

25. De Jonghe B, Bastuji-Garin S, Durand MC, et al. Respiratory weakness is associated with limb weakness and delayed weaning in critical illness. Crit Care Med 2007;35(9):2007–15.

26. Barr J, Fraser GL, Puntillo K, et al. Clinical practice guidelines for the management of pain, agitation, and delirium in adult patients in the intensive care unit. Crit Care Med 2013;41(1):263–306.

27. de Letter M-ACJ, Schmitz PIM, Visser LH, et al. Risk factors for the development of polyneuropathy and myopathy in critically ill patients. Crit Care Med 2001; 29(12):2281–6.

28. Leijten FSS, Weerd JEH-d, Poortvliet DCJ, et al. The role of polyneuropathy in motor convalescence after prolonged mechanical ventilation. JAMA 1995; 274(15):1221–5.

29. Ali NA, O'Brien JM Jr, Hoffmann SP, et al. Acquired weakness, handgrip strength, and mortality in critically ill patients. Am J Respir Crit Care Med 2008;178(3):261–8.

30. Fan E, Cheek F, Chlan L, et al. An official American Thoracic Society Clinical Practice guideline: the diagnosis of intensive care unit-acquired weakness in adults. Am J Respir Crit Care Med 2014;190(12):1437–46.

31. Bailey P, Thomsen GE, Spuhler VJ, et al. Early activity is feasible and safe in respiratory failure patients. Crit Care Med 2007;35(1):139–45.

32. Morris PE, Goad A, Thompson C, et al. Early intensive care unit mobility therapy in the treatment of acute respiratory failure. Crit Care Med 2008;36(8):2238–43.

33. National Institute for Health and Care Excellence. Rehabilitation after critical illness in adults. Updated March 25, 2009. CG83 Available at: https://www.nice.org.uk/guidance/cg83.

34. Needham DM, Davidson J, Cohen H, et al. Improving long-term outcomes after discharge from intensive care unit: report from a stakeholders' conference. Crit Care Med 2012;40(2):502–9.

35. Dinglas VD, Aronson Friedman L, Colantuoni E, et al. Muscle weakness and 5-year survival in acute respiratory distress syndrome survivors. Crit Care Med 2017;45(3):446–53.

36. Pfoh ER, Wozniak AW, Colantuoni E, et al. Physical declines occurring after hospital discharge in ARDS survivors: a 5-year longitudinal study. Intensive Care Med 2016;42(10):1557–66.

37. Fan E, Dowdy DW, Colantuoni E, et al. Physical complications in acute lung injury survivors: a 2-year longitudinal prospective study. Crit Care Med 2014; 42(4):849–59.

38. Herridge MS, Tansey CM, Matte A, et al. Functional disability 5 years after acute respiratory distress syndrome. N Engl J Med 2011;364(14):1293–304.

39. Brodsky MB, Huang M, Shanholtz C, et al. Recovery from dysphagia symptoms after oral endotracheal intubation in acute respiratory distress syndrome

survivors. A 5-Year Longitudinal Study. Annals of the American Thoracic Society 2017;14(3):376–83.

40. Lord RK, Mayhew CR, Korupolu R, et al. ICU early physical rehabilitation programs: financial modeling of cost savings. Crit Care Med 2013;41(3):717–24.

41. Hodgson CL, Stiller K, Needham DM, et al. Expert consensus and recommendations on safety criteria for active mobilization of mechanically ventilated critically ill adults. Crit Care 2014;18(6):658.

42. Nydahl P, Sricharoenchai T, Chandra S, et al. Safety of patient mobilization and rehabilitation in the intensive care unit. systematic review with meta-analysis. Annals of the American Thoracic Society 2017;14(5):766–77.

43. Ely EW. The ABCDEF bundle: science and philosophy of how ICU liberation serves patients and families. Crit Care Med 2017;45(2):321–30.

44. Devlin JW, Skrobik Y, Gelinas C, et al. Clinical practice guidelines for the prevention and management of pain, agitation/sedation, delirium, immobility, and sleep disruption in adult patients in the ICU. Crit Care Med 2018;46(9):e825–73.

45. Thomas P, Baldwin C, Beach L, et al. Physiotherapy management for COVID-19 in the acute hospital setting and beyond: an update to clinical practice recommendations. J Physiother 2022;68(1):8–25.

46. Thomas P, Baldwin C, Bissett B, et al. Physiotherapy management for COVID-19 in the acute hospital setting: clinical practice recommendations. J Physiother 2020;66(2):73–82.

47. Rousseau A-F, Prescott HC, Brett SJ, et al. Long-term outcomes after critical illness: recent insights. Crit Care 2021;25(1):108.

48. Kamdar BB, Suri R, Suchyta MR, et al. Return to work after critical illness: a systematic review and meta-analysis. Thorax 2020;75(1):17–27.

49. Muscedere J, Waters B, Varambally A, et al. The impact of frailty on intensive care unit outcomes: a systematic review and meta-analysis. Intensive Care Med 2017;43(8):1105–22.

50. Connolly B, Milton-Cole R, Adams C, et al. Recovery, rehabilitation and follow-up services following critical illness: an updated UK national cross-sectional survey and progress report. BMJ Open 2021;11(10):e052214.

51. Twose P, Terblanche E, Jones U, et al. Therapy professionals in critical care: a UK wide workforce survey. Journal of the Intensive Care Society. 0(0):17511437221100332. doi:10.1177/17511437221100332.

52. Twose P, Jones U, Cornell G. Minimum standards of clinical practice for physiotherapists working in critical care settings in the United Kingdom: a modified delphi technique. Journal of the Intensive Care Society 2019;20(2):118–31.

53. Skinner EH, Thomas P, Reeve JC, et al. Minimum standards of clinical practice for physiotherapists working in critical care settings in Australia and New Zealand: a modified Delphi technique. Physiother Theory Pract 2016;32(6):468–82.

54. Schweickert WD, Pohlman MC, Pohlman AS, et al. Early physical and occupational therapy in mechanically ventilated, critically ill patients: a randomised controlled trial. Lancet 2009;373(9678):1874–82.

55. Needham DM. Mobilizing patients in the intensive care unit: improving neuromuscular weakness and physical function. JAMA Oct 8 2008;300(14):1685–90.

56. Truong AD, Fan E, Brower RG, et al. Bench-to-bedside review: mobilizing patients in the intensive care unit–from pathophysiology to clinical trials. Crit Care 2009;13(4):216.

57. Hopkins RO, Spuhler VJ, Thomsen GE. Transforming ICU culture to facilitate early mobility. Crit Care Clin 2007;23(1):81–96.

58. Schweickert WD, Hall J. ICU-acquired weakness. Chest 2007;131(5):1541–9.

59. Bailey PP, Miller RR 3rd, Clemmer TP. Culture of early mobility in mechanically ventilated patients. Crit Care Med 2009;37(10 Suppl):S429–35.

60. Hopkins RO, Spuhler VJ. Strategies for promoting early activity in critically ill mechanically ventilated patients. AACN Adv Crit Care 2009;20(3):277–89.

61. Ferrante LE, Pisani MA, Murphy TE, et al. The association of frailty with post-ICU disability, nursing home admission, and mortality: a longitudinal study. Chest 2018;153(6):1378–86.

62. Puthucheary ZA, Rawal J, McPhail M, et al. Acute skeletal muscle wasting in critical illness. JAMA 2013;310(15):1591–600.

63. Pandharipande PP, Girard TD, Ely EW. Long-term cognitive impairment after critical illness. N Engl J Med 9 2014;370(2):185–6.

64. Iwashyna TJ, Ely EW, Smith DM, et al. Long-term cognitive impairment and functional disability among survivors of severe sepsis. JAMA 2010;304(16):1787–94.

65. Kayambu G, Boots R, Paratz J. Physical therapy for the critically ill in the ICU: a systematic review and meta-analysis. Crit Care Med 2013;41(6):1543–54.

66. Tipping CJ, Harrold M, Holland A, et al. The effects of active mobilisation and rehabilitation in ICU on mortality and function: a systematic review. Intensive Care Med 2017;43(2):171–83.

67. Li Z, Peng X, Zhu B, et al. Active mobilization for mechanically ventilated patients: a systematic review. Arch Phys Med Rehabil 2013;94(3):551–61.

68. Reid JC, Unger J, McCaskell D, et al. Physical rehabilitation interventions in the intensive care unit: a scoping review of 117 studies. J Intensive Care 2018;6:80.

69. Connolly B, O'Neill B, Salisbury L, et al. Physical rehabilitation interventions for adult patients during critical illness: an overview of systematic reviews. Thorax 2016;71(10):881–90.

70. Worraphan S, Thammata A, Chittawatanarat K, et al. Effects of inspiratory muscle training and early mobilization on weaning of mechanical ventilation: a systematic review and network meta-analysis. Arch Phys Med Rehabil 2020; 101(11):2002–14.

71. Burtin C, Clerckx B, Robbeets C, et al. Early exercise in critically ill patients enhances short-term functional recovery. Crit Care Med 2009;37(9):2499–505.

72. Gerovasili V, Stefanidis K, Vitzilaios K, et al. Electrical muscle stimulation preserves the muscle mass of critically ill patients: a randomized study. Crit Care 2009;13(5):R161.

73. Schaller SJ, Anstey M, Blobner M, et al. Early, goal-directed mobilisation in the surgical intensive care unit: a randomised controlled trial. Lancet 2016; 388(10052):1377–88.

74. Moss M, Nordon-Craft A, Malone D, et al. A randomized trial of an intensive physical therapy program for patients with acute respiratory failure. Am J Respir Crit Care Med 2016;193(10):1101–10.

75. Denehy L, Skinner EH, Edbrooke L, et al. Exercise rehabilitation for patients with critical illness: a randomized controlled trial with 12 months of follow-up. Crit Care 2013;17(4):R156.

76. TEAM Study Investigators, Hodgson C, Bellomo R, et al. Early mobilization and recovery in mechanically ventilated patients in the ICU: a bi-national, multi-centre, prospective cohort study. Crit Care 2015;19:81.

77. Kho ME, Molloy AJ, Clarke FJ, et al. Multicentre pilot randomised clinical trial of early in-bed cycle ergometry with ventilated patients. BMJ Open Respir Res 2019;6(1):e000383.

78. Iwashyna IJ, Netzer G. The burdens of survivorship: an approach to thinking about long-term outcomes after critical illness. Semin Respir Crit Care Med 2012;33(4):327–38.

79. Parry SM, Granger CL, Berney S, et al. Assessment of impairment and activity limitations in the critically ill: a systematic review of measurement instruments and their clinimetric properties. Intensive Care Med 2015;41(5):744–62.

80. Parry SM, Huang M, Needham DM. Evaluating physical functioning in critical care: considerations for clinical practice and research. Crit Care 2017; 21(1):249.

81. Needham DM, Sepulveda KA, Dinglas VD, et al. Core outcome measures for clinical research in acute respiratory failure survivors. an international modified delphi consensus study. Am J Respir Crit Care Med. Nov 1 2017;196(9): 1122–30.

82. Heyland DK, Day A, Clarke GJ, et al. Nutrition and Exercise in Critical Illness Trial (NEXIS Trial): a protocol of a multicentred, randomised controlled trial of combined cycle ergometry and amino acid supplementation commenced early during critical illness. BMJ Open 2019;9(7):e027893.

83. Crowe JM, Bradley CA. The effectiveness of incentive spirometry with physical therapy for high-risk patients after coronary artery bypass surgery. Phys Ther 1997;77(3):260–8.

84. Maffiuletti NA. Physiological and methodological considerations for the use of neuromuscular electrical stimulation. Eur J Appl Physiol 2010;110(2):223–34.

85. Alves IGN, da Silva ESCM, Martinez BP, et al. Effects of neuromuscular electrical stimulation on exercise capacity, muscle strength and quality of life in COPD patients: a systematic review with meta-analysis. Clin Rehabil 2022;36(4):449–71.

86. Zayed Y, Kheiri B, Barbarawi M, et al. Effects of neuromuscular electrical stimulation in critically ill patients: a systematic review and meta-analysis of randomised controlled trials. Aust Crit Care 2020;33(2):203–10.

87. Segers J, Hermans G, Bruyninckx F, et al. Feasibility of neuromuscular electrical stimulation in critically ill patients. J Crit Care 2014. https://doi.org/10.1016/j.jcrc.2014.06.024.

88. Lamontagne F, Rowan KM, Guyatt G. Integrating research into clinical practice: challenges and solutions for Canada. CMAJ (Can Med Assoc J) 2021;193(4): E127–31.

89. Morris PE, Berry MJ, Files DC, et al. Standardized rehabilitation and hospital length of stay among patients with acute respiratory failure: a randomized clinical trial. JAMA 2016;315(24):2694–702.

90. Wright SE, Thomas K, Watson G, et al. Intensive versus standard physical rehabilitation therapy in the critically ill (EPICC): a multicentre, parallel-group, randomised controlled trial. Thorax 2017. https://doi.org/10.1136/thoraxjnl-2016-209858.

91. Berney S, Hopkins RO, Rose JW, et al. Functional electrical stimulation in-bed cycle ergometry in mechanically ventilated patients: a multicentre randomised controlled trial. Thorax 2021;76(7):656–63.

92. Waldauf P, Hrušková N, Blahutova B, et al. Functional electrical stimulation-assisted cycle ergometry-based progressive mobility programme for mechanically ventilated patients: randomised controlled trial with 6 months follow-up. Thorax 2021;76(7):664–71.

93. World health organization and the world bank. World report on disability 2011, 2011. Available at: https://www.who.int/teams/noncommunicable-diseases/

sensory-functions-disability-and-rehabilitation/world-report-on-disability. Accessed date October 14, 2019.

94. Parry SM, Berney S, Granger CL, et al. A new two-tier strength assessment approach to the diagnosis of weakness in intensive care: an observational study. Crit Care 2015;19(1):52.

95. Reid JC, McCaskell DS, Kho ME. Therapist perceptions of a rehabilitation research study in the intensive care unit: a trinational survey assessing barriers and facilitators to implementing the CYCLE pilot randomized clinical trial. Pilot and Feasibility Studies 2019;5:131.

96. Adler J, Malone D. Early mobilization in the intensive care unit: a systematic review. Cardiopulm Phys Ther J 2012;23(1):5–13.

97. Guyatt GH, Oxman AD, Kunz R, et al. GRADE guidelines 6. Rating the quality of evidence–imprecision. J Clin Epidemiol 2011;64(12):1283–93.

98. Waldauf P, Gojda J, Urban T, et al. Functional electrical stimulation-assisted cycle ergometry in the critically ill: protocol for a randomized controlled trial. Trials 2019;20(1):724.

99. Brummel NE, Girard TD, Fly EW, et al. Feasibility and safety of early combined cognitive and physical therapy for critically ill medical and surgical patients: the Activity and Cognitive Therapy in ICU (ACT-ICU) trial. Intensive Care Med 2014; 40(3):370–9.

100. Connolly B, Denehy L, Hart N, et al. Physical rehabilitation core outcomes in critical illness (PRACTICE): protocol for development of a core outcome set. Trials 2018;19(1):294.

101. Hodgson CL, Fulcher B, Mariajoseph FP, et al. A core outcome set for research in patients on extracorporeal membrane oxygenation. Crit Care Med 2021; 49(12):e1252–4.

102. Wang YT, Lang JK, Haines KJ, et al. Physical Rehabilitation in the ICU: a systematic review and meta-analysis. Crit Care Med Aug 18 2021. https://doi.org/10. 1097/ccm.0000000000005285.

103. Waldauf P, Jiroutkova K, Krajcova A, et al. Effects of rehabilitation interventions on clinical outcomes in critically ill patients: systematic review and meta-analysis of randomized controlled trials. Crit Care Med 2020;48(7):1055–65.

104. Reid JC, Molloy A, Strong G, et al. Research interrupted: applying the CONSERVE 2021 Statement to a randomized trial of rehabilitation during critical illness affected by the COVID-19 pandemic. Trials 2022;23(1):735.

105. Duffett M, Cook DJ, Strong G, et al. The effect of COVID-19 on critical care research during the first year of the pandemic: a prospective longitudinal multinational survey. medRxiv 2021. https://doi.org/10.1101/2020.10.21.20216945.

106. Cook DJ, Kho ME, Duan EH, et al. Principles guiding nonpandemic critical care research during a pandemic. Crit Care Med 2020;48(10):1403–10.

107. Pun BT, Badenes R, Heras La Calle G, et al. Prevalence and risk factors for delirium in critically ill patients with COVID-19 (COVID-D): a multicentre cohort study. Lancet Respir Med 2021. https://doi.org/10.1016/S2213-2600(20) 30552-X.

108. Helms J, Kremer S, Merdji H, et al. Delirium and encephalopathy in severe COVID-19: a cohort analysis of ICU patients. Crit Care 2020;24(1):491.

109. Courcelle R, Gaudry S, Serck N, et al. Neuromuscular blocking agents (NMBA) for COVID-19 acute respiratory distress syndrome: a multicenter observational study. Crit Care 2020;24(1):446.

110. Tong A, Baumgart A, Evangelidis N, et al. Core outcome measures for trials in people with coronavirus disease 2019: respiratory failure, multiorgan failure, shortness of breath, and recovery. Crit Care Med 2021;49(3):503–16.
111. Sigfrid L, Drake TM, Pauley E, et al. Long Covid in adults discharged from UK hospitals after Covid-19: a prospective, multicentre cohort study using the ISA-RIC WHO Clinical Characterisation Protocol. medRxiv 2021. https://doi.org/10.1101/2021.03.18.21253888.
112. Michelen M, Manoharan L, Elkheir N, et al. Characterising long COVID: a living systematic review. BMJ Global Health 2021;6(9):e005427.
113. Park JJH, Detry MA, Murthy S, et al. How to use and interpret the results of a platform trial: users' guide to the medical literature. JAMA 2022;327(1):67–74.
114. Luker JA, Craig LE, Bennett L, et al. Implementing a complex rehabilitation intervention in a stroke trial: a qualitative process evaluation of AVERT. BMC Med Res Methodol 2016;16:52.
115. Van Stan JH, Dijkers MP, Whyte J, et al. The rehabilitation treatment specification system: implications for improvements in research design, reporting, replication, and synthesis. Arch Phys Med Rehabil 2019;100(1):146–55.
116. Mehta S, Rose L, Cook D, et al. The speaker gender gap at critical care conferences. Crit Care Med 2018;46(6):991–6.
117. Wojkowski S, Unger J, McCaughan M, et al. Development, implementation, and outcomes of an acute care clinician scientist clinical placement: case report. Physiother Can 2017. https://doi.org/10.3138/ptc.2016-45E.
118. Sepsis Canada. Sepsis Canada & LifTING research training programs. Available at: https://www.sepsiscanada.ca/training-programs. Accessed August 15, 2022.

Critical Care Pharmacists
A Focus on Horizons

Andrea Sikora, PharmD, MSCR, BCCCP, FCCM[a,b,*]

KEYWORDS

- Critical care • Intensive care unit • Patient safety • Quality • Pharmacy
- Pharmacists

KEY POINTS

- Critical care pharmacists are essential members of the interprofessional health care team when caring for critically ill patients.
- Critical care pharmacists care for patients through three domains: direct patient care via comprehensive medication management services, indirect patient care via quality improvement, and professional service including research and education.
- The evolution of the critical care pharmacist parallels the advancement of the discipline of critical care medicine and is fueled by the importance of safe and effective medication use practices.
- Harnessing Big Data to make precision-oriented predictions that influence medication decision-making and predict pharmacist workload are elements of the future of critical care pharmacy.

Only he who keeps his eye fixed on the far horizon will find the right road.
— *Dag Hammarskjöld*

INTRODUCTION

The critical care pharmacist (CCP) is essential to the high-quality care of critically ill patients. CCPs provide dedicated medication expertise at the bedside, drive quality improvement (QI) initiatives, and serve in a myriad of other professional roles. However, this image of a highly trained pharmacotherapeutic expert integrated into the care of the hospital's sickest patients is in striking contrast to the 1939 Rockwellian depiction of the feverish child waiting at the apothecary. This transformation is a response to the demands on clinical providers generated by the explosion in the understanding of critical illness over the last 100 years. The history of medicine and pharmacy are

[a] Department of Clinical and Administrative Pharmacy, University of Georgia College of Pharmacy, 120 15th Street, HM-118, Augusta, GA 30912, USA; [b] Department of Pharmacy, Augusta University Medical Center, Augusta, GA, USA
* University of Georgia College of Pharmacy, 120 15th Street, HM-118, Augusta, GA 30912.
E-mail address: sikora@uga.edu

Crit Care Clin 39 (2023) 503–527
https://doi.org/10.1016/j.ccc.2023.01.006
0749-0704/23/Published by Elsevier Inc.
criticalcare.theclinics.com

interwoven, and like the story of critical care medicine, the story of critical care pharmacy remains in its first articles. Despite the extraordinary advancements in life-saving technology, our discipline faces a plethora of growing pains: soaring health care costs, poor long-term outcomes of intensive care unit (ICU) survivors, and concerns for both clinician burn-out and patient safety.[1] Reflecting on our shared history is essential to chart our course to the next horizon. The purpose of this review was to envision the future of critical care pharmacy by first placing the pharmacist into the broader story of critical care medicine.

Critical Care Pharmacists: A Snapshot

CCPs are clinical pharmacists with a specialty in critical care medicine. Clinical pharmacists "collaborate directly in the decision-making of a patient's care with other health-system professionals to ensure optimal medication management (**Box 1**)." Today, a CCP in the United States has earned a 4-year Doctor of Pharmacy degree, followed by 2 years of intensive, postgraduate clinical residency training (a first year geared toward the breadth of inpatient care and the second year focused on the depth of critical care). Finally, a CCP earns Board Certification in Critical Care Pharmacotherapy (BCCCP) (**Table 1**).[7] Beyond direct and indirect patient care, CCPs provide education to all professions and serve in organizations that contribute broadly to the advancement of critical care medicine.[8] CCPs can be found leading the highest levels of federally-funded research and international organization-led guideline development. A percentage even pursue graduate degrees in public health, clinical research, or health care administration, along with obtaining fellowships in interprofessional, critical-care-oriented organizations (**Fig. 1**). Indeed, two pharmacists have served as President of the Society of Critical Care Medicine (SCCM) in recent years.[9]

HISTORY

As the complexity of medicine increases so does the value of pharmacists. The history of landmark critical care treatment modalities and the evolution of CCPs is depicted in **Fig. 2**. The changes in critical care pharmacy over the last century are products of this exponential rate of knowledge growth—the doubling time of medical knowledge in 1950 took 50 years compared with in the modern day of less than a year.[10] Similar to SCCM (which celebrated its 50th birthday in 2020)[9] and the modern positive pressure ventilator (developed in the 1940s and 50s),[11] a vast majority of the

---

Box 1
Outcomes showed in studies to improve critical care pharmacists' involvement in the ICU

Adverse drug events

Medication errors

Antimicrobial stewardship

Quality indicators (eg, head of bed and removal of catheters)

ICU-related complications

Duration of mechanical ventilation

ICU and hospital length of stay

Hospital mortality

Cost savings

Table 1 Definitions and background	
Training Terminology	
Doctor of Pharmacy (PharmD)	A 4-year professional doctorate program (following appropriate years of undergraduate schooling) consisting of didactic and experiential education that meets the standards set by the Accreditation Council for Pharmacy Education (ACPE)[2]
Licensed Pharmacist (RPh)	A licensed pharmacist, per a state Board of Pharmacy, whose been granted the right to practice pharmacy after obtaining a PharmD and completing the law and competency-based examination[2]
Post-Graduate Year One (PGY1) Pharmacy Residency	An accredited program following an accredited professional pharmacy degree program that focuses on enhancing general competencies of optimizing medication therapy outcomes in a broad range of disease states[3]
Post-Graduate Year Two (PGY2) Specialty Pharmacy Residency	An accredited program following a PGY1 residency that focuses on enhancing the knowledge, skills, and expertise in a specific area of practice[3]
Board of Pharmacy Specialties Certification	A certification recognizing advanced practice levels gained through the Board of Pharmaceutical Specialties (BPS) after completion of a validated examination[2]
Professional Role Terminology	
Staff/Operations Pharmacist	A licensed pharmacist in an inpatient or outpatient hospital pharmacy who is involved in pharmaceutical operations related to medication education, verification, compounding, monitoring, administration, and distribution[4]
Pharmacy Resident	A licensed pharmacist in a PGY1 or PGY2 program who is being trained as a clinical practitioner under the supervision of an experienced preceptor[3]
Clinical Pharmacist	A pharmacist who collaborates directly in the decision-making of a patient's care with other health-system professionals to ensure optimal medication management[5]
Clinical Pharmacist Specialist	A pharmacist with advanced clinical expertise generally obtained through residency training and specialized board certification[5]
Privileging	A written collaborative drug therapy management (CDTM) agreement within a health care system expanding practice privileges to clinical pharmacists; mostly associated with inpatient practice[5]
Credentialing	Documented evidence of professional qualifications often denoting expertise in a particular disease or knowledge domain[6]

pharmacotherapy used today did not exist 100 years ago.[12] For perspective, the US Food and Drug Administration has approved over 20,000 prescription drug products since its inception in 1906.

The first use of penicillin in the United States to treat a septic patient was followed 10 years later by the establishment of the first formal ICU in Copenhagen by the

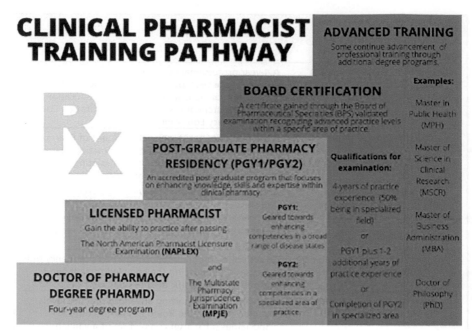

Fig. 1. Critical care pharmacist training pathway. Training pathway of a critical care pharmacist.

anesthesiologist Bjørn Ibsen after the 1952 polio epidemic.[13,14] The first critical care fellowship program was developed at the University of Pittsburgh in the early 1960s.[15] The groundwork for modern clinical pharmacy services in the ICU also began in the 1960s with the highly successful University of California San Francisco's "Ninth-Floor Pharmacy Project."[16] This project marked the use of decentralized pharmacist services (ie, pharmacists in the same physical location as the physicians, nurses, and patients) and had the goal to oversee all aspects of the medication distribution process and provide a source of high-quality drug information. In 1990, the first critical care pharmacy residency accreditation standards were published.[17] Board certification for pharmacists in critical care became available in 2015.[18] This certification is accredited by the same independent accrediting organizations (International Accreditation Service and the National Commission for Certifying Agencies) as other professions, including physicians.[19] An inter-professionally endorsed Position Statement on Critical Care Pharmacy services states the "essential" nature of CCPs to ICU patient care. Published in 2000 (and updated in 2020), this statement is the culmination of

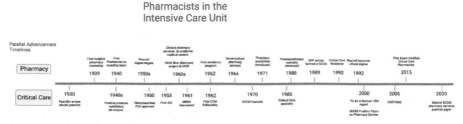

Fig. 2. Timeline of critical care medicine and pharmacy.

these many years of efforts to ensure appropriate recognition for the role of pharmacists in the ICU.[20]

CRITICAL CARE PHARMACISTS IMPROVE OUTCOMES

CCPs are integrally involved in the delivery of high-quality patient care and advancement of medical knowledge. CCPs improve patient outcomes and improve health care value through three domains (**Table 2**). This Triple Domain of Critical Care Pharmacists includes direct patient care (eg, rounding), indirect patient care (eg, institutional [QI]), and professional service (eg, scholarship, teaching, leadership) (**Fig. 3**). These activities are delineated in the Position Statement that discusses foundational and desirable levels of CCP professional activity.[8] Services are organized into pharmacy practice models, which are defined as the systems in which pharmacists are deployed within a given institution to provide pharmacotherapeutic care. These practice models include components like shifts (eg, weekday day-time), clinical expectations (eg, rounding with the interprofessional team, pharmacokinetic consults), and patient coverage (eg, by medical service, by physical ICU location).[21–23] The current state of critical care pharmacy practice is rapidly evolving, as evidenced by two national surveys of CCP activities from 2006 and 2019.[21,24,25] Owing to the rapid growth, pharmacy services are heterogeneous and vary widely by institution.[23,24]

Patient-centered outcomes: CCPs have been shown to improve patient outcomes in nearly every domain that has been evaluated in the direct patient care environment.[8]

Table 2
Triple domain of critical care pharmacists

Domain[26]	Definition/Scope	Examples
Direct Patient Care	Any activity related to the delivery of comprehensive medication management and generally in concordance with the five rights of pharmacy care (right patient, drug, time, dose, route) occurring in the presence of direct patient care delivery	Participation in multiprofessional rounds, optimizing treatment regimens, medication reconciliation, and counseling, avoiding adverse events, therapeutic drug monitoring recommendations made on rounds
Indirect Patient Care	Any activity related to optimizing patient care downstream of a process or logistic strategy designed to improve quality, effectiveness, safety, and cost of care	Quality improvement projects, clinical protocols (eg, treatment algorithms, institutional guidance documents), cost mitigation measures
Professional	Activities related to scholarship, education, and service ranging from the local to an international level that benefit the critical care community through creating new knowledge, developing practitioners though enhanced training, and advocating for the discipline	Clinical Research (retrospective to prospective RCTs), translational research (bench to bedside), in-service presentations to medical services, nursing education, conduct training, and certification programs didactic lectures to health-care students, precept health-care students, professional organization leadership, and professional activism

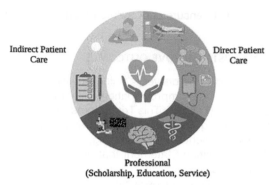

Indirect Patient Care

Direct Patient Care

Professional
(Scholarship, Education, Service)

Fig. 3. Triple domain of critical care pharmacists. Critical care pharmacists enhance the quality and value of health care delivered through three primary domains: direct patient care, indirect patient care, and scholarship, education, and service. Direct patient care includes multiprofessional rounds and comprehensive medication management. Indirect patient care includes quality improvement initiatives like protocolized care and medication use evaluations. The final category of professional service includes education of fellow health care workers and trainees, research, and leadership positions (eg, supervisory roles) that contributes to the culture of evidence-based medication use. (Created with BioRender.com.)

Increasing the number of clinical pharmacists per occupied patient bed has been negatively associated with hospital mortality for patients.[27] A 2019 meta-analysis showed that CCPs attending interprofessional rounds in the ICU were associated with a 22% reduction in mortality and a 1.33-day reduction in the length of ICU stay.[28] Notably, this study showed a 74% reduction in adverse drug events (ADEs), in line with approximately 70% ADE reduction first observed in 1999 in a landmark article in the *Journal of the American Medical Association (JAMA)*.[29] Beyond direct patient care, pharmacists play an integral role in the indirect patient care realm, specifically related to QI initiatives that improve the safety and value of health care.[30,31] Targeted studies have evaluated pharmacist-driven QI at the bedside, including initiatives that improved outcomes in infections/sepsis,[32,33] heparin-induced thrombocytopenia,[34] thromboembolisms,[35] anti-coagulation management[36] sedation and mechanical ventilation weaning,[37–39] pain, agitation, and delirium,[40] spontaneous breathing trials,[41] stress-ulcer prophylaxis,[42] QTc prolongation,[43] and deresucitation.[30]

Health care costs: Economic analyses have repeatedly pointed to a high return on investment, with cost-avoidance to CCP salary predicted between $3.3:1 and $9.6:1.[32,44–48] Furthermore, ICUs lacking CCPs were found to have significantly higher mortality rates and longer ICU lengths of stay in critically ill infected patients, and the economic return on investment for a CCP was estimated at 25:1.[32] The evidence suggests that CCPs improve outcomes in a highly cost-effective manner, in line with the concept that high quality, interprofessional, team-based care is often the most cost-effective care. **Box 2** provides an annotated bibliography of studies representative of this extensive body of literature.

EVIDENCE-BASED MEDICINE: QUALITY DRIVES THE NEED FOR CRITICAL CARE PHARMACISTS

Globally, it is important to acknowledge that "quality" is a relatively novel concept in health care. Physician writers have repeatedly recounted that the advances in medicine have come with associated risks to patient safety. Atul Gawande has highlighted the historic barriers to focusing on safety and quality in medicine, including the

Box 2
Seminal literature of CCP influence on economic and clinical outcomes

Leape LL, et al. Pharmacist participation on physician rounds and adverse drug events in the intensive care unit. *JAMA*. 1999;282(3):267-270.[29]
- Before-after study of CCP participation on the multiprofessional rounding team and providing medication interventions and consulting services in a medical and coronary ICU
- Preventable ADEs decreased by 66% from 10.4 to 3.5 per 1000 patient days with more than 99% of pharmacist recommendations were accepted by physicians
- Impact: Shows a significant improvement in medication safety through CCP involvement in direct patient care in the ICU

Buckley MS, et al. Impact of a clinical pharmacist stress ulcer prophylaxis management program on inappropriate use in hospitalized patients. *Am J Med*. 2015;128(8):905-913.[42]
- Retrospective pre–post evaluation of the clinical and economic impact of pharmacist-directed stress ulcer prophylaxis program in the ICU and medical ward
- Pharmacist-managed SUP program decreased the rate of inappropriate SUP use and resulted in significant cost savings (est. annual savings of > $200,000)
- Impact: Shows an example of a quality improvement imitative that resulted in significant cost savings and improvement in appropriate medication use

Stollings JL, et al. Pharmacist leadership in ICU quality improvement: coordinating spontaneous awakening and breathing trials. *Ann Pharmacother*. 2015;49(8):883-891.[41]
- Evaluation of a pharmacist-implemented awakening and breathing coordination quality improvement (QI) program compared with a previous protocol without pharmacists
- The rates of passing spontaneous awakening trial (SAT) safety screen improved from 63% to 78% ($p = 0.03$) and the overall rates of SATs among eligible patients on continuous infusions improved from 53% to 85% ($p = 0.0001$)
- Impact: Associated studies showed similar QI initiatives reduced the duration of mechanical ventilation[49] and show that CCPs have a role beyond "medication use" to improve overall value of care provided

Leguelinel-Blache G, et al. Impact of Quality Bundle Enforcement by a Critical Care Pharmacist on Patient Outcome and Costs. *Crit Care Med*. 2018;46(2):199-207.[31]
- Evaluated the effect of pharmacists interventions on patient outcomes and costs in two ICUs
- CPP intervention was associated with reductions in length of stay in the hospital (−3.7 days) and ICU (−1.4 days), mechanical ventilation duration (−1.2 days), and CCP intervention was associated with cost-savings (approx. $12,000 per month)
- Impact: This protocol shows that CCPs are active participants in multiprofessional care delivery that goes beyond medications

Lee H, et al. Impact on Patient Outcomes of Pharmacist Participation in Multidisciplinary Critical Care Teams: A Systematic Review and Meta-Analysis. *Crit Care Med*. 2019;47(9):1243-1250.[28]
- Meta-analysis of 14 randomized and non-randomized studies evaluating patient outcomes compared with the presence or absence of a CCP
- Intervention of CCP as part of a multiprofessional ICU team was associated with lower mortality odds compared with no CCP (OR, 0.78; 95% CI, 0.73 to 0.83; $p < 0.00001$) and associated with shorter ICU length of stay (−1.12 days)
- Impact: Shows the overall impact of CCPs on mortality and significant reductions to ADEs, providing a link between improving medication safety and reducing mortality in the ICU via CCP-delivered care

Bissell BD, et al. Impact of protocolized diuresis for de-resuscitation in the intensive care unit. *Crit Care*. 2020;24(1):70-70.[30]
- Pre–post single-center pilot study evaluating the impact of a pharmacy-driven de-resuscitation protocol in mechanically ventilated ICU patients where protocolized diuresis was associated with decreased 72-h fluid balance post-shock (median reduction 2257 mL, $p < 0.0001$) and decreased in-hospital mortality (5.5% vs 16.1%, $p = 0.008$)
- Impact: Shows nuanced medication therapy management that highlights the unique training and experience of a CCP to provide assessment and intervention in critically ill patients

Rech MA, et al. PHarmacist Avoidance or Reductions in Medical Costs in CRITically Ill Adults: PHARM-CRIT Study. *Critical Care Explorations.* 2021;3(12).[50]
- Multicenter prospective observational study of 215 CCPs' interventions and their association with cost-avoidance over six months.
- Mean cost-avoidance was $845 per patient day with annualized cost-avoidance of $1,784,302 for a CCP
- Impact: Shows cost avoidance through optimization of medication therapy management

Sikora A, et al. Impact of pharmacists to improve patient care in the critically ill: A large multicenter analysis using meaningful metrics with the MRC-ICU. *Critical Care Medicine.* 2022. 2022 Sep 1;50(9):1318-1328.[51]
- Multi-center prospective observational study of 28 centers evaluating CCP interventions, length of stay, mortality, and a novel medication regimen complexity prediction metric
- Observed that for every one-point increase in medication regimen complexity, mortality increases by 9%. Increased patient:pharmacist ratio (indicating more patients per clinician) was significantly associated with increased ICU length of stay and reduced quantity and intensity of interventions.
- Impact: Shows a strong link between medication regimen complexity and mortality, indicating the need for pharmacotherapeutic expertise in ICU medication management. This study is the first to show that overburdened CCPs are unable to provide the same level of care, which deleteriously impacts length of stay.

examples of obstetricians denying the relationship between hand washing and puerperal fever in the 1800s[52] and surgeons' resistance to the adoption of anesthesia, aseptic technique, and QI measures such as checklists. But even in modern times, studies show some of the same barriers. For example, health care professionals still do not always wash their hands before entering a patient's room.[53,54] The abuses during the early stages of medicine and device development that lacked regulatory and professional oversight are notable. Pope Brock's recount of Morris Fishbein (a physician and editor of *JAMA*) and his crusade for improved regulation of medical practices (including debunking that transplantation of glands from male goats into the human body to improves virility, a common practice at the turn of the century) is a fascinating account and vivid counterfactual to our present focus on evidence-based medicine and emphasis on regulatory oversight.[55] Humble appreciation for the life-saving nature of safe medication practices—spanning the spectrum from drug development to bedside administration—is the lifeblood of a clinical pharmacist.

The disjointed nature of providing medical care means that health care professionals are often unaware of the long-term impact of their interventions. Thus, a situation arises where the perils of "eminence-based medicine" are present. Eminence-based medicine has been defined as "the more senior the colleague, the less importance he or she placed on the need for anything as mundane as evidence. Experience...is worth any amount of evidence...which has been defined as 'making the same mistakes with increasing confidence over an impressive number of years.'" In addition, errors in prediction can occur in a field characterized by professional judgment from "respect experts."[1,12,53] Recently, Nobel-prize-winning Daniel Kahneman discussed sources of prediction error when a judgment is not verifiable, as can be the case in medicine: "Yet some professionals in these domains come to be called experts. The confidence we have in these experts' judgment is entirely based on the respect they enjoy from their peers. We call them respect-experts."[56] As noted in the book *Deep Medicine*, many health care professionals make judgments without necessarily knowing the long-term outcomes of those decisions, and the health care system suffers from this lack of feedback.[57-59] This early era of rapid development of medical knowledge and technology was plagued by a blind-spot in medicine characterized by pushing the limits of medical knowledge as opposed to the patient-centered, high-quality delivery of that knowledge.

The realization that the safe and effective use of medications is tightly interwoven with ICU outcomes is thus still novel, in part due to the relative youth of evidence-based medicine. The Agency for Healthcare Quality and Research (AHRQ) was established in 1989, and The Institute of Medicine (IOM) published its chilling report "To Err is Human" in 2000. The ICU has been described as the most medication error-prone in medicine, with estimates for medication errors ranging from 1.2 to 947 per 1000 ICU-patient days (medication errors in the form of severe ADEs can double the mortality risk).[60] Notably, the IOM report coincided with the seminal study demonstrating that CCPs on interprofessional rounds reduced ADEs by 66%.[61–63] Owing to these events, the past two decades have shown an increased focus on medication safety and the quality and value of health care, fueling the growth of CCPs as they have repeatedly showed value in these domains.

A salient example of CCP importance in optimizing ICU pharmacotherapy comes with the advent of FAST-HUG, the ICU mnemonic developed in 2005 to address essential elements of daily ICU care (and updated to FAST-HUGS BID), of which nine of the eleven elements are distinctly drug-related.[64] Wes Ely's 2021 book, *Every Deep-Drawn Breath,* chronicles the history of the use and misuse of medications in critically ill patients and is an important reminder that medications are not just "treatment" for a disease but can in fact be independent causes of new disease.[65] Interestingly, implementation of the other components of FAST-HUGS BID which are not drug related (eg, head of the bed elevation for mechanical ventilation, assessment of the need for indwelling catheters) have also been shown to be associated with improved outcomes for patients when managed by the quality oriented CCP.[31] The importance of dedicated pharmacotherapeutic expertise to improve ICU outcomes cannot be understated.

THE GAP: NOT EVERY CRITICALLY ILL PATIENT RECEIVES THE CARE OF A CRITICAL CARE PHARMACIST

Interprofessional care is repeatedly cited as part of the solution to the challenges of managing critically ill patients, yet gaps in CCP access are still present.[66–68] The exact number of pharmacists practicing in the ICU is unknown. There are approximately 3,600 pharmacists with BCCCP, and SCCM reports 6,000 pharmacists caring for patients in over 100,000 ICU beds in the United States.[69] For reference, there are approximately 20,000 intensivists and 512,000 critical care nurses.[70] Expert opinion on the ideal CCP-to-patient ratio has placed the value around 1:15,[71] but approximately one-quarter of CCPs self-reported a CCP-to-patient ratio of 1:18, and another quarter reported working at a ratio greater than 1:30.[72] One survey of 441 US hospitals observed a median ratio of 1:17 (interquartile range, 1:12 to 1:26), but only 70% reported having a CCP present for multiprofessional rounds. Further, only 15% had weekend rounding services, and it appears that a 24 h a day, 365-days-a-year model, whereas the standard of practice for physicians and nurses in the ICU, is rare for CCPs.[24] Supply is a significant issue given that every year qualified trainees to go unmatched because there are only 171 accredited critical care residency programs. Despite these apparent gaps, position justification and national recognition remains a perennial challenge for CCPs.[73–79]

DISCUSSION OF THE FUTURE

The gap in CCP services is a significant, yet underappreciated, public health concern.[71] To date, the primary focus of the profession has been the implementation of clinical pharmacy services into the direct patient care environment. When one reads the 2020 Position Statement, it is a veritable laundry list of activities a pharmacist can perform to improve outcomes.[8] Yet, the major drawback of this focus on individual services is that the Position Statement has almost no commentary on the infrastructure and processes for how to optimally deploy a CCP (eg, pharmacist-to-patient ratio, pharmacy practice models, quality tracking). Thus, although a necessary component of the literature to document the details of how a pharmacist specifically improves a component of patient care (eg, a protocolized means of diuresis following sepsis resuscitation), taking a step back from these efforts to a broader discussion of future directions is warranted.

Factors that have contributed to the lack of CCPs include.

1. Department of Pharmacy budgets combining drug costs with personnel costs (eg, if drug costs go up for independent reasons it may still necessitate personnel losses)
2. Not enough Critical Care Pharmacy Residencies (Ie, current supply cannot meet demand)
3. Lack of compensation for services rendered (also known as "provider status," CCPs cannot bill for services like physicians, nurse practitioners, etc.)
4. No minimum staffing regulations from major accrediting and oversight bodies such as The Joint Commission, or Centers for Medicare and Medicaid Services
5. Antiquated ICU culture (eg, lack of awareness by the health care team regarding the potential of CCP to improve outcomes for patients)
6. Minimal public awareness (eg, although it would be cause for media attention and concern if a patient was treated in the ICU without a physician or nurse, this would not be the same for CCPs)
7. Pharmacy's siloed approach to management and clinicians. When clinical management roles are filled by pharmacists who have completed health-system administration residency programs, the clinical foundation required for many aspects of ICU-related QI and staffing needs is lacking. Identifying meaningful ways for CCP advancement into leadership roles or thoughtful pairing of complementary skillsets between clinicians and administrators is needed.

Mapping a New Horizon

A vision of the future state of critical care includes CCPs embedded into every interprofessional ICU care team to provide real-time optimization of pharmacotherapy. Just as a patient in the ICU would never be without an attending physician and a dedicated nurse, they should never be without a CCP. In this vision, interprofessional team discussions would incorporate the respective expertise and the focus of each professional to devise a proactive treatment plan. These recommendations would be documented, and services rendered billable under major insurance providers. Beyond this, minimum CCP staffing requirements for ICU patients would be incorporated into health care quality and safety standards.

Four steps toward bridging this gap include.

Acknowledging the inherent dangers of intensive care unit care

Despite best intentions, care provided in the ICU is often accompanied by significant long-term harms.[1] To *acknowledge* this reality, it is helpful to conceptualize the Three Principles of Critical Care (**Fig. 4**). The First Principle is "Treat the underlying cause." The Second Principle is "Provide supportive care." The Third Principle is "Minimize iatrogenic harm caused by the first two principles." In essence, the Third Principle

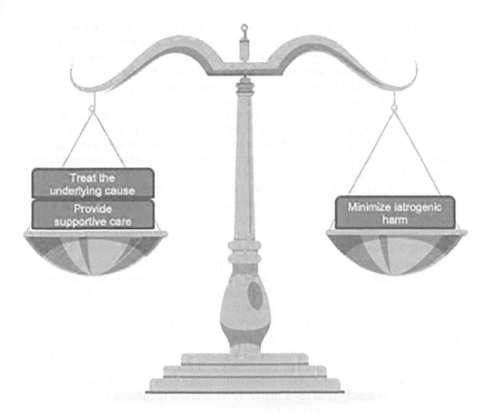

Fig. 4. The three principles of critical care. The Three Principles of Critical Care are (1) treat the underlying cause, (2) provide supportive care, and (3) minimize iatrogenic harm. Maximizing the benefit of treatment-oriented and supportive-care-oriented pharmacotherapy while minimizing iatrogenic harm is the cornerstone of critical care pharmacy direct patient care.

counterbalances the first two. Each new intervention must be carefully examined such that its benefits outweigh its harms. Using this construct, medications, and those who manage them, must be viewed as vital elements to obtaining this fine balance of benefits and harms of ICU care.

Re-thinking the paradigm of medication use in the intensive care unit

Traditionally, medication safety has been synonymous with operational safety: right patient, right drug, right dose, right route. In fact, ICU medications are notorious for their high-risk nature that demand systems to guide safe, operational use (eg, ordering, dispensing, administration). The Institute for Safe Medication Practices (ISMP) publishes a list of High Alert Medications, a majority of which are primarily used in the ICU, and stories of deadly errors from "look alike sound alike" drugs have highlighted the need for individuals focused on this operational aspect of medication use. Historically, CCPs have focused primarily on operational safety, intending to reduce medication errors by ensuring appropriate ordering, dispensing, and administration. This focus was bred from necessity due to the lack of information technology (IT) solutions like computerized provider order entry (CPOE) systems, clinical decision support systems (CDSS), barcoding, and drug-drug interaction (DDI) and dose-range checking software. Fortunately, technologies have evolved automating many safe practices. Moreover, health care informatics teams from all professions that focus specifically on optimizing these IT systems have evolved. In the modern era, CCPs serve as essential liaisons and consultants to these teams; however, medications used in the ICU are dangerous not only from a standpoint of operational errors but from long-term sequalae. Herein lies the primary role of the modern CCP.

In 1968, Donald E. Francke, founder of the peer-reviewed journal *The Annals of Pharmacotherapy* explained this paradigm shift from operational to clinical expertise stating, "The dispensing function of the pharmacist, while important and even vital, is essentially a superficial practice of the profession which, by itself, does not require knowledge or skills sufficiently basic to merit professional recognition."[80] ICU medications require high-level consideration from the standpoint of evidence-based medicine, which necessitates comprehensive medication management provided by CCPs well above and beyond the operational expertise. Inappropriate medication therapy, even If deployed "safely" from an operational perspective, is associated with various ICU complications that worsen patient-centered outcomes: fluid overload, mechanical ventilation, acute kidney injury, continuous renal replacement therapy, delirium, and superinfections. Using an ineffective therapy (or misusing an effective therapy) is ultimately a safety concern that violates the Third Principle of Critical Care. For example, although neuromuscular blockade agents (NMBAs) have a role in diseases like acute respiratory distress syndrome, they also play a significant role in ICU-acquired muscle weakness and post-traumatic stress disorder in ICU survivors.[81] Historically, a CCP might focus on key operational safety concerns: DDI or dosing in end-organ dysfunction. Although these elements are still part of the CCP role, IT solutions and integrated multiprofessional care have off-loaded some of these concerns to create time for a higher-level analysis to identify how to deploy a therapy in individualized clinical contexts that come with the risk of causing as much, or more, harm than benefit. For example, with NMBAs the goals might be 1. to determine the best practice for monitoring (eg, train of four versus bispectral index); 2. Identify how optimal sedation and analgesia can be delivered seamlessly via protocols; 3. Assess guidelines that can be developed to guide the most appropriate indications for this therapy, and 4. Develop such protocols and guidelines to optimize use is a primary role of the modern-day CCP. Although seemingly subtle, this shift in focus from minimizing medication errors to *optimizing pharmacotherapeutic care* marks a key evolution not only in the role of the CCP but in how all of the pharmacotherapy is viewed by the interprofessional care team. These positive changes have allowed for an evolution of the CCP to higher-level pharmacotherapy considerations regarding both safety *and* efficacy. We describe this paradigm shift of viewing medications within the Patient-Medication Optimization-Outcome Pathway in **Fig. 5**.

Prioritizing optimizing health care systems that optimize clinician workload

Clinician workload plays a key role in the quality of care.[82–84] Quality of care maximizes the four key components of medical ethics: non-maleficence, beneficence, autonomy, and justice. Overburdened and fatigued clinicians are more likely to fail in all of these domains (eg, at the end of a shift, health care professionals are less likely to wash their hands before going to the next patient room, and physicians are more likely to prescribe opioids). These factors indicate that fatigue plays a role in decision-making.[56] In this way, overburdening critical care health care professionals directly impacts the Three Principles of Critical Care (**Fig. 6**) because such health care professionals are more likely to cause iatrogenic harm via medical errors or other poor judgments.

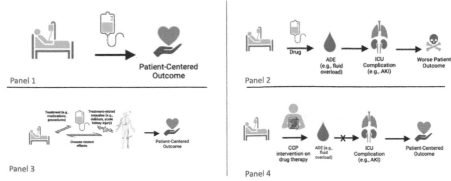

Fig. 5. Patient-medication optimization-outcome pathway. The Patient-Medication Optimization-Outcome Pathway is a theoretical construct that supports investigation into how medication optimization is an independent factor in ultimate patient outcomes. Moreover, it allows for careful analysis of the *relative* efficacy and safety differences among therapies. Panel 1 shows the historical construct: a patient is treated with a medication that leads to recovery. However, this construct does not include how medications are independent risk factors for adverse patient outcomes. Panel 2 incorporates medications as independent risk factors by showing that patients treated with a medication may develop an ADE that increases the risk for an ICU complication that can then lead to worse patient outcomes. However, this expansion upon Panel 1 does not do justice to the complex interplay between disease–treatment–treatment-related adverse effects. Panel 3 incorporates this complex interplay of factors that lead to patient-centered outcomes, with the star denoting the key zone where optimized health care systems can improve outcomes. Finally, Panel 4 incorporates the specific role of CCPs in this medication use pathway, indicating how medications, optimized by CCPs, can reduce ADEs that reduce ICU complications, and ultimately improve patient-centered outcomes. (Created with BioRender.com.)

In addition, overburdened health care professionals suffer from higher rates of burn-out, which is also known to adversely affect patient safety.[85–88] However, although the relationship between overwork, burn-out, and medical errors is often discussed, lack of care optimization is just as concerning.

Overburdened CCPs have less potential to both prevent harm (ie, non-maleficence) and optimize the efficacy of therapies provided (ie, beneficence). With lack of medication optimization, a therapy that may not be actively causing harm or be "a mistake" may still not be the "best" choice. That "best" choice may reduce ICU length of stay and therefore "unseen harms" that are associated with prolonged ICU stays. Put simply, the systems of care in which individuals work cannot be extricated from the quality of care those individuals provide.

Although investigations of workload and care quality have been conducted for nurses and physicians demonstrating that lower workloads reduce mortality, much less investigation has been conducted for CCPs.[82,83,87,89–93] Ultimately, these investigations must focus not just on the addition of the first pharmacist, but on the incremental increase in staff in relation to outcomes (ie, the workload ratio). In the first study of its kind, a multi-center trial of 3,908 patients showed that increasing the number of patients a CCP cared for resulted in fewer medication interventions per patient (and less intensity or complexity of those interventions) and a longer length of stay.[57] More studies of this nature are needed.

Burn-out has been well documented to occur at higher rates in critical care,[94–96] and the rate of burn-out has ranged up to 60% for CCPs (and 80% for clinical

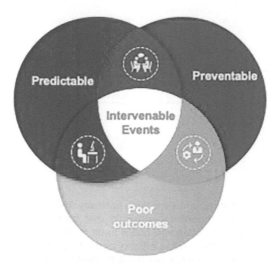

Fig. 6. CCPs target intervenable medication events. Intervenable medication events have three characteristics: (1) predictable based on known characteristics of the patient and medications, (2) associated with poor outcomes when they occur, and (3) preventable via timely medication interventions. Targeting intervenable events (as opposed to Adverse Drug Events) is a key goal of critical care pharmacist-driven outcome improvement.

pharmacists).[24,97–101] **Fig. 7** depicts how workload must be calibrated for the Stakeholder Triad that seeks to optimize patient-centered outcomes, health care worker wellness, and institutional needs. A sustainable workload indicates high-quality care is being provided in a way that protects the health care workers and elevates value. Priority must be placed on establishing profession-specific safe workloads for health care workers caring for critically ill patients.

Critical care pharmacist-specific workload factors. CCP shifts are unique for both physician and nursing counterparts. Traditionally, ICU nurses work shifts focused on delivering patient care to specifically assigned patients in an ICU, with minimal responsibilities for non-direct patient care activities during those shifts. (Indirect patient care activities are instead assigned to designated nurses in supervisor and QI positions). Intensivists work in an on-service, off-service model with the on-service aspect similar to the ICU nurses, where the primary responsibility is providing direct patient care. During off-service periods, direct patient care is limited to scheduled clinic hours or other specialty responsibilities (such as a surgeon) and is filled with other professional and administrative obligations. In contrast, CCPs usually have a mixture of responsibilities in both the direct and indirect patient care realms that must be juggled on a daily basis. Though painting broadly, this set-up often means that CCPs deliver a majority of their direct patient care in the morning in conjunction with interprofessional rounds, with afternoons left for follow-up and as-needed consultation, with a primary focus on indirect patient care and professional service responsibilities. In settings of high patient care workload, indirect patient care activities (while still essential to overall care) are not performed, or the pharmacist must work beyond the scheduled shift, likely without compensation due to the salaried nature of pharmacist positions. Notably, because of the integral role that CCPs play with QI, lack of dedicated time has implications for patient-centered outcomes.

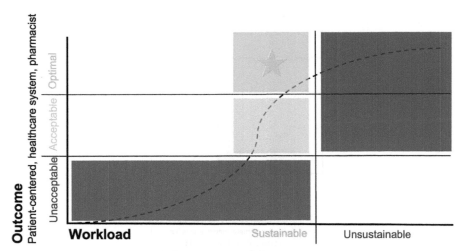

Fig. 7. Optimization of workload based on the Stakeholder Triad for Pharmacy Practice Models: patients, health care providers, institutions. Critical care pharmacist workload must be optimized for the Stakeholder Triad: providing excellent patient care to patients, sustainably managing health care worker wellness for critical care pharmacists, and maximizing return on investment for institutions. The green zone depicts a sustainable workload that achieves these outcomes.

A key issue with asking a professional (regardless of profession) to take care of more patients than is reasonable in a given shift is that the consequences of poor perfor- mance directly impact a patient's life. Moreover, this professional has taken an oath regarding the provision of high-quality care up to an ethical standard: put simply, a health care professional is unlikely to "clock out" at the designated shift end time if they perceive patients still need their care (**Fig. 8**). They are aware of the differences in the quality of care they can provide when the workload is reasonable versus unrea- sonable (and overwork can result in sustained moral distress and/or fatigue).[102–105] Interestingly, indirect patient care activities like QI are associated with reduced burn-out among CCPs.[101] Although the survey-based nature of this finding prohibits causal inference, a hypothesis worthy of consideration is that CCPs recognize the value of QI and education efforts to improve the quality of care, and lack of protected time reduces feelings of efficacy and/or increases feelings of moral distress.

CCPs frequently "cross-cover" colleagues' paid-time off or sick leave. Here, a CCP is required to care for their usual service in addition to another CCP's usual service, essentially doubling the volume of patient care required on that particular day. In addi- tion, cross-coverage implies different levels of care provided: for example, if the med- ical ICU pharmacist is on vacation, the surgical ICU pharmacist may care for the medical ICU patients in their absence; however, if rounds occur at the same time, this surgical ICU pharmacist can only attend one set of rounds, likely limiting the comprehensiveness of the care delivered. A key ramification is that CCPs are frequently placed in a "reactive" role where therapies are started without their direct involvement and must then "intervene" upon the medication regimen. This reactive model is in contrast to a proactive model, where CCPs are incorporated during the initial decision-making process to have the optimal therapy started at the time of diag- nosis, as opposed to the time of the CCP shift. Although the costs of inappropriate therapies initiated and later modified to CCPs on the health care system and patient have not been evaluated, there is reason to believe that significant improvements could be realized by incorporating CCPs proactively.

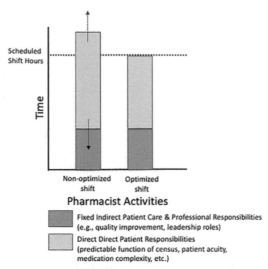

Fig. 8. Ramifications of non-optimized CCP workload. When CCP workload is not optimized, the result is the poor quality of direct patient care, inability to complete indirect patient care responsibilities, and/or overworking the pharmacist attempting to fulfill unrealistic workload burden.

Updating the paradigm of a critical care pharmacist

A video produced by United Nations Educational, Scientific and Cultural Organization (UNESCO) discussed how the education system must prepare trainees for jobs that do not exist yet, due to the rapidly changing nature of today's workforce.[106] Increased emphasis is less on technical skills but on the metacognitive and emotional intelligence skillsets that allow for high rates of adaptability and team-oriented work.[107,108] Indeed, Cal Newport discusses "Two Core Abilities for Thriving in the New Economy: 1. The ability to quickly master hard things; 2. The ability to produce at an elite level, in terms of both quality and speed."[109] CCP training unequivocally meets this call. When the COVID-19 pandemic hit, ICU pharmacists worked alongside their fellow health care professionals to serve as key drivers of pharmacotherapy protocols, research efforts, and vaccination programs.[110] Their efforts were immediately apparent and showed the ability of the profession to pivot rapidly when needed. This experience showed that a pharmacist is a multi-tool of readily adaptable, meta-cognitive abilities who can solve problems regarding the optimization of pharmacotherapy. As such, pharmacists' scope of practice should not be limited based on prior studies. Put simply, complex questions of optimizing pharmacotherapy are best solved by a team with a pharmacist. The question should thus be, "How do we deploy pharmacists to optimally improve the outcomes in this disease state?" The baseline assumption is that pharmacists improve patient outcomes. This assumption has already been adopted by physicians and nurses, as no disease state is managed without these individuals, and it is time to include CCPs in this conceptualization of care.

Table 3 depicts the thought shifts necessary to achieve this vision. Medication regimens must be viewed as requiring expert management to optimize outcomes. Moreover, the transition must ultimately be made from individuals to a comprehensive view of the systems in which this interprofessional team works. Box 3 provides actionable steps for current clinicians and administrators.

Table 3
Paradigm shifts in the future vision of critical care pharmacist services

Domain	Historical View		Future Vision
CCPs provide a:	Commodity	→	Service
CCPs are responsible for a:	Task	→	Patient
Workload is measured by:	Frequency of tasks	→	Intensity of patient needs
The value of CCPs is based on:	Error catching	→	Pharmacotherapy optimization
Medication changes occur via:	Reactive intervention	→	Proactive decision making
Optimal outcomes are achieved by the:	Individual professional	→	Systems of clinician care

A DATA-DRIVEN FUTURE

Improving outcomes via optimization of CCP workload is the next horizon. The core gap is a lack of quantifiable means to benchmark the care provided: no metrics that describe and predict CCP workload have been universally accepted. Similarly, dashboards to benchmark the value and quality of CCPs are lacking. Alone, ICU census and patient acuity do not reliably correlate with CCP workload (which is unsurprising, as pharmacists provide comprehensive medication therapy management across the continuum of patient acuity and each patient requires a precision-approach to their care). The relationship among CCP workload, quality of CCP care, and resulting patient-centered outcomes is also poorly delineated. Moreover, CCPs influence and mold the culture of evidence-based medication use in the ICU. Over time, their presence can impart important values of evidence-based decision-making. For example, a regular practice of participating in the 30-min lectures during morning teaching in the medical ICU or participating in interprofessional QI efforts like the ABCDEF bundle likely has a more durable impact on culture and prescribing practices, yet often this service goes unaccounted for in productivity dashboards. Novel solutions are required for this complex problem. Owing to technology that integrates electronic health record data with advanced statistical and even artificial-intelligence-based modeling, clinician-designed dashboards that use metrics-based, data-driven approaches are a promising strategy (**Fig. 9**).

Box 3
Actionable steps to increasing patient access to CCP care

Multiprofessional advocacy of team-based care
1. Identifying institutional gaps of CCPS on rounding and QI teams
2. Advocacy for incorporation of CCPs into staffing standards for ICUs

Data-driven approaches to CCP workload optimization
1. Clinician-designed dashboards that focus on patient-centered outcomes
2. CCP-oriented prediction workload metrics
3. Analysis of pharmacist-to-patient ratio against meaningful outcomes
4. Incorporation of the Stakeholder Triad to personnel decisions
5. Innovation in practice models for the unique nature of CCP roles

Improving access to CCP care
1. Increasing the number of residency training programs
2. Consideration of expanded institutional privileging
3. Identifying means to improve billable services (including advocacy)
4. Institutional support for professional development (eg, BCCCP and training courses)

Developing models to predict patient needs for CCP care (ie, CCP workload) is essential. A CCP's direct patient care workload derives from the patient's medication regimens, therefore broadly describing the intensity of effort required to optimally manage these regimens is a first step. The medication regimen complexity-ICU (MRC-ICU) Scoring Tool is the first metric proposed with the intention of connecting the components of patient-centered outcomes, health care costs, pharmacist welfare, and pharmacist resources. This metric has been externally validated to reliably characterize the complexity of an individual patient medications. To calculate a patient's MRC-ICU score, each medication prescribed is assigned a weighted value ranging from 0 to 3. These values are summed to provide a total score. For example, a patient receiving cefepime (2 points), vancomycin (3 points), norepinephrine (1 point), and dopamine (1 point) on ICU day 1, would have a day 1 MRC-ICU score of 7. In preliminary studies, the MRC-ICU has been correlated to patient acuity, outcomes including mortality and length of stay, ICU-related complications including fluid overload and drug-drug interactions, and pharmacist workload via documented pharmacist interventions. It has shown a stronger correlation to pharmacist interventions than the Sequential Organ Failure Assessment (SOFA) score and has been successfully incorporated into the electronic health record.[111–118] In the largest evaluation to date, for every one-point increase in MRC-ICU score, the odds of mortality increased by 7%. Total pharmacist interventions, and composite intensity of pharmacist interventions,

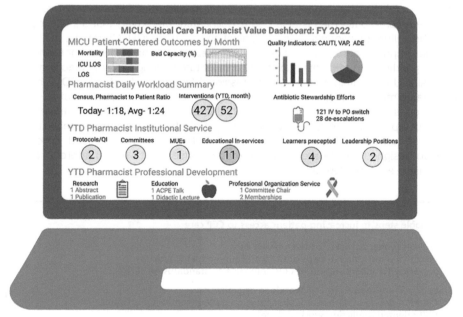

Fig. 9. Wireframe of clinician-designed dashboard. Dashboards serve several key functions: (1) enhance CCP care delivery at the bedside through patient-specific predictions, (2) describe CCP workload for resource allocation and position justification, and (3) benchmark CCP care quality and value. This wireframe incorporates the Triple Aim of the Critical Care Pharmacist and denotes tracking measures that incorporate The Stakeholder Triad. It visualizes the paradigm shifts described in **Box 3** with CCP care oriented to patients (instead of tasks) and describes the intensity and complexity of care (instead of frequency of interventions). It incorporates three key qualities of pharmacy practice models: data-driven, metrics-based, clinician-oriented. (Created with BioRender.com.)

also significantly increased. This ability to meaningfully describe a holistic picture of CCP care with one number holds promise for the ability to conduct meaningful prospective workload studies; however, further investigation is required.

SUMMARY

Ella Maillart wrote, "The wideness of the horizon has to be inside us, cannot be anywhere but inside us, otherwise what we speak about is geographic distances." Similarly, the horizon of critical care medicine is within the individuals that comprise this discipline. As critical care has developed over time, it has become apparent that the highest quality of care cannot be provided to critically ill patients without a pharmacist; an interprofessional health care team in the ICU is incomplete without a CCP. Improving patient outcomes will come through the advancement of the professions that work together as a team to care for the hospital's sickest patients.

CLINICS CARE POINTS

- The modern-day training pathway for a critical care pharmacist has evolved to include a Doctor of Pharmacy, 2 years of postgraduate residency training, board-certification in critical care pharmacotherapy, and opportunities to pursue advanced training in health care administration or clinical research
- Critical care pharmacists improve patient-centered outcomes and reduce costs through direct patient care (via comprehensive medication therapy management), indirect patient care (via QI), and professional service (via organizational leadership, education, and research)
- Critical care pharmacists who round with the interprofessional care team reduce mortality, length of stay, and adverse drug events
- Strategizing ways to improve access to critical care pharmacists (via institutional credentialing, nationally recognized provider status, and increasing training programs) is vital to optimizing patient-centered outcomes
- Improving patient-centered outcomes via optimizing critical care pharmacy services will involve an interprofessional, data-driven, metrics-based approach to workload allocation that ensures that each critically ill patient receives the care of a critical care pharmacist

CONFLICTS OF INTEREST

The authors have no conflicts of interest to disclose.

FUNDING

Dr A. Sikora has received funding through the Agency for Health care Research and Quality through 1R21HS028485.

ACKNOWLEDGMENTS

Kaitlin Blotske, Timothy W. Jones.

REFERENCES

1. Ely EW. Every deep-drawn breath: a critical care doctor on healing, recovery, and transforming medicine in the ICU. First Scribner hardcover edition. ed. Scribner: New York, NY, 2021:1 online resource.

2. Knoer SJ, Eck AR, Lucas AJ. A review of American pharmacy: education, training, technology, and practice. Journal of Pharmaceutical Health Care and Sciences 2016;2(1):32.

3. ACCP. (n.d.). Residency training programs . American college of clinical pharmacy. Available at: https://www.accp.com/resandfel/resandfel.aspx. Accessed March 24, 2022.

4. Smith Y. (2019, february 27). Types of pharmacy. News medical and life science. Available at: https://www.news-medical.net/health/Types-of-Pharmacy.aspx. Accessed March 24, 2022.

5. About clinical pharmacists. American college of clinical pharmacy (ACCP). Available at: https://www.accp.com/about/clinicalpharmacists.aspx. Accessed March 24, 2022.

6. Credentialing and privileging of pharmacists: a resource paper from the Council on Credentialing in Pharmacy. J Am Pharmaceut Assoc 2003;54(6):e354–64.

7. Critical care pharmacy. BPS. Available at: https://www.bpsweb.org/bps-specialties/critical-care-pharmacy/. Accessed March 25, 2022.

8. Lat I, Paciullo C, Daley MJ, et al. Position paper on critical care pharmacy services: 2020 update. Crit Care Med 2020;48(9):e813–34.

9. Kleinpell R, Grabenkort WR, Boyle WA 3rd, et al. The society of critical care medicine at 50 years: interprofessional practice in critical care: looking back and forging ahead. Crit Care Med 2021;49(12):2017–32.

10. Densen P. Challenges and opportunities facing medical education. Trans Am Clin Climatol Assoc 2011;122:48–58.

11. Kacmarek RM. The mechanical ventilator: past, present, and future. Respir Care 2011;56(8):1170–80.

12. Mukherjee S. The emperor of all maladies : a biography of cancer. 1st Scribner trade paperback. Scribner 2011;573:12, 8 p. of plates.

13. Berthelsen PG, Cronqvist M. The first intensive care unit in the world: Copenhagen 1953. Acta Anaesthesiol Scand 2003;47(10):1190–5.

14. Grossman CM. The first use of penicillin in the United States. Ann Intern Med 2008;149(2):135–6.

15. Grenvik A, Pinsky MR. Evolution of the intensive care unit as a clinical center and critical care medicine as a discipline. Crit Care Clin 2009;25(1):239–50, x.

16. Day RL, Goyan JE, Herfindal ET, et al. The origins of the clinical pharmacy program at the university of California, san Francisco. DICP 1991;25(3):308–14.

17. ASHP supplemental standard and learning objectives for residency training in critical-care pharmacy practice. American Society of Hospital Pharmacists. Am J Hosp Pharm 1990;47(3):609–12.

18. Benedict N, Hess MM. History and future of critical care pharmacy practice. Am J Health Syst Pharm 2015;72(23):2101–5.

19. Board of pharmacy specialties: accreditation. BPS.. Available at: https://www.bpsweb.org/about-bps/accreditation/. Accessed March 27, 2022.

20. Rudis MI, Brandl KM. Position paper on critical care pharmacy services. Society of critical care medicine and American college of clinical pharmacy task force on critical care pharmacy services. Crit Care Med 2000;28(11):3746–50.

21. Executive summary. Am J Health Syst Pharm 2011;68(12):1079–85.

22. Jacobi J, Ray S, Danelich I, et al. Impact of the pharmacy practice model initiative on clinical pharmacy specialist practice. Pharmacotherapy 2016;36(5):e40–9.

23. Al-Jazairi A, Hijazi H, Samarkandi H, et al. What is the ideal clinical pharmacy practice model? A satisfaction comparative study. Journal of the American College of Clinical Pharmacy 2021;4(4):441–9.

24. MacLaren R, Roberts RJ, Dzierba AL, et al. Characterizing critical care pharmacy services across the United States. Crit Care Explor 2021;3(1):e0323.

25. Maclaren R, Devlin JW, Martin SJ, et al. Critical care pharmacy services in United States hospitals. Ann Pharmacother 2006;40(4):612–8.

26. Wong D, Feere A, Yousefi V, et al. How hospital pharmacists spend their time: a work-sampling study. Can J Hosp Pharm. Fall 2020;73(4):272–8.

27. Bond CA, Raehl CL. Clinical pharmacy services, pharmacy staffing, and hospital mortality rates. Pharmacotherapy 2007;27(4):481–93.

28. Lee H, Ryu K, Sohn Y, et al. Impact on patient outcomes of pharmacist participation in multidisciplinary critical care teams: a systematic review and meta-analysis. Crit Care Med 2019;47(9):1243–50.

29. Leape LL, Cullen DJ, Clapp MD, et al. Pharmacist participation on physician rounds and adverse drug events in the intensive care unit. JAMA 1999; 282(3):267–70.

30. Bissell BD, Laine ME, Thompson Bastin ML, et al. Impact of protocolized diuresis for de-resuscitation in the intensive care unit. Crit Care 2020;24(1):70.

31. Leguelinel-Blache G, Nguyen TL, Louart B, et al. Impact of quality bundle enforcement by a critical care pharmacist on patient outcome and costs. Crit Care Med 2018;46(2):199–207.

32. MacLaren R, Bond CA, Martin SJ, et al. Clinical and economic outcomes of involving pharmacists in the direct care of critically ill patients with infections. Crit Care Med 2008;36(12):3184–9.

33. Beardsley JR, Jones CM, Williamson J, et al. Pharmacist involvement in a multidisciplinary initiative to reduce sepsis-related mortality. Am J Health Syst Pharm 2016;73(3):143–9. https://doi.org/10.2146/ajhp150186.

34. To L, Schillig JM, DeSmet BD, et al. Impact of a pharmacist-directed anticoagulation service on the quality and safety of heparin-induced thrombocytopenia management. Ann Pharmacother 2011;45(2):195–200.

35. MacLaren R, Bond CA. Effects of pharmacist participation in intensive care units on clinical and economic outcomes of critically ill patients with thromboembolic or infarction-related events. Pharmacotherapy 2009;29(7):761–8.

36. Bond CA, Raehl CL. Pharmacist-provided anticoagulation management in United States hospitals: death rates, length of stay, Medicare charges, bleeding complications, and transfusions. Pharmacotherapy 2004;24(8):953–63.

37. Marshall J, Finn CA, Theodore AC. Impact of a clinical pharmacist-enforced intensive care unit sedation protocol on duration of mechanical ventilation and hospital stay. Crit Care Med 2008;36(2):427–33.

38. Devlin JW, Holbrook AM, Fuller HD. The effect of ICU sedation guidelines and pharmacist interventions on clinical outcomes and drug cost. Ann Pharmacother 1997;31(6):689–95.

39. Forni A, Skehan N, Hartman CA, et al. Evaluation of the impact of a tele-ICU pharmacist on the management of sedation in critically ill mechanically ventilated patients. Ann Pharmacother 2010;44(3):432–8.

40. Louzon P, Jennings H, Ali M, et al. Impact of pharmacist management of pain, agitation, and delirium in the intensive care unit through participation in multidisciplinary bundle rounds. Am J Health Syst Pharm 2017;74(4):253–62.

41. Stollings JL, Foss JJ, Ely EW, et al. Pharmacist leadership in ICU quality improvement: coordinating spontaneous awakening and breathing trials. Ann Pharmacother 2015;49(8):883–91.

42. Buckley MS, Park AS, Anderson CS, et al. Impact of a clinical pharmacist stress ulcer prophylaxis management program on inappropriate use in hospitalized patients. Am J Med 2015;128(8):905–13.

43. Ng TM, Bell AM, Hong C, et al. Pharmacist monitoring of QTc interval-prolonging medications in critically ill medical patients: a pilot study. Ann Pharmacother 2008;42(4):475–82.

44. Hammond DA, Flowers HJC, Meena N, et al. Cost avoidance associated with clinical pharmacist presence in a medical intensive care unit. Journal of the American College of Clinical Pharmacy 2019;2(6):610–5.

45. Hammond DA, Gurnani PK, Flannery AH, et al. Scoping review of interventions associated with cost avoidance able to be performed in the intensive care unit and emergency department. Pharmacotherapy 2019;39(3):215–31.

46. Claus BO, Robays H, Decruyenaere J, et al. Expected net benefit of clinical pharmacy in intensive care medicine: a randomized interventional comparative trial with matched before-and-after groups. J Eval Clin Pract 2014;20(6):1172–9.

47. Kopp BJ, Mrsan M, Erstad BL, et al. Cost implications of and potential adverse events prevented by interventions of a critical care pharmacist. Am J Health Syst Pharm 2007;64(23):2483–7.

48. Rech MA, Gurnani PK, Peppard WJ, et al. PHarmacist avoidance or reductions in medical costs in CRITically Ill adults: PHARM-CRIT Study. Critical Care Explorations 2021;3(12):e0594.

49. Hahn L, Beall J, Turner RS, et al. Pharmacist-developed sedation protocol and impact on ventilator days. J Pharm Pract 2013;26(4):406–8.

50. Rech MA, Gurnani PK, Peppard WJ, et al. PHarmacist avoidance or reductions in medical costs in CRITically Ill adults: PHARM-CRIT study. Crit Care Explor 2021;3(12):e0594.

51. Sikora A, Ayyala D, Rech MA, et al. Impact of pharmacists to improve patient care in the critically ill: a large multicenter analysis using meaningful metrics with the medication regimen complexity-ICU (MRC-ICU) Score. Crit Care Med 2022;50(9):1318–28.

52. Ataman AD, Vatanoğlu-Lutz EE, Yıldırım G. Medicine in stamps-ignaz semmelweis and puerperal fever. J Turk Ger Gynecol Assoc 2013;14(1):35–9.

53. Gawande A. 1st edition. The checklist manifesto : how to get things right, 209. New York, NY: Metropolitan Books; 2010. p. x.

54. Aptowicz COK. Dr. Mutter's marvels : a true tale of intrigue and innovation at the dawn of modern medicine. Sheridan, WY: Gotham Books; 2014. p. 371.

55. Brock P. 1st edition. Charlatan : America's most dangerous huckster, the man who pursued him, and the age of flimflam, 324. New York, NY: Crown Publishers; 2008. p. 8–p.

56. Kahneman D, Sibony O, Sunstein CR. 1st edition. Noise : a flaw in human judgment, ix. New York, NY: Random House; 2021. p. 454.

57. Topol EJ. Deep medicine : how artificial intelligence can make healthcare human again, 1st edition, 2019, Basic Books, New York, NY, 1, online resource.

58. Lepore J. *The mansion of happiness : a history of life and death*, xxxiii. 1st edition. New York, NY: Alfred A. Knopf; 2012. p. 282.

59. Mukherjee S. The gene : an intimate history. First Scribner hardcover edition, 2016, Scribner, New York, NY, 592, 8 pages of plates.

60. Kane-Gill S, Weber RJ. Principles and practices of medication safety in the ICU. Crit Care Clin 2006;22(2):273–90. https://doi.org/10.1016/j.ccc.2006.02.005, vi.

61. Institute of Medicine (US) Committee on. In: Quality of Health Care in America. To Err is Human: Building a Safer Health System. Washington DC: National Academies Press US; 2000.

62. Stelfox HT, Palmisani S, Scurlock C, et al. The "To Err is Human" report and the patient safety literature. Qual Saf Health Care 2006;15(3):174–8.

63. Rothschild JM, Landrigan CP, Cronin JW, et al. The Critical Care Safety Study: the incidence and nature of adverse events and serious medical errors in intensive care. Crit Care Med 2005;33(8):1694–700.

64. Vincent JL. Give your patient a fast hug (at least) once a day. Crit Care Med 2005;33(6):1225–9.

65. Ely EW. Every deep-drawn breath: a critical care doctor on healing, recovery, and transforming medicine in the ICU. First Scribner hardcover edition. ed. Scribner, 2021:1 online resource. New York, NY.

66. Kim MM, Barnato AE, Angus DC, et al. The effect of multidisciplinary care teams on intensive care unit mortality. Arch Intern Med 2010;170(4):369–76.

67. Flannery AH, Thompson Bastin ML, Montgomery-Yates A, et al. Multidisciplinary prerounding meeting as a continuous quality improvement tool: leveraging to reduce continuous benzodiazepine use at an academic medical center. J Intensive Care Med 2019;34(9):707–13.

68. Al Khalfan A, Al Ghamdi A, De Simone S, et al. The impact of multidisciplinary team care on decreasing intensive care unit mortality. Review Article. Saudi Critical Care Journal 2021;5(2):13–8.

69. Specialities BoP. Critical care pharmacotherapy specialist board certification 7/4/22. Available at: https://www.bpsweb.org/bps-specialties/critical-care-pharmacy/#:~:text=Currently%20there%20are%20more%20than%203%2C500%20BPS%20Board%20Certified%20Critical%20Care%20Pharmacists.

70. Medicine SoCC. Critical care statistics. . Accessed 7 4, 2022, Available at: https://www.sccm.org/Communications/Critical-Care-Statistics.

71. Newsome AS, Murray B, Smith SE, et al. Optimization of critical care pharmacy clinical services: a gap analysis approach. Am J Health Syst Pharm 2021; 78(22):2077–85.

72. Newsome AS, Smith SE, Jones TW, et al. A survey of critical care pharmacists to patient ratios and practice characteristics in intensive care units. Journal of the American College of Clinical Pharmacy 2019;3:68–74.

73. Jones TW, Newsome AS, Smith SE, et al. Interprofessional shared decision-making: who is at the table? Crit Care Med. Feb 2020;48(2):e158–9.

74. Forehand CC, Fitton K, Keats K, et al. Productivity tracking: a survey of critical care pharmacist practices and satisfaction. Hosp Pharm 2022;57(2):273–80.

75. Murray B, Buckley MS, Newsome AS. Action plan for successful implementation of optimal ICu pharmacist activities: next steps for the critical care pharmacist position paper. Crit Care Med 2021;49(2):e199–200.

76. Barlow B, Barlow A, Newsome AS. Comment on Gross and MacDougall "Roles of the clinical pharmacist during the COVID-19 pandemic". Journal of the American college of Clinical Pharmacy 2020;3(4):829.

77. Newsome AS, Jones TW, Smith SE. Pharmacists are associated with reduced mortality in critically ill patients: now what? Crit Care Med 2019;47(12):e1036–7.

78. Erstad BL. Justification of the value of critical care pharmacists: still a work in progress? Am J Health Syst Pharm 2020;77(22):1906–9.

79. Murray B, Newsome AS. Avoiding cost avoidance. Am J Health Syst Pharm 2022;79(2):14–5.
80. Francke D. The new role of pharmacy. Drug Intell 1968;2(11):291.
81. deBacker J, Hart N, Fan E. Neuromuscular blockade in the 21st century management of the critically ill patient. Chest 2017;151(3):697–706.
82. Chang LY, Yu HH, Chao YC. The relationship between nursing workload, quality of care, and nursing payment in intensive care units. J Nurs Res 2019;27(1):1–9.
83. Almenyan AA, Albuduh A, Al-Abbas F. Effect of nursing workload in intensive care units. Cureus 2021;13(1):e12674.
84. Michtalik HJ, Yeh HC, Pronovost PJ, et al. Impact of attending physician workload on patient care: a survey of hospitalists. JAMA Intern Med 2013;173(5):375–7.
85. Pastores SM, Kvetan V, Coopersmith CM, et al. Workforce, workload, and burnout among intensivists and advanced practice providers: a narrative review. Crit Care Med 2019;47(4):550–7.
86. Kerlin MP, McPeake J, Mikkelsen ME. Burnout and joy in the profession of critical care medicine. Crit Care 2020;24(1):98.
87. Ward NS, Afessa B, Kleinpell R, et al. Intensivist/patient ratios in closed ICUs: a statement from the society of critical care medicine taskforce on ICU staffing. Crit Care Med 2013;41(2):638–45.
88. Lilly CM, Cucchi E, Marshall N, et al. Battling intensivist burnout: a role for workload management. Chest 2019;156(5):1001–7.
89. Lilly CM, Oropello JM, Pastores SM, et al. Workforce, workload, and burnout in critical care organizations: survey results and research agenda. Crit Care Med. Nov 2020;48(11):1565–71.
90. Moss M, Good VS, Gozal D, et al. A critical care societies collaborative statement: burnout syndrome in critical care health-care professionals. A Call for Action. Am J Respir Crit Care Med 2016;194(1):106–13.
91. Sakr Y, Moreira CL, Rhodes A, et al. The impact of hospital and ICU organizational factors on outcome in critically ill patients: results from the Extended Prevalence of Infection in Intensive Care study. Crit Care Med 2015;43(3):519–26.
92. Haegdorens F, Van Bogaert P, De Meester K, et al. The impact of nurse staffing levels and nurse's education on patient mortality in medical and surgical wards: an observational multicentre study. BMC Health Serv Res 2019;19(1):864.
93. Sikora A. Impact of pharmacists to improve patient care in the critically ill: a large multicenter analysis using meaningful metrics with the MRC-ICU. Crit Care Med 2022;50(9):1318–28.
94. Chuang CH, Tseng PC, Lin CY, et al. Burnout in the intensive care unit professionals: a systematic review. Medicine (Baltim) 2016;95(50):e5629.
95. Guntupalli KK, Wachtel S, Mallampalli A, et al. Burnout in the intensive care unit professionals. Indian J Crit Care Med 2014;18(3):139–43.
96. Saravanabavan L, Sivakumar MN, Hisham M. Stress and burnout among intensive care unit healthcare professionals in an indian tertiary care hospital. Indian J Crit Care Med 2019;23(10):462–6.
97. Smith SESA, Butler SA, Buckley MS, et al. Examination of critical care pharmacist work activities and burnout. Journal of the American College of Clinical Pharmacy 2021;4(5):554–69.
98. Ball AM, Schultheis J, Lee HJ, et al. Evidence of burnout in critical care pharmacists. Am J Health Syst Pharm 2020;77(10):790–6.
99. Smith SEBM, MacClaren R, Newsome AS. Examination of critical care pharmacist work activities and burnout. Journal of the American College of Clinical Pharmacy 2021. https://doi.org/10.1002/jac5.1408.

100. Newsome A, Smith SE, Jones TW, et al. A survey of critical care pharmacists to patient ratios and practice characteristics in intensive care units. J Am Coll Clin Pharm 2020;3:68–74.
101. Smith S, Slaughter A, Buckley M, et al. 41: relationship between critical care clinical pharmacist activities and burnout syndrome. Crit Care Med 2021;49(1):21.
102. LeClaire M, Poplau S, Linzer M, et al. Compromised integrity, burnout, and intent to leave the job in critical care nurses and physicians. Crit Care Explor 2022; 4(2):e0629.
103. Romero-Garcia M, Delgado-Hito P, Galvez-Herrer M, et al. Moral distress, emotional impact and coping in intensive care unit staff during the outbreak of COVID-19. Intensive Crit Care Nurs 2022;70:103206.
104. Reith TP. Burnout in United States healthcare professionals: a narrative review. Cureus 2018;10(12):e3681.
105. 1974;30:159–165. Sb-oFHJSI.
106. UNESCO. Education and training in a changing world: what skills do we need? 6/7/22, Available at: https://www.youtube.com/watch?v=Ui_rzJ8OYNc&ab_channel=UNESCO. Accessed May 31, 2022.
107. Goleman D. Emotional intelligence, *Bantam 10th anniversary hardcover*, xxiv. New York, NY: Bantam Books; 2006. p. 358.
108. Donovan AL, Aldrich JM, Gross AK, et al. Interprofessional care and teamwork in the ICU. Crit Care Med 2018;46(6):980–90.
109. Newport C. Deep work : rules for focused success in a distracted world. First Edition. Grand Central Publishing; 2016. p. 295.
110. Ferguson NC, Quinn NJ, Khalique S, et al. Clinical pharmacists: an invaluable part of the coronavirus disease 2019 frontline response. Crit Care Explor 2020;2(10):e0243.
111. Gwynn ME, Poisson MO, Waller JL, et al. Development and validation of a medication regimen complexity scoring tool for critically ill patients. Am J Health Syst Pharm 2019;76(Supplement_2):S34–40.
112. Newsome AS, Anderson D, Gwynn ME, et al. Characterization of changes in medication complexity using a modified scoring tool. Am J Health Syst Pharm 2019;76(Supplement_4):S92–5.
113. Newsome A, Smith SE, Olney WJ, et al. Medication regimen complexity is associated with pharmacist interventions and drug-drug interactions: a use of the novel MRC-ICU scoring tool. J Am Coll Clin Pharm 2020;3(1):47–56.
114. Newsome AS, Smith SE, Olney WJ, et al. Multicenter validation of a novel medication-regimen complexity scoring tool. Am J Health Syst Pharm 2020;77(6):474–8.
115. Al-Mamun MA, Brothers T, Newsome AS. Development of machine learning models to validate a medication regimen complexity scoring tool for critically ill patients. Ann Pharmacother 2021;55(4):421–9.
116. Olney WJ, Chase AM, Hannah SA, et al. Medication regimen complexity score as an indicator of fluid balance in critically ill patients. J Pharm Pract 2021. https://doi.org/10.1177/0897190021999792. 897190021999792.
117. Smith SE, Shelley R, Newsome AS. Medication regimen complexity vs patient acuity for predicting critical care pharmacist interventions. Am J Health Syst Pharm 2021. https://doi.org/10.1093/ajhp/zxab460.
118. Webb AJ, Rowe S, Sikora Newsome A. A descriptive report of the rapid implementation of automated MRC-ICU calculations in the EMR of an academic medical center. Am J Health Syst Pharm 2022. https://doi.org/10.1093/ajhp/zxac059.

Palliative Care in the Intensive Care Unit: Past, Present, and Future

James Downar, MDCM, MHSc (Bioethics)[a,b,*], May Hua, MD, MS[c,d],
Hannah Wunsch, MD, MSc[e,f]

KEYWORDS

- Palliative care • Critical care • Advance care planning • Review
- History of medicine

KEY POINTS

- Intensive Care Units (ICUs), first created in the 1950s, were initially viewed solely as places to save lives, with little focus on the challenges of end-of-life care in the context of sophisticated, organ supporting technology.
- The term "palliative care" was coined in 1974 by Dr Balfour Mount, a surgical oncologist from McGill University. The discussion of palliative care as it relates to ICU naturally begins at this point.
- By the 2000s, the concept of integrating palliative care principles in the ICU became mainstream.
- Palliative care in the ICU can be delivered using a consultative or integrative model, but studies of interventions to improve the quality of palliative care in the ICU have yielded mixed results to date.
- Some individuals are now dual certified in critical care and palliative care, which may lead to more integrated models of care in some ICUs.

PRE-PALLIATIVE CARE

Until 1928, all "critical care" was essentially palliative care. Understanding of resuscitation techniques was still in its infancy, penicillin and other antibiotics were not yet

The authors have no relevant conflicts of interest to disclose.
[a] Division of Palliative Care, Department of Medicine, University of Ottawa, 43 Rue Bruyere, Suite 268J, Ottawa K1N 5C8, Canada; [b] Department of Critical Care, The Ottawa Hospital, 1053 Carling Avenue, Ottawa, ON K1Y 4E9, Canada; [c] Department of Anesthesiology, Columbia University, 622 West 168th Street, New York, NY 10032, USA; [d] Department of Epidemiology, Mailman School of Public Health, Columbia University, 722 West 168th Street, New York, NY 10032, USA; [e] Department of Critical Care Medicine, Sunnybrook Health Sciences Centre, 2075 Bayview Avenue, Toronto, ON M4N 3M5, Canada; [f] Department of Anesthesiology and Pain Medicine and Interdepartmental Division of Critical Care Medicine, University of Toronto, 2075 Bayview Avenue, Room D1.08, Toronto, Ontario M4N 3M5, Canada
* Corresponding author. 43 Rue Bruyere, Suite 268J, Ottawa K1N 5C8.
E-mail address: jdownar@toh.ca

Crit Care Clin 39 (2023) 529–539
https://doi.org/10.1016/j.ccc.2023.01.007   criticalcare.theclinics.com
0749-0704/23/© 2023 Elsevier Inc. All rights reserved.

available, and no organ support existed. Therefore, as an individual transitioned from moderate illness to critical illness, the primary focus would have been on alleviation of symptoms, often with the administration of morphine or other sedatives.

In 1928, Philip Drinker and Louis Agassiz Shaw invented the first "respirator."[1] The iron lung, as it was dubbed, was designed to provide negative pressure ventilation, primarily for patients with respiratory paralysis from poliomyelitis. The concept was to provide transient support while an individual recovered strength from paralytic polio, although it was also used occasionally in other situations of respiratory failure. The development of the iron lung was one of the first steps toward modern critical care and is of particular note because it represented the first time that humans became dependent on machines for their lives. Up until that moment, there was no ability to prolong life through the mechanical support of individual organs.

From 1928 to the mid-1950s, the use of iron lungs became routine. In the United States, centers were created where there was expertise in the care of individuals who required this respiratory support due to polio. Over the same period, particularly during World War II, understanding of resuscitation of shock improved, and the first dialysis machines were introduced into use. The 1952 polio epidemic in Copenhagen then provided the turning point for the development of critical care, as it was the first large-scale demonstration of the utility of positive pressure ventilation outside of the operating room.[2] Bjørn Ibsen, an anesthesiologist, proposed the use of tracheostomies and hand ventilation for the care of severe polio patients. The following year he established the first "modern" ICU in Copenhagen at the Municipal Hospital (Kommunehospitalet).[3]

Bjorn Ibsen saw himself as the manager of the body's response to illness—respiration, circulation, and temperature control—giving the body time to heal from the underlying problem. He described these fundamental aspects of the body's function as the handle of an umbrella that he held and saw the individual diseases as the different spokes.[4] In those early years, the goal was to prove the utility of critical care by demonstrating how an individual, who previously would have solely received some rudimentary form of palliative care, could now receive full life support and survive. Ibsen even went so far as to require an admitting surgeon to acknowledge that there was nothing more standard medicine could provide. Ibsen explained that whenever a patient was transferred to him, "the chief surgeon made a written statement in the record that the patient was moribund [near death], before I would receive him for [intensive therapy] ... I wanted to make sure that if the patient recovered, it would be recognised to be due to our treatment, and that if he did not recover, our treatment would not be blamed."[5] The idea of providing comprehensive critical care to individuals slowly gained traction in hospitals throughout the world, and by the late 1960s and early 1970s, most major centers in the United States had ICUs. However, with this newfound ability to stave off death and allow people to recover from reversible diseases that were previously terminal, the focus was firmly on recovery.

Yet Philip Drinker and one of his colleagues in Boston, James L Wilson, had worried as far back as 1928 regarding the consequences for humanity of prolonging life with machines. Wilson wrote..."we would be forced to use the respirator indefinitely or until someone should turn executioner by stopping the machine."[6] This, of course, did happen. However, these individuals were otherwise healthy (aside from being paralyzed) and able to lead active lives, albeit wedded to iron lungs for support. However, as critical care took hold, the potential for indefinite support of individuals who were moribund became a reality for the first time. After proving the utility of the care he offered, Bjørn Ibsen himself became uncomfortable with the direction critical care had gone, as he expressed in a radio interview in 1974 with a journalist, Christian Stentoft:

Stentoft: Do we prolong the death process?

Ibsen: Yes and oftentimes it would be much more humane to give morphine, peace, and comfort to patients with no hope of surviving.

Stentoft: Have you done that?

Ibsen: Yes I have.[7]

This caused an uproar in the Danish newspapers, with concern that he might be charged for murder. The situation was smoothed over but highlights the lack of conversation in the field regarding the role of palliative care in units that were seen as places to "save" lives.

PARADIGM SHIFT: 1970S TO 2010S

The concept that we now call "palliative care" was not widely discussed in the literature until quite recently, although it seemed in articles in the 1940s (**Fig. 1**). The term "palliative care" was coined in 1974 by Dr Balfour Mount, a surgical oncologist from McGill University. The discussion of palliative care as it relates to ICU naturally begins at this point (**Fig. 2**). We cannot pinpoint the precise origins of palliative care within critical care, but with the benefit of hindsight, we can describe a profound shift in end-of-life and palliative practices in the ICU between the 1970s and the 1990s.

Modern care planning, and the model of "shared decision-making" used in much of the world, depends on a *medicolegal framework* that seeks to balance the *wishes of the patient* with the *capabilities of medical science*, often through a process of *informed consent* that requires some degree of *communication* between clinical staff, patients, and/or their families.[8] These are all concepts that formed and developed in the 1970s and 1980s. In the early 1970s, physicians in the United States had no professional obligation to disclose a serious diagnosis or communicate a limited prognosis—the American Medical Association Code of Ethics only included a vague reference to veracity for the first time in 1980. Paternalistic medical decision-making was nearly universal, and patients and family members were not seen as partners in decision-making. The American Heart Association Guidelines for cardiopulmonary

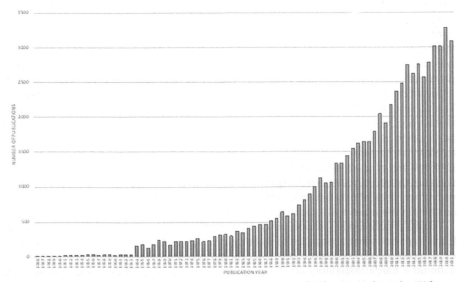

Fig. 1. Number of publications in Pubmed under the Medical Subject Headings (MeSH) term "Palliative Care," through 2021.

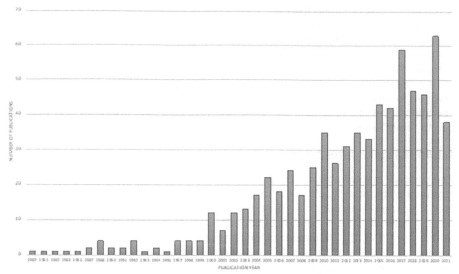

Fig. 2. Number of publications in Pubmed under the combined MeSH terms of "Palliative Care" and "Critical Care," through 2021. Note that the first article was published in 1980.

resuscitation (CPR) in 1974 indicated that there were situations where CPR would not offer benefit and should be electively withheld (ie, a "Do-not-resuscitate" order), but made no mention of including patients or family members in the decision-making process or even communicating the decision to them after it had been made.[9]

Advance directives are commonplace today, but the legal framework for a person to leave a binding instruction not to receive CPR, life-support, or other therapies that might otherwise be indicated was only created for the first time in California in 1975.[10] By 1990, interest in advance directives had grown to the point that the US Congress passed the Patient Self-Determination act, which required many health care facilities in the United States to ensure that patients were aware of their rights to create advance directives, to ask about any existing advance directives, and record them in the patient's medical record. However, this Golden Age of advance directives was short lived. The SUPPORT study (1995) revealed not only the poor state of patient–physician communication but also the inability of even an intensive, high-resource intervention to improve communication and align patient care with their directives.[11] The subsequent efforts have struggled to improve on the results of SUPPORT, and studies and meta-analyses of advance directives and advance care planning in general continue to show disappointing outcomes.[12] However, the growing and sustained interest in advance directives and advance care planning is a reflection of a societal shift toward shared decision-making, and a recognition that "palliative" priorities such as symptom management, quality of life, and family support should be integrated with other medical priorities that arise in cases of serious or incurable illness where life-sustaining therapies available in ICUs are an option.

Today, a substantial proportion of ICU deaths in many parts of the world occur following a consensual decision to withdraw life support. However, the legality of withdrawing life support is also a relatively recent development. In 1975, Karen Quinlan suffered a cardiorespiratory arrest, whereas she was resuscitated, she was left in a vegetative state. Her family requested the withdrawal of her ventilator, but physicians refused on the grounds that they considered it tantamount to murder, and the trial judge agreed with the physicians. The following year, the New Jersey Supreme Court overturned that decision and Ms Quinlan's ventilator was withdrawn. In Canada, it was only in 1992 that the case of Nancy B established the right of a competent patient to stop their own life-sustaining measures. The right to stop artificial nutrition and hydration in the United States was affirmed by the Supreme Court in 1990 in the case of Nancy Cruzan.[10] As these decisions have become commonplace in ICUs across North America, Europe, Australia, New Zealand, and other jurisdictions, it is easy to forget how recently they were considered illegal or controversial. We must also recognize that legal decisions do not always lead to immediate changes in practice; ICU practices are not homogenous in any country or region, even at one point in time. In 1998, Prendergast and colleagues[13] looked at end-of-life care in 131 ICUs across the United States and found a wide range of practices. In six ICUs, life-sustaining measures were withdrawn in more than 70% of cases. In six others, life-sustaining measures were not withdrawn in even a single case over a 5-month period. In the early 2000s, the ETHICUS study found substantial variability in end-of-life practices across Europe, with some Southern European countries performing CPR in almost half of all ICU deaths and some Northern European countries withholding or withdrawing life-sustaining measures in more than 80% of cases.[14] Twenty years later, ETHICUS 2 showed that practices had changed; unsuccessful CPR had become less frequent in southern Europe, and withholding and withdrawing life-sustaining measures were more common.[15] ETHICUS 2 also included data from other parts of the world, showing a similar range in worldwide practices to that seen in Europe in ETHICUS. It is logical to assume that a repeated survey in 2040 (ETHICUS 3?) would reveal a similar evolution in practice.

By the 2000s, the concept of integrating palliative care principles in the ICU had become mainstream enough that a series of highly read textbooks and articles began to appear on the subject. The first textbook focusing solely on this topic was *Managing Death in the ICU: The Transition from Cure to Comfort*, which was published in 2000 and covered a range of topics from symptom management to ethical issues.[16] This was soon followed by *End of Life Care in the ICU: From Advanced Disease to Bereavement*, and others. Specialized clinical roles began to appear, such as palliative care consultation teams whose practice was focused on the intensive care setting.[17]

Guidelines for palliative care management in the ICU were also published around this time. In 1997, in the New England Journal of Medicine, Brody and colleagues[18] published guidelines specific for withdrawal of life-sustaining treatment. In 2001, the American Thoracic Society released a set of clinical recommendations for providing end-of-life care in the ICU.[19] These recommendations have been updated multiple times since and others have developed consensus clinical guidelines as well.[20] Also in 2001, Rubenfeld and Curtis published a research agenda for improving end-of-life care in the ICU.[21] This agenda, developed by an interprofessional working group, identified important issues to be overcome and proposed the solutions and means of evaluating these potential solutions and ways to overcome existing barriers.

In 2003, Cook and colleagues[22] published a multicenter observational study of end-of-life care in Canadian ICUs in the New England Journal of Medicine, indicating the degree to which this issue was viewed as important to the medical community at large. Soon after, prospective interventional studies of palliative care (or elements of palliative care) in the ICU began to appear in the highest tier of medical journals. In 2007, Lautrette and colleagues[23] demonstrated that a specific communication strategy and brochure improved bereavement outcomes among French relatives of ICU decedents. In 2010, Curtis and colleagues[24] showed that a multicomponent quality improvement intervention on end-of-life care did not improve the quality of dying reported by nurses and family members. In 2016, Carson and colleagues[25] reported that palliative care-led meetings with family members of chronic critically ill patients did not reduce the symptoms of anxiety or depression and actually worsened the symptoms of post-traumatic stress disorder. In 2018, White and colleagues[26] reported that a family-support intervention improved the quality of communication and perceived patient-centeredness in a cluster-randomized trial. A systematic review by Aslakson and colleagues[27] published in 2014 already identified 37 published studies of either integrative or consultative palliative care in the ICU. Not every high-impact publication showed positive results. However, these negative studies have not dampened interest in further investigations, and the number of studies has only increased since then.

By the 2010s, another important shift was occurring. Although much of the early research on palliative care in the ICU had been led by ICU-based clinicians, a new generation of clinicians and researchers with dual training and certification in palliative care and critical care emerged. The evidence base for palliative care practice continues to evolve, and the role for dual-trained clinicians is varies across centers, but this growing population of experts will form an important core of clinicians and researchers with wide expertise in the years to come.

THE FUTURE OF PALLIATIVE CARE IN THE ICU

Although the importance of palliative care delivery as part of the practice of critical care is well accepted, the optimal way to provide palliative care to critically ill patients remains unknown. Palliative care may be delivered by ICU clinicians or by specialty-trained palliative care clinicians. Existing evidence does not clearly point to the superiority of one approach or the other. Currently, in places with hospital-based palliative care services, palliative care is delivered in a "mixed" model where the burden of palliative care delivery is shared between the primary ICU team and consultants.[28] Several pressing questions remain regarding how this model may be best operationalized.

The mixed model of palliative care delivery necessarily requires that particular patients be identified as having a need for specialty palliative care. Conceptually, basic needs regarding communication, goals of treatment, and symptom management may be provided by the ICU team, whereas complex needs regarding symptom control, medical decision-making, and management of conflict requiring further expertise should be reserved for specialists.[29] It is estimated that approximately 15% of critically ill patients meet common criteria for specialty palliative care involvement,[30] but in practice, only 2% to 10% of patients actually receive this specialty care.[31] However, two factors complicate the sustainability of the mixed model. First, there is an ongoing shortage of specialty-trained palliative care clinicians.[32,33] Second, there is growing interest in expanding use of palliative care specialists for a variety of serious illnesses. ICU consults already represent up to 25% of a hospital-based palliative care service's consult volume, placing a large demand on such teams.[31] As up to 30% of older adults receive intensive care within the last 30 days of life,[34] the need for both primary and specialty palliative care delivery will only increase in the future.

Multiple methods to integrate palliative care specialists into the flow of care for critically ill patients have been described, including proactive screening, inclusion of palliative care specialists in ICU rounds, and the use of triggers (or specific clinical criteria) to identify potential patients with specialty palliative care needs. Most methods have been associated with an increase in palliative care consultation and have been associated with a decrease in ICU length of stay and a decrease in prolonged use of life-sustaining therapies without affecting mortality.[35–37] The concept of triggers for specialty palliative care has been most prominent, and many common triggers relate to the need for ongoing life-sustaining therapy or simply having a particular diagnosis with a poor prognosis.[30] Although recommendations for how to choose and use triggers have been published,[38] several aspects of using triggers in practice lack consensus. Clinicians often differ on which criteria are most appropriate, and the most acceptable criteria may not easily be operationalized (eg, need for complex decision-making, unrealistic goals of care).[39] Clinicians also have concerns that common triggers may not be specific enough, with overuse of specialists, leading to a wasting of resources on patients who may not benefit, or that triggers may lack sensitivity and miss patients for whom there is true need.[40] These concerns have merit, as a recent study comparing palliative care needs among patients who did and did not meet common triggers demonstrated that needs were not different according to a patient's trigger status, and common triggers did not reliably identify patients with the most serious needs.[41] In addition, clinicians hold differing views on how the logistics of how trigger systems should be implemented (eg, through the electronic health record or through interdisciplinary rounds) and whether triggers should lead to an automatic consult or a discussion between clinicians.[40] Thus, although triggers are a potentially promising strategy for integrating palliative care specialists into ICU care, the substantive details of how they should be implemented to ensure adequate buy-in and equitable distribution of services have yet to be determined. Other methods of integration like routine rounds or embedded palliative care clinicians overcome many of the drawbacks of a trigger-based strategy but are highly resource intensive and may not be generalizable or implementable across different practice settings.

Regardless of the model, specialists must be used in the most efficient manner possible to maximize the benefit to those with the most complex needs. Critically ill patients receiving specialty palliative care are a heterogeneous population with a variety of palliative care needs, and certain needs may require more expertise, or time, than others. A single-center study aiming to phenotype patients identified four "classes" of palliative care need among critically ill patients receiving consultation: patients requiring help primarily with (1) goals of care and advance directives, (2) symptom management, (3) supportive care, and (4) patients who had multiple needs.[42] Patients in the "goals of care and advance directives" class were less likely to be "high utilizers" of specialty palliative care (with respect to the number of visits) in comparison to other classes. Also, patients in certain classes were more or less likely to be seen by different types of palliative care clinicians; for example, patients requiring supportive care were more likely to be seen by social workers and chaplains and less likely to be seen by a physician or nurse practitioner. Similarly, a recent study that used a screening tool specifically designed to measure all facets of palliative care need identified four different phenotypes critically ill patients. Most of the patients (65%) fell into a class with lower need severity, but there were measurable differences between classes with respect to the quality of communication and the perception that care was patient-centered (Fig. 3).[43] These data suggest that even among patients with serious palliative care needs, care delivery can be adaptable, and there may be innovative ways to use a variety of staffing models to best match resources to needs.

Given resource constraints on specialty palliative care services, it is likely that most of the palliative care for critically ill patients will always be delivered by the ICU team. Yet, the training and comfort level of intensivists in delivering primary palliative care varies, and it is unclear what the components of high-quality primary palliative care in the ICU are. Core competencies in palliative care have increasingly become a part of critical care training, and specific curricula have been shown to improve primary palliative care skills.[44] As this process may take time to impact the ICU

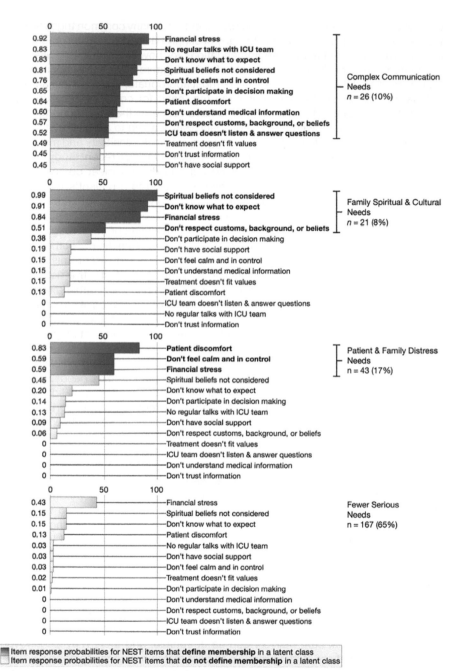

Fig. 3. Example of classification using latent class analysis of serious palliative care needs, demonstrating four latent classes identified from responses to the needs at the End-of-Life Screening Tool (NEST). (*From* Cox CE, Olsen MK, Parish A, et al. Palliative care phenotypes among critically ill patients and family members: intensive care unit prospective cohort study [published online ahead of print, 2022 Sep 27]. BMJ Support Palliat Care. 2022;bmjspcare-2022-003622; with permission.)

community as a whole, palliative care "champions" may help improve the quality of palliative care delivery in the interim.[45] In addition, various primary ICU palliative care interventions have been studied and have largely centered on improving communication between clinicians and surrogates through enhanced communication pathways and providing supportive services to surrogates. These interventions have had mixed results with respect to outcomes, with some showing a significant decrease in ICU length of stay, but no consistent differences in surrogate psychological symptomatology and distress.[24,26,46,47] Consequently, improving primary palliative care delivery in the ICU remains an active area of investigation.

CLINICS CARE POINTS

- Studies of interventions to improve the quality of palliative care in the ICU have yielded inconsistent results in terms of quality of death and dying, symptom control, length of stay, family satisfaction, and mental health outcomes in family members.

- Future studies could help identify the ideal model of providing palliative care in the ICU; the population that could most benefit from palliative care; and the ideal timing of a palliative care intervention.

REFERENCES

1. Markel H. The genesis of the iron lung. Early attempts at administering artificial respiration to patients with poliomyelitis. Arch Pediatr Adolesc Med 1994; 148(11):1174–80.
2. Lassen HC. A preliminary report on the 1952 epidemic of poliomyelitis in Copenhagen with special reference to the treatment of acute respiratory insufficiency. Lancet 1953;1(6749):37–41.
3. Berthelsen P, Cronqvist M. The first intensive care unit in the world: Copenhagen 1953. Acta Anaesthesiol Scand 2003;47(10):1190–5.
4. Ibsen B. Causeri om alvorligt emne, foredrag holdt I københavns rotary klub den 21. Maj 1969. NYT Nordisk Forlag Arnold Busck; 1969. p. 17.
5. Ibsen B. From Anaesthesia to Anaesthesiology. Personal experiences in Copenhagen during the past 25 years. Acta Anaesthesiol Scand Suppl 1975;61:33.
6. Wilson JL. Respiratory failure in poliomyelitis: treatment with the Drinker respirator. Am J Dis Child 1932;43(6):1445.
7. Wertheim BM. How a polio outbreak in copenhagen led to the invention of the ventilator. Smithsonian Magazine; 2020.
8. White DB, Braddock CH 3rd, Bereknyei S, et al. Toward shared decision making at the end of life in intensive care units: opportunities for improvement. Arch Intern Med 2007;167(5):461–7.
9. Standards for cardiopulmonary resuscitation (CPR) and emergency cardiac care (ECC). JAMA 1974;227(7):833–68.
10. Fine RL. From Quinlan to Schiavo: medical, ethical, and legal issues in severe brain injury. SAVE Proc 2005;18(4):303–10.
11. A controlled trial to improve care for seriously ill hospitalized patients. The study to understand prognoses and preferences for outcomes and risks of treatments (SUPPORT). The SUPPORT Principal Investigators. JAMA 1995;274(20):1591–8.
12. Morrison RS, Meier DE, Arnold RM. What's wrong with advance care planning? JAMA 2021;326(16):1575–6.

13. Prendergast TJ, Claessens MT, Luce JM. A national survey of end-of-life care for critically ill patients. Am J Respir Crit Care Med 1998;158(4):1163–7.

14. Sprung CL, Cohen SL, Sjokvist P, et al. End-of-life practices in European intensive care units: the Ethicus Study. JAMA 2003;290(6):790–7.

15. Avidan A, Sprung CL, Schefold JC, et al. Variations in end-of-life practices in intensive care units worldwide (Ethicus-2): a prospective observational study. Lancet Respir Med 2021;9(10):1101–10.

16. Curtis JR, Rubenfeld GD. Managing death in the ICU: the transition from cure to comfort. OXFORD University press; 2000.

17. Campbell ML, Guzman JA. A proactive approach to improve end-of-life care in a medical intensive care unit for patients with terminal dementia. Crit Care Med 2004;32(9):1839–43.

18. Brody H, Campbell ML, Faber-Langendoen K, et al. Withdrawing intensive life-sustaining treatment – recommendations for compassionate clinical management. N Engl J Med 1997;336(9):652–7.

19. Truog RD, Cist AF, Brackett SE, et al. Recommendations for end-of-life care in the intensive care unit: the Ethics committee of the society of critical care medicine. Crit Care Med 2001;29(12):2332–48.

20. Downnar J, Delaney JW, Hawryluck L, et al. Guidelines for the withdrawal of life-sustaining measures. Intensive Care Med 2016;42(6):1003–17.

21. Rubenfeld GD, Curtis JR. End-of-Life Care in the ICUWG. End-of-life care in the intensive care unit: a research agenda. Crit Care Med 2001;29(10):2001–6.

22. Cook D, Rocker G, Marshall J, et al. Withdrawal of mechanical ventilation in anticipation of death in the intensive care unit. N Engl J Med 2003;349(12):1123–32.

23. Lautrette A, Darmon M, Megarbane B, et al. A communication strategy and brochure for relatives of patients dying in the ICU. N Engl J Med 2007;356(5):469–78.

24. Curtis JR, Nielsen EL, Treece PD, et al. Effect of a quality-improvement intervention on end-of-life care in the intensive care unit: a randomized trial. Am J Respir Crit Care Med 2011;183(3):348–55.

25. Carson SS, Cox CE, Wallenstein S, et al. Effect of palliative care-led meetings for families of patients with chronic critical illness: a randomized clinical trial. JAMA 2016;316(1):51–62.

26. White DB, Angus DC, Shields AM, et al. A randomized trial of a family-support intervention in intensive care units. N Engl J Med 2018;378(25):2365–75.

27. Aslakson R, Cheng J, Vollenweider D, et al. Evidence-based palliative care in the intensive care unit: a systematic review of interventions. J Palliat Med 2014;17(2):219–35.

28. Hua M, Wunsch H. Integrating palliative care in the ICU. Curr Opin Crit Care 2014;20(6):673–80.

29. Quill TE, Abernethy AP. Generalist plus specialist palliative care–creating a more sustainable model. N Engl J Med 2013;368(13):1173–5.

30. Hua MS, Li G, Blinderman CD, et al. Estimates of the need for palliative care consultation across United States intensive care units using a trigger-based model. Am J Respir Crit Care Med 2014;189(4):428–36.

31. Stix B, Wunsch H, Clancy C, et al. Variability in frequency of consultation and needs assessed by palliative care services across multiple specialty ICUs. Intensive Care Med 2016;42(12):2104–5.

32. Kamal AH, Wolf SP, Troy J, et al. Policy changes key to promoting sustainability and growth of the specialty palliative care workforce. Health Aff 2019;38(6):910–8.

33. Lupu D, American Academy of H, Palliative Medicine Workforce Task F. Estimate of current hospice and palliative medicine physician workforce shortage. J Pain Symptom Manage 2010;40(6):899–911.
34. Teno JM, Gozalo P, Trivedi AN, et al. Site of death, place of care, and health care transitions among US medicare beneficiaries, 2000-2015. JAMA 2018;320(3): 264–71.
35. O'Mahony S, McHenry J, Blank AE, et al. Preliminary report of the integration of a palliative care team into an intensive care unit. Palliat Med 2010;24(2):154–65.
36. O'Mahony S, Johnson TJ, Amer S, et al. Integration of palliative care advanced practice nurses into intensive care unit teams. Am J Hosp Palliat Care 2017; 34(4):330–4.
37. Norton SA, Hogan LA, Holloway RG, et al. Proactive palliative care in the medical intensive care unit: effects on length of stay for selected high-risk patients. Crit Care Med 2007;35(6):1530–5.
38. Nelson JE, Curtis JR, Mulkerin C, et al. Choosing and using screening criteria for palliative care consultation in the ICU: a report from the Improving Palliative Care in the ICU (IPAL-ICU) Advisory Board. Crit Care Med 2013;41(10):2318–27.
39. Wysham NG, Hua M, Hough CL, et al. Improving ICU-based palliative care delivery: a multicenter, multidisciplinary survey of critical care clinician attitudes and beliefs. Crit Care Med 2017;45(4):e372–8.
40. Murali KP, Fonseca LD, Blinderman CD, et al. Clinicians' views on the use of triggers for specialist palliative care in the ICU: a qualitative secondary analysis. J Crit Care 2022;71:154054.
41. Cox CE, Ashana DC, Haines KL, et al. Assessment of clinical palliative care trigger status vs actual needs among critically ill patients and their family members. JAMA Netw Open 2022;5(1):e2144093.
42. Wang D, Ing C, Blinderman CD, et al. Latent class analysis of specialized palliative care needs in adult intensive care units from a single academic medical center. J Pain Symptom Manage 2019;57(1):73–8.
43. Cox CE, Olsen MK, Parish A, et al. Palliative care phenotypes among critically ill patients and family members: intensive care unit prospective cohort study. BMJ Support Palliat Care 2022. https://doi.org/10.1136/spcare-2022-003622.
44. Zante B, Schefold JC. Teaching end-of-life communication in intensive care medicine: review of the existing literature and implications for future curricula. J Intensive Care Med 2019;34(4):301–10.
45. Kamal AH, Bowman B, Ritchie CS. Identifying palliative care champions to promote high-quality care to those with serious illness. J Am Geriatr Soc 2019; 67(S2):S461–7.
46. Curtis JR, Treece PD, Nielsen EL, et al. Randomized trial of communication facilitators to reduce family distress and intensity of end-of-life care. Am J Respir Crit Care Med 2016;193(2):154–62.
47. Cox CE, White DB, Hough CL, et al. Effects of a personalized web-based decision aid for surrogate decision makers of patients with prolonged mechanical ventilation: a randomized clinical trial. Ann Intern Med 2019;170(5):285–97.

Evolution of Visiting the Intensive Care Unit

Kerry A. Milner, DNSc, APRN, FNP-BC, EBP-C

KEYWORDS

- Open visitation • Intensive care unit • Family presence • Patient-centered care
- Family-centered care • COVID-19 visitor restrictions

KEY POINTS

- Open visitation, defined as anyone of the patient's choosing can visit any time, has had sluggish adoption in intensive care units (ICUs) worldwide over the past 50 years.
- The COVID-19 pandemic halted global progress for in-person visiting and family presence in the ICU.
- Virtual visitation is a newer concept, and research is needed to evaluate its effect on family presence and engagement and patient and family outcomes.
- In the United States, some states responded to COVID-19 no-visitation hospital policies by enacting laws that make it a patient's right to a visitor while receiving hospital care.
- Health care systems should consider adopting family presence policies to support and maintain a family presence, including open visitation, in hospitals under any circumstance.

INTRODUCTION

Visitation to the intensive care unit (ICU) has been discussed and debated since the creation of the first ICUs in the 1950s in Europe[1] and the United States (US).[2] The past 60 years of expert opinions and research suggests a consensus that family presence is needed for patient- and family-centered care (PFCC). However, in practice, ICU visiting policies are variable and tend toward restrictive policies. This article gives a historical perspective of ICU visitation and summarizes the current issues and research needs.

Evolution of Visitation in the Intensive Care Unit

Early versions of restrictive visiting policies and reference to family waiting rooms in ICUs in the US can be found in the 1962 and 1965 US Public Health Service (USPHS) reports. The first report suggested visiting periods of 5 minutes every hour and a designated room near the ICU for the family to be close without interfering with patient

Sacred Heart University, Dr. Susan L. Davis, RN & Richard J. Henley College of Nursing, 5151 Park Avenue, Fairfield, CT 06825, USA
E-mail address: milnerk@sacredheart.edu
Twitter: @ProfKerryMilner (K.A.M.)

Crit Care Clin 39 (2023) 541–558
https://doi.org/10.1016/j.ccc.2023.01.005
0749-0704/23/© 2023 Elsevier Inc. All rights reserved.

care.[3] The second report declared that the acute coronary patient should not be denied visitors and their number and length of stay should be based on the patient's condition and the needs of the unit.[4] Nearly a decade after hospitals adopted the USPHS recommendations, nurses and physicians began questioning the justification for such strict visiting policies.[5,6]

A movement to liberalize ICU visiting policies began in the late 1970s with nurses and physicians recognizing the importance of family support that could not happen with restrictive visitation policies.[5,7–9] Several studies[10,11] debunked earlier findings from small-scale, single-setting studies where family visits to the ICU caused physiological changes for patients with cardiac problems.[12–14] Rationales for restrictive visiting included the ideas that visitors interfered with unit routine, drained staff time and energy, and might transmit infection were no longer justified. Instead, some began to believe that in the high-technology critical care environment, opening visiting was an important part of humanizing ICU processes.[6] Open visitation was defined as a family allowed to visit a patient any time during the 24 hours and as often and as long as they like.[7] Family referred to anyone related by birth, or not, who was of significance to the patient.

Table 1 is a historical perspective of visitation policies in ICUs from more than 40 countries since the 1980s. Researchers used telephone interviews, questionnaires, and later Web sites to identify visiting policies in ICUs. The type of visitor restrictions in the ICU has been similar over time and comparable among countries. Restrictions in the US and other countries include the number and duration of visits, number and age of visitors, and hours of visits. Early reasons for restricting adults from visiting were psychological (upsets visitor), physiological (disruptive to the patient), and infection control (patient or visitor may spread infection).[6] Similar reasons appear in the literature for restricting children.[31–33] There has been little evidence to support restricting children from visiting the ICU, and restricting may be harmful to a child's coping process.[33] Rather, the preparation before and the support during the visit are critical to the success of the child's visit to the adult ICU.[34]

Open visitation has been consistently low in the US, with 18% of coronary care units in teaching hospitals in 1985 reporting this practice,[16] 14% of critical care units in 2006,[20] and 18.5% of ICUs in "Magnet or Pathway to Excellence" recognized hospitals in 2020.[28] Reports of open visitation in other countries are variable. A systematic review of studies on visiting hours published between 2002 and 2011 found the highest percentage of open visitation in ICUs in Sweden (70%) and the lowest rate in Italy (1%),[25] and a survey of Canadian ICUs showed 69% of ICUs had open visitation before the COVID-19 pandemic.[30] In the largest study to date on the global practice of open visitation in ICUs, 39.6% of respondents reported this practice, and among 28 countries at least one survey respondent from each country reported fully adopting open visitation.[27] In a recent survey of pediatric ICUs in Latin American countries, 63% allowed parental open visitation.[29] These data suggest that the global adoption of open visitation has been slow to advance in the past 40 years even in pediatric ICUs. Moreover, the COVID-19 pandemic has derailed the progress of open visitation in the ICU worldwide, with most hospitals enacting no visitation policies in the first wave.[30,35]

Open Visitation, Family Presence, and Family Engagement Within the Family-Centered Care Approach

"Open visiting" as a concept appeared in the literature in 1979 yet only meant visiting the ward between 2 PM and 8 PM daily.[5] "Open visitation,"[6] defined as allowing any one of the patient's choosing to visit at any time, appeared in the literature in 1985 and

Table 1
Historical perspective of visitation policies in intensive care units

Author, Year Title	Design	Subjects	Results	Trends
Garton,[5] 1979 In praise of open visiting	Descriptive	Ward sister, Oldchurch Hospital, UK	Ward visiting hours for hospital 19:00–19:45 Monday to Friday and 14:00–15:30 weekends changed to visitors could call at their convenience between 14:00 and 19:00 daily	First use of open visiting
Kirchhoff,[15] 1982 Visiting policies for patients with myocardial infarction: a national survey	Cross-sectional national survey	Visiting policies for patients with myocardial infarction in ICU or Coronary Care Unit	Bed capacity, average daily census, geographic location correlates of visitation Nurses' highest level of education negative correlate of importance of restrictive visitation Smaller hospitals (<200 beds) have hourly visits Large hospitals have more scheduled visits	Restrictive visitation
Youngner et al[6] 1984 ICU visiting policies	Telephone survey	Head nurses in 37 hospitals in a 5-county area northeast Ohio with 78 medical, surgical, neonatal, cardiac, and pediatric ICUs	91% restricted family visiting to structured time blocks of 10–20 minutes, 30–45 minutes, or 1–2 hours. Age and number of visitors restricted	Restrictive visitation
Heater,[16] 1985 Nursing responsibilities in changing visiting restrictions in the intensive care unit	Survey	50 coronary care units in 10 midwestern states	18% of teaching hospitals allowed open or negotiated visitation and 0% among nonteaching hospitals	Restrictive visitation

(continued on next page)

Table 1
(continued)

Author, Year Title	Design	Subjects	Results	Trends
Stockdale & Hughes,[17] 1988 Critical care unit visiting policies: a survey	Survey	240 nurses attending AACN NTI representing 197 ICU	Limited number of visits per day (73.1%), number and type of visitor (94.4%), duration of visit (84.4%), age of visitor (89.3%) Nurses believed number of visits (38%) and length of visit (27%) should be unlimited	Restrictive visitation Disconnect between policy and what nurses believed
Simon et al,[18] 1997 Current practices regarding visitation policies in critical care units	Survey	201 nurses at 5 metropolitan hospitals in a midwestern city	70% of official policies were restrictive 78% of nurses were nonrestrictive in visitation in practice	Decrease in restrictive visitation Regardless of visitation policy, most nurses report they do not restrict visitation
Carlson et al,[19] 1998 Visitation: policy versus practice	National survey	Nurses who care for AMI patients during the first few days of hospitalization Response rate 34.8% (n = 882)	Visitation policy from most common to least was 10-minute visits every 2 hours (53.5%, n = 470), open visiting with some limitations (not described) (39.2%, n = 344), and <4% reported open visiting. Differences in policies were independent of hospital size or teaching status.	Restrictive visitation

Kirchhoff & Dahl,[20] 2006 American Association of Critical-Care Nurses' survey of facilities and units providing critical care	American Association of Critical-Care Nurses randomized national survey	118 of 658 (18.2%) eligible facilities in US participated representing 576 critical care units	14% (n = 16) open visitation always; 31% open except for rounds or shift changes; 44% (n = 52) open visitation on a scheduled basis	Decrease in restrictive visitation
Lee et al,[21] 2007 Visiting hours policies in New England intensive care units: strategies for improvement	Survey and focus groups	ICU visitation policies in 6 New England states. Response rate 96% (171 of 177 hospitals) representing 195 ICUs	32% (n = 62) had unrestricted, open visiting hours but had restrictions for age and number of visitors. Restrictions included number and duration of visits, number and age of visitors, hours of visits	Decrease in restricted visitation
Vandijck et al,[22] 2010 An evaluation of family-centered care services and organization of visiting policies in Belgian intensive care units: a multicenter survey	Multicenter survey	57 (75%) Belgian ICUs completed survey	100% reported restricting visiting hour policies and limited numbers of visitors. Restrictions included immediate relatives only in 11 (19.3%), no children in 5 (8.8%), and age of visitor in 46 (80.7%)	Restricted visitation issue outside the US
Haghbin,[23] 2011 Visiting Hour Policies in intensive care units, Southern Iran	Descriptive cross-sectional study	Phone interviews with head nurses of 71 ICUs in Southern Iran	39.4% (n = 28) no visitation. Restrictions on hours, visits per week, number of visitors, age of visitor	Largest percentage of no visitors allowed
Liu et al,[24] 2013 Visitation policies and practice in US ICUs	Telephone survey	ICUs stratified by US region and hospital type (community, federal, or university), between 2008 and 2009; n = 606	89.6% (n = 543) restrictive visitation policies. ICUs $\geq$ 3 restrictions (n = 375; 61.9%), with most common restrictions of visiting hours and visitor number or age. 94.8% allowed visitation exceptions (n = 474; 94.8%)	Increase in restricted visitation

(continued on next page)

Table 1
(continued)

Author, Year Title	Design	Subjects	Results	Trends
Cappellini et al,[25] 2014 Open Intensive Care Units a Global Challenge for Patients, Relatives, and Critical Care Teams	Systematic review	ICUs in Italy, Greece, France, Belgium, US, United Kingdom, Spain, Holland, Sweden	Open visiting policies reported by 70% (Sweden), 32% (US), 23% (France), 20% (United Kingdom), and 1% (Italy). Visiting hours policy and number of visitors varied from precise segments of time to unrestricted access 24 h/d but 2 visitors per patient was standard across most studies Access to children under 12 y was restricted in most ICUs in US and European countries	Large variation in restrictive visitation globally
Noordermeer et al,[26] 2013 Visiting policies in the adult intensive care units in the Netherlands: survey among ICU directors	Survey	85 (83.3%) medical directors of Dutch ICUs	74 (87.1%) restrictive visitation policies, 2 (2.4%) unrestricted 80 (94.1%) adaptation of visiting hours if patients is dying	Restricted visitation
Kleinpell et al,[27] 2018 Patient and family engagement in the ICU: report from the task force of the World Federation of Societies of Intensive and Critical Care Medicine	Cross-sectional survey	345 responses from 40 countries	Open visitation reported by 39.6% (n = 136) representing 28 countries	Restricted visitation is a global issue. Open visitation practiced in 28 countries

Study	Design	Methods	Findings	Conclusion
Milner et al,[28] (2020) Is open visitation really "open" in adult intensive care units in United States?	Descriptive	Review of 536 Magnet or Pathway to Excellence hospital Web sites and follow-up telephone calls to confirm adult ICU visitation policies to hospitals that reported open visitation on their Web site	51% (n = 274) indicated open visitation policy per Web site. Follow-up phone calls revealed only 18.5% (n = 99) followed AACN-recommended practice of unrestricted visitation. Restrictions in adult ICUs without open visitation were 68.2% (n = 116) number of visitors, 59.5% (n = 94) visitor age, 19.8% (n = 33) visiting hours, 4.4% (n = 7) visitor type	Restricted visitation in a sample of hospitals known for nursing excellence
González-Dambrauskas et al,[29] 2021 Family presence and visitation practices in Latin American PICUs: an international study	Cross-sectional survey	47 pediatric ICUs across 11 Latin American countries (97.9% response rate)	All pediatric ICUs had some form of parental visitation. Unrestricted (24 h/d) parental visitation 63% Siblings 23%	Parental and sibling visitation restricted in pediatric ICUs in Latin American countries
Fiest et al,[30] 2021 An environmental scan of visitation policies in Canadian ICUs during first wave of COVID	Environmental scan	Visitor restrictions before and during COVID; 257 visitation policy documents from 230 Canadian hospitals with 38/257 (15%) ICU-specific no visitor policy	Pre-COVID ICU-specific visiting policy; 69% (24/35) were open with 24-h visiting Mid-COVID ICU-specific no-visitor policy with exceptions (end-of-life) 86% (61/71) Late-COVID ICU-specific no visitor policy with exceptions 76% (65/85)	COVID-19 pandemic has halted progress of family presence in ICU via open visiting

has been used interchangeably with the term "unrestricted visitation" (eg, no restrictions on visit time, duration, visitor type, age, or number)[36] but has a different meaning from "flexible visitation" (eg, flexibility in the number of hours allowed to visit).[37] In 2019 the Society of Critical Care Medicine (SCCM) family-centered care (FCC) guideline contributors suggested that the term "family presence" replace the term "visiting" and should be open and flexible to meet the needs of the family and not the staff or physicians.[38]

Fig. 1 depicts the potential relationship between open visitation, family presence, and family engagement under the FCC approach to health care. This author hypothesizes that open visitation is a strategy to facilitate family presence and engagement. Research is needed, specifically randomized control trials, to test the effect of open visitation on family presence and engagement in the ICU.

Historically, personal or family pets have been also restricted from visiting the ICU despite some evidence showing a decrease in patient anxiety, depression, loneliness, and sadness.[39] In the 1990s the idea of pets as family members appeared in the literature[40] and the practice of personal pet visitation was considered a psychological support intervention.[41,42] An informal survey of the SCCM FCC guideline coauthors found wide variation in pet visitation globally.[38] More research is needed on the efficacy of personal/family pet visitation.

Recommendations from Organizations for Open Visitation in the Intensive Care Unit

Fig. 2 displays the timeline of recommendations and position statements from organizations to support family presence via open visitation in the ICU. The Institute for Healthcare Improvement challenged hospitals to implement open visitation in their ICUs in 2004.[43] From 2007 to 2017 nursing and medicine critical care practice organizations released recommendations for PFCC that included open or unrestricted visitation in the adult ICU.[44-48] Based on the percentages of open visitation in the US and other countries in **Table 1**, explicit statements from these organizations did not change practice and other factors may explain the slow uptake.

Barriers and Facilitators to Open Visitation

Several barriers and facilitators of open visitation have been identified that have not changed much over time. In 1979 identified barriers were that visitors interfered with physicians' and nurses' work, visitors were a nuisance and pester staff, and the ward appears untidy with lots of visitors.[5] Facilitators at this time were the idea

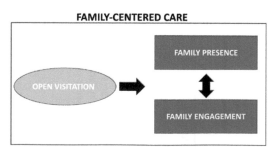

Fig. 1. Relationship between open visitation, family presence, and family engagement. Hypothesized relationship of open visitation as a strategy to facilitate family presence and family engagement under a family-centered care approach in the intensive care unit. Family presence may influence family engagement and vice versa.

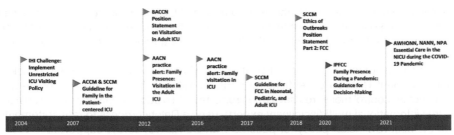

Fig. 2. Timeline of recommendations from organizations for open visitation in the ICU. In 2004 the Institute for Healthcare Improvement (IHI) challenged the United States intensive care units (ICU) to implement unrestricted visitation. In 2007 the Anesthesiology & Critical Care Medicine (ACCM) and the Society for Critical Care Medicine (SCCM) published their guideline for family-centered care that included open visitation. In 2012 the British and American Associations of Critical Care Nursing (BACCN, ACCN) released statements that included open visitation in the ICU and the AACN issued a follow-up position on ICU family visitation in 2016. In 2017 the SCCM updated its 2007 guideline and called for family presence in the ICU. The SCCM released its position on family presence and engagement during outbreaks in 2018. In response to no visitation or severely restricted visitation during the COVID-19 pandemic, the Institute for Patient- and Family-Centered Care (IPFCC) released their iterative process for decision-making for family presence. Similarly, the Association of Women's Health, Obstetrics, and Neonatal Nurses (AWHONN), the National Association of Neonatal Nurses (NANN), and the National Perinatal Association (NPA) released their position on parents being allowed unrestricted access to hospitalized infant regardless of circumstance.

that the nurse-family relationship is strengthened and this improves communication regarding a patient's condition and family needs, and open visiting was important for the terminal patient and their loved ones to help process their grief. Fast forward 40 years and the barriers to open visitation in the ICU continue to be provider-centric with reports of increased workload, perceived loss of control, interruption of care, and skepticism about the benefits.[49,50] Other barriers include the belief that it compromises patient safety and protection, visitors are demanding, and there is no physical space for visitors.[50] Nurses have reported inadequate preparation on effective communication and interaction with visitors,[50,51] variation among nurses in following the visiting policy, and discomfort with family watching them work.[49] Current facilitators of open visitation include improving staffing; creating new roles dedicated to assisting families (eg, relative caregiver specialist)[49]; providing adequate education and training to staff and visitors;[49,51] creating structured, clear visitor guidelines that are communicated widely[51]; and visitation legislation.[25] Unforeseen was the worldwide COVID-19 pandemic that became a barrier for open visitation in the ICU.

Status of Visiting in Intensive Care Units During the COVID-19 Pandemic

In a review of the literature on visitation during the first wave of the COVID-19 pandemic, no visitation to hospitals was the norm, with some hospitals granting exceptions for children and end-of-life and childbirth patients.[52–55] The public health rationale for strict visitor policies globally was based on the precautionary principle where the interests of the individual patient were weighed against the societal responsibility to mitigate the transmission of COVID-19 to, from, and within hospitals.[56] There was a large prepandemic body of evidence on the positive impact of family presence on the patient's psychological and physical well-being in ICUs.[37,50,57–60] Yet, no visitation policies continued in the second and third COVID-19 waves when there was sufficient personal protective equipment, testing, and vaccines and available research supporting the fact that visitors to the ICU were not a source of transmission of the virus.[61–64]

The clinical practice of infection control in ICUs has also affected visiting policies. Variability in ICU visitor exceptions for patients with COVID-19 at the end-of-life due to infection control measures have been reported.[65] To address infection control measures international multidisciplinary experts used a Delphi process to rate statements on the best ICU visitor policy for patients with COVID-19; 85.3% supported reduced visitation (limit timing, visits, visitors, or exceptions considered for end-of-life, pediatric) and 29.4% supported a uniform visitation policy regardless of patient COVID-19 status.[66] With the availability of vaccines, PPE, and a better understanding of COVID-19 transmission, 29.4% of experts still believed visitation restrictions should continue, suggesting that the harm to patients, families, and staff was not well understood.

Fig. 2 includes the 2018 prepandemic SCCM position statement for FCC during international public health outbreaks that includes respect for family presence and engagement using e-visit and e-presence and recommends physical structures that have a window for family and patient to see each other.[67] It is likely that the investigators did not envision a situation like the COVID-19 pandemic with widespread "no visitor" policies, even in cases of dying patients, and an updated position statement is needed. The Institute for PFCC[68] and the Association of Women's Health, Obstetrics, Neonatal Nurses (AWHONN), the National Association of Neonatal Nurses (NANN), and the National Perinatal Association (NPA)[69] released guidelines for family presence during the COVID-19 pandemic that called on health systems around the world to balance the risks and benefits of visitation with the holistic needs of the family. Guidelines recommend that parents be defined as essential caregivers with unrestricted access to their infant and visitation be allowed for cases of life-threatening conditions that arise in the parent (eg, infant/child can visit a parent in adult ICU) or infant (eg, parent can visit infant in neonatal ICU).

The concept of the essential caregiver may be traced to the Centers for Disease Control (CDC) guideline for visitation to non-US health care settings in the context of COVID-19.[70] In this situation the CDC recommended visitors be limited to those that are essential to helping provide care to the patient or caring for pediatric patients. Thus, there have been calls for reversal of strict visitation[71] and the assertion that the existing literature does not support any scenario where complete restriction of essential caregivers across all patient subtypes from hospitals is required.[56]

Virtual Visitation: a Newer Concept

Virtual visitation (VV) was born out of necessity during the COVID-19 pandemic to connect patients with their loved ones, facilitate decision-making, and support PFCC in the absence of in-person visits to the ICU. Survey data show from 69%[72] to 97%[73] of ICUs during the pandemic had some form of VV. Technological supports used for VV have been reported such as cyber-secure platforms, ICU-supplied tablets or iPads,[72,74–76] and adapted virtual ICUs with cameras in the patient's room.[77] VVs have been described as lasting 10 to 30 minutes[74,75,77]; administered by nurses, social workers, or specialty-specific coordinators[72,75,77]; and prescheduled or on-demand.[78]

The available evidence evaluating VV is from descriptive studies. Commonly reported benefits of VV include decreasing patient psychological stress, reorienting patients with delirium,[73] allowing for more visitors from different geographic areas and including pets, and shielding visitors from busy, noisy ICU environments and other critical patients.[76] For families with no ICU experience VV allowed them to see their loved one, and this helped with processing the patient condition and making informed care decisions that could not be done by traditional phone calls.[76] Studies of VV demonstrate that families had a positive experience and were appreciative that they had this option to see their loved ones when visiting was banned.[74,75,77] Clinicians and families believed phone calls were useful for information sharing and brief updates and video communication/VV for aligning clinician and family perspectives when in-person was not possible. But both methods were viewed as inferior to in-person communication and visitation.[79]

Common barriers associated with VV include technological glitches such as Internet lag, audio and video quality problems, visitor having difficulty getting connected,[73,74,77] and not enough devices (tablets, iPads).[75] Communication challenges were encountered when patients were intubated, staff wore PPE, or background noise levels made it difficult to hear.[74,77] Some settings did not have enough staff,[73] or staff was unprepared to handle the VV when families were unaware of the patient's condition and this caused emotional strain,[74,75] and staff were frustrated when the family did not show up for the scheduled VV.[74]

VV is likely to stay postpandemic because of its numerous benefits, and families liked it as an alternative. Research is needed to evaluate its place in the hierarchy of options for visitation that may include in-person or VV. Platforms, software, and other technical entities that support VV should also be evaluated.

Consequences of Visitor Restriction Policies During the COVID-19 Pandemic

Reports of patient stress and trauma due to "no visitor" policies during the pandemic have been well documented.[80-83] Patients who experienced visitation restrictions were more likely to have delays in care requests (eg, toileting, call light response, hospital discharge),[35,84] medication management errors,[54] higher fall and sepsis rates,[35] less understanding of medical status,[72] and increased anxiety due to hospitalization and separation from family.[56,80,81,84]

Effects of ICU visitation restrictions on family have also been documented in the literature.[80] Decreased involvement in care, delays in conversations about goals of care,[85,86] decreased family comprehension of disease progression, and inadequate preparation for end-of-life decision-making such as discussions of do-not-resuscitate orders or withdrawing life-sustaining measures have been reported.[87,88] Mental health consequences included a heightened sense of distrust of medical staff,[89] traumatic response to separation,[81] and complex bereavement responses for families who could not visit their loved ones before they died.[90]

Numerous effects on frontline health care workers related to visitation restrictions have also been documented.[55,60,91] Mental health consequences for health care workers included symptoms of posttraumatic stress disorder, regret about enforcing restrictive visitation and desire for the family to return to ICU,[92,93] burnout, intention to leave their jobs due to their roles enforcing no visitation policies,[94] and moral distress from telling families they cannot visit their dying loved ones.[85]

Going forward, decision-makers need to be mindful of the consequences of "no visitation" on patients, families, and health care workers during the COVID-19 pandemic. Lessons learned must be incorporated into postpandemic visitation policies. In the US 8 states have passed legislation called the No Patient Left Alone Act.[95] Under this law a child or adult admitted to the hospital has the right to a parent or designated family member who may be present while the patient is receiving hospital care.[96] As with any legislation, loopholes or unforeseen consequences may not be immediately obvious. Florida, North Carolina, and Oklahoma laws have provisions where hospitals can limit or restrict visitation.[96-100] It is possible that a future public health emergency may result in similar COVID-19 visitor restrictions despite these laws. It is up to the frontline health care workers, patients, family, and practice organizations to develop an evidence-informed, data-driven PFCC policy that maintains a family presence in the ICU, and other units, whatever the circumstances.

Recommendations for Intensive Care Unit Visitor Policies During and After COVID-19

In response to visitor restrictions during the COVID-19 pandemic, organizations have developed decision-making frameworks to support and maintain a family presence in hospitals for now and during future public health emergencies. The Institute for Patient- and Family-Centered Care (IPFCC) developed an iterative process for decision-making within a PFCC ethical framework.[68] Planetree International (PI) and the American Nurses Foundation (ANF) developed the Family Presence Policy Decision-Making Toolkit for nurse leaders.[101] The Canadian Foundation for Healthcare Improvement (CFHI) created policy guidance for reintegrating family caregivers as essential partners in care.[102] Taken together, these frameworks include many factors that should be considered when developing a family presence policy, and they are displayed in **Table 2**. Ultimately, ICU visitation decisions should honor the core concepts of PFCC and fundamental principles of bioethics, and family presence cannot continue to be restricted.[68]

Table 2
Factors to consider in the development of family presence policy

Factor	Organization
Use evidence to guide decisions that may include local conditions, research, and/or expressed needs of patients, families, staff, and experts like CDC and WHO	CFHI, IPFCC, PI/ANF
Include key stakeholders in the policy process like patient, family, nurses	CFHI, IPFCC, PI/ANF
Differentiate between visitor and essential family caregivers who play a significant role in providing physical, psychological, and emotional support and support decision-making and care coordination	CFHI
Review previous policy	CFHI, IPFCC
Apply patient- and family-centered care principles	CFHI, IPFCC, PI/ANF
Apply ethical principles	IPFCC
Conduct a balanced, comprehensive risk/benefit assessment	CFHI, IPFCC, PI/ANF
Communicate policy decision to stakeholders	IPFCC
Create a rapid appeal process for visitors who are denied	CFHI
Use Family Presence Decision Aid that generates risk/benefit score that considers current environment including evidence base, local conditions, resource availability, and equity	PI/ANF
Define workflow for policy	CFHI, PI/ANF
Education for staff, patient, and family/visitors of roles and safety protocols	CFHI
Evaluate the policy change	IPFCC
Generate evidence to guide decisions on family caregiver presence	CFHI

Abbreviations: CDC, Centers for Disease Control; CFHI, Canadian Foundation for Healthcare Improvement; IPFCC, Institute for Patient- and Family-Centered Care; PI/ANF, Planetree International/American Nurses Foundation; WHO, World Health Organization.

Directions for Future Research

Open visitation where anyone of the patient's choosing can visit any time is a strategy to support PFCC and family presence in the ICU. It is important to recognize that the work needed to advance open visitation must be done globally because what is found to work in one country may not be generalizable to another. Research priorities for the future study of visitation in the ICU are as follows.

- Theoretical testing of relationship among open visitation, family presence, and family engagement.
- Development and testing of implementation and sustainment strategies to support open visitation.
- Effect of open visitation on patient, family, and staff/health system outcomes.
- Effect of personal/family pet visitation on patient, family, children, ICU staff, and the environment.
- Investigating the long-term consequences of restrictive visitation on patients, family, and health care staff.
- The effect of legislation such as the No Patient Left Alone Act on visitation in the ICU.
- Development and testing of real-time decision aid that supports and sustains visitation/family presence in the ICU.
- Evaluating the efficacy of virtual visitation.
- Comparison of in-person open visitation and virtual visitation on patient, family, and staff/health system outcomes.

SUMMARY

Visitation policies in ICUs have evolved over time from very restrictive in the 1960s to more open. The COVID-19 pandemic shone a spotlight on the importance of family presence and visitation in the ICU. The belief that no visitation or being severely restricted during this public health crisis benefits the patient, family, and health care staff is not supported by the evidence. Global visitation policies that honor PFCC and bioethical principles, which are created by patients, families, clinicians, practice organizations, and health systems, are a must.

CLINICS CARE POINTS

- Open visitation is an intervention to promote family presence and engagement within a family-centered care approach.
- In public health crises ICUs and health systems must balance the risk and benefits of visitation with the holistic needs of the family and allow for at least one visitor to be physically present.
- Virtual visitation can be used as an adjunct to in person visitation if selected by the family but not as a replacement.

DISCLOSURE

The author has nothing to disclose.

REFERENCES

1. Berthelsen PG, Cronqvist M. The first intensive care unit in the world: copenhagen 1953. Acta Anaesthesiol Scand 2003;47(10):1190–5.

2. Weil MH, Tang W. From intensive care to critical care medicine: a historical perspective. Am J Respir Crit Care Med 2011;183(11):1451–3.

3. United States Public Health Service. Elements of progression and patient care US Gov Print Off. Washington, DC: USPHS Publ; 1962.

4. United States Public Health Service. A facility designed for coronary care. Washington, DC: US Gov Print Off; 1965.

5. Garton EJ. In praise of open visiting. Nurs Times 1979;75(41):1747.

6. Youngner SJ, Coulton C, Welton R, et al. ICU visiting policies. Crit Care Med 1984;12(7):606–8.

7. Kirchhoff KT, Hansen CB, Evans P, et al. Open visiting in the ICU: a debate. Dimens Crit Care Nurs 1985;4(5):296–306.

8. Woellner DS. Flexible visiting hours in the adult critical care unit. Focus Crit Care 1988;15(2):66–9.

9. Pearlmutter DR, Locke A, Bourdon S, et al. Models of family-centered care in one acute care institution. Nurs Clin North Am 1984;19(1):173–88.

10. Krapohl GL. Visiting hours in the adult intensive care unit: using research to develop a system that works. Dimens Crit Care Nurs 1995;14(5):245–58.

11. Poole EL. The visiting needs of critically ill patients and their families. J Post Anesth Nurs 1992;7(6):377–86.

12. Lynch JJ, Thomas SA, Mills ME, et al. The effects of human contact on cardiac arrhythmia in coronary care patients. J Nerv Ment Dis 1974;158(2):88–99.

13. Brown AJ. Effect of family visits on the blood pressure and heart rate of patients in the coronary-care unit. Heart Lung 1976;5(2):291–6.

14. Theorell T, Wester PO. The significance of psychological events in a coronary care unit. Preliminary report. Acta Med Scand 1973;193(3):207–10.

15. Kirchhoff KT. Visiting policies for patients with myocardial infarction: a national survey. Heart Lung 1982;11(6):571–6.

16. Heater BS. Nursing responsibilities in changing visiting restrictions in the intensive care unit. Heart Lung 1985;14(2):181–6.

17. Stockdale LL, Hughes JP. Critical care unit visiting policies: a survey. Focus Crit Care 1988;15(6):45–8.

18. Simon SK, Phillips K, Badalamenti S, et al. Current practices regarding visitation policies in critical care units. Am J Crit Care 1997;6(3):210–7.

19. Carlson B, Riegel B, Thomason T. Visitation: policy versus practice. Dimens Crit Care Nurs 1998;17(1):40–7.

20. Kirchhoff KT, Dahl N. American Association of Critical-Care Nurses' national survey of facilities and units providing critical care. Am J Crit Care 2006;15(1): 13–27.

21. Lee MD, Friedenberg AS, Mukpo DH, et al. Visiting hours policies in New England intensive care units: strategies for improvement. Crit Care Med 2007; 35(2):497–501.

22. Vandijck DM, Labeau SO, Geerinckx CE, et al. An evaluation of family-centered care services and organization of visiting policies in Belgian intensive care units: a multicenter survey. Heart Lung 2010;39(2):137–46.

23. Haghbin S, Tayebi Z, Abbasian A, et al. Visiting-hour policies for intensive care units in southern Iran. Iran Red Crescent Med J 2011;13(9). https://doi.org/10.5812/kowsar.20741804.2242.

24. Liu V, Read JL, Scruth E, et al. Visitation policies and practices in US ICUs. Crit Care 2013;17(2):R71.

25. Cappellini E, Bambi S, Lucchini A, et al. Open intensive care units: a global challenge for patients, relatives, and critical care teams. Dimens Crit Care Nurs 2014;33(4):181–93.
26. Noordermeer K, Rijpstra TA, Newhall D, et al. Visiting policies in the adult intensive care units in The Netherlands: survey among ICU directors. ISRN Crit Care 2013;2013:1–6.
27. Kleinpell R, Heyland DK, Lipman J, et al. Patient and family engagement in the ICU: report from the task force of the world federation of societies of intensive and critical care medicine. J Crit Care 2018;48:251–6.
28. Milner KA, Goncalves S, Marmo S, et al. Is open visitation really "open" in adult intensive care units in the United States? Am J Crit Care 2020;29(3):221–5.
29. González-Dambrauskas S, Mislej C, Vásquez-Hoyos P, et al. Family presence and visitation practices in Latin American PICUs: an international survey. J Pediatr Intensive Care 2021;10(4):276–81.
30. Fiest KM, Krewulak KD, Hiploylee C, et al. An environmental scan of visitation policies in Canadian intensive care units during the first wave of the COVID-19 pandemic. Can J Anesth Can d'anesthésie 2021;68(10):1474–84.
31. Desai PP, Flick SL, Knutsson S, et al. Practices and perceptions of nurses regarding child visitation in adult intensive care units. Am J Crit Care 2020; 29(3):195–203.
32. Johnstone M. Children visiting members of their family receiving treatment in ICUs: a literature review. Intensive Crit Care Nurs 1994;10(4):289–92.
33. Hanley JB, Piazza J. A visit to the intensive cares unit. Crit Care Nurs Q 2012; 35(1):113–22.
34. Laurent A, Leclerc P, Nguyen S, et al. The effect visiting relatives in the adult ICU has on children. Intensive Care Med 2019;45(10):1490–2.
35. Silvera GA, Wolf JA, Stanowski A, et al. The influence of COVID-19 visitation restrictions on patient experience and safety outcomes: a critical role for subjective advocates. Patient Exp J 2021;8(1):30–9.
36. McAdam JL, Puntillo KA. Open visitation policies and practices in US ICUs: can we ever get there? Crit Care 2013;17(4):171.
37. Nassar Junior AP, Besen BAMP, Robinson CC, et al. Flexible versus restrictive visiting policies in ICUs. Crit Care Med 2018;46(7):1175–80.
38. Davidson JE, McDuffie M, Mitchell K. International best practices in critical care nursing. In: Goldsworthy S, Kleinpell R, Williams G, editors. World federation of critical care nurses. 2nd edition. NSW Australia: World Federation of Critical Care Nurses; 2019. p. 96–112.
39. Sehr J, Eisele-Hlubocky L, Junker R, et al. Family pet visitation. Am J Nurs 2013; 113(12):54–9.
40. Cain AO. Pets and the family. Holist Nurs Pract 1991;5(2):58–63.
41. Cullen L, Titler M, Drahozal R. Family and pet visitation in the critical care unit. Crit Care Nurse 1999;19(3):84–7.
42. Giuliano KK, Bloniasz E, Bell J. Implementation of a pet visitation program in critical care. Crit Care Nurse 1999;19(3):43–50.
43. Berwick DM, Kotagal M. Restricted visiting hours in ICUs: time to change. JAMA 2004;292(6):736–7.
44. Davidson JE, Powers K, Hedayat KM, et al. Clinical practice guidelines for support of the family in the patient-centered intensive care unit: American College of Critical Care Medicine Task Force 2004-2005. Crit Care Med 2007;35(2):605–22.
45. Davidson JE, Aslakson RA, Long AC, et al. Guidelines for family-centered care in the neonatal, pediatric, and adult ICU. Crit Care Med 2017;45(1):103–28.

46. Gibson V, Plowright C, Collins T, et al. Position statement on visiting in adult critical care units in the UK. Nurs Crit Care 2012;17(4):213–8.
47. Family presence. Visitation in the adult ICU. Crit Care Nurse 2012;32(4):76–8.
48. Family visitation in the adult intensive care unit. Crit Care Nurse 2016;36(1): e15–8.
49. Monroe M, Wofford L. Open visitation and nurse job satisfaction: an integrative review. J Clin Nurs 2017;26(23–24):4868–76.
50. Ning J, Cope V. Open visiting in adult intensive care units – a structured literature review. Intensive Crit Care Nurs 2020;56:2–8.
51. Kozub E, Scheler S, Necoechea G, et al. Improving nurse satisfaction with open visitation in an adult intensive care unit. Crit Care Nurs Q 2017;40(2):144–54.
52. Jaswaney R, Davis A, Cadigan RJ, et al. Hospital policies during COVID-19: an analysis of visitor restrictions. J Public Health Manag Pract 2022;28(1): E299–306.
53. Weiner HS, Firn JI, Hogikyan ND, et al. Hospital visitation policies during the SARS-CoV-2 pandemic. Am J Infect Control 2021;49(4):516–20.
54. Siddiqi H. To suffer alone: hospital visitation policies during COVID-19. J Hosp Med 2020;15(11):694–5.
55. Moss SJ, Krewulak KD, Stelfox HT, et al. Restricted visitation policies in acute care settings during the COVID-19 pandemic: a scoping review. Crit Care 2021;25(1):347.
56. Munshi L, Odutayo A, Evans GA, et al. Impact of Hospital Visitor Restrictions during the COVID-19 Pandemic. Science Briefs of the Ontario COVID-19 Science Advisory Table 2021;2(31). https://doi.org/10.47326/ocsat.2021.02.31.1.0.
57. Fumagalli S, Boncinelli L, Lo Nostro A, et al. Reduced cardiocirculatory complications with unrestrictive visiting policy in an intensive care unit: results from a pilot, randomized trial. Circulation 2006;113(7):946–52.
58. da Silva Ramos F, Fumis RR, Azevedo LC, et al. Perceptions of an open visitation policy by intensive care unit workers. Ann Intensive Care 2013;3(1):34.
59. Rosa RG, Tonietto TF, da Silva DB, et al. Effectiveness and safety of an extended ICU visitation model for delirium prevention. Crit Care Med 2017;45(10):1660–7.
60. Shulkin D, O'Keefe T, Visconi D, et al. Eliminating visiting hour restrictions in hospitals. J Healthc Qual 2014;36(6):54–7.
61. Zhou Q, Gao Y, Wang X, et al. Nosocomial infections among patients with COVID-19, SARS and MERS: a rapid review and meta-analysis. Ann Transl Med 2020;8(10):629.
62. Rhee C, Baker M, Vaidya V, et al. Incidence of nosocomial COVID-19 in patients hospitalized at a large US academic medical center. JAMA Netw Open 2020; 3(9):e2020498.
63. Wee LE, Conceicao EP, Sim JX-Y, et al. The impact of visitor restrictions on health care-associated respiratory viral infections during the COVID-19 pandemic: experience of a tertiary hospital in Singapore. Am J Infect Control 2021;49(1):134–5.
64. Passarelli VC, Faico-Filho K, Moreira LVL, et al. Asymptomatic COVID-19 in hospital visitors: the underestimated potential of viral shedding. Int J Infect Dis 2021;102:412–4.
65. Marmo S, Milner KA. From open to closed: COVID-19 restrictions on previously unrestricted visitation in adult intensive care units. Am J Crit Care 2023;32(1): 31–41.

66. Nasa P, Azoulay E, Chakrabarti A, et al. Infection control in the intensive care unit: expert consensus statements for SARS-CoV-2 using a Delphi method. Lancet Infect Dis 2022;22(3):e74–87.

67. Papadimos TJ, Marcolini EG, Hadian M, et al. Ethics of outbreaks position statement. Part 2. Crit Care Med 2018;46(11):1856–60.

68. Dokken DL, Johnson BH, Markwell HJ. Family presence during a pandemic: Guidance for decision-making. Institute for Patient-and Family-Centered Care. 2021

69. Awhonn NANN. NPA. Essential care in the NICU during the COVID-19 pandemic. 2021. Available at: https://www.ipfcc.org/resources/visiting.pdf. Accessed June 17, 2022.

70. Management of visitors to healthcare facilities in the context of COVID-19: non-US healthcare settings | CDC. Available at: https://www.cdc.gov/coronavirus/2019-ncov/hcp/non-us-settings/hcf-visitors.html. Accessed June 17, 2022.

71. Curley MAQ, Broden EG, Meyer EC. Alone, the hardest part. Intensive Care Med 2020;46(10):1974–6.

72. Valley TS, Schutz A, Nagle MT, et al. Changes to visitation policies and communication practices in Michigan ICUs during the COVID-19 Pandemic. Am J Respir Crit Care Med 2020;202(6):883–5.

73. Rose L, Yu L, Casey J, et al. Communication and virtual visiting for families of patients in intensive care during the COVID-19 pandemic: a UK National survey. Ann Am Thorac Soc 2021;18(10):1685–92.

74. Dhahri AA, De Thabrew AU, Ladva N, et al. The benefits and risks of the provision of a hospital-wide high-definition video conferencing virtual visiting service for patients and their relatives. Cureus 2021. https://doi.org/10.7759/cureus.13435.

75. Mendiola B, Gomez C, Furst C, et al. Facilitating virtual visitation in critical care units during a pandemic. Holist Nurs Pract 2021;35(2):60–4.

76. Xyrichis A, Pattison N, Ramsay P, et al. Virtual visiting in intensive care during the COVID-19 pandemic: a qualitative descriptive study with ICU clinicians and non-ICU family team liaison members. BMJ Open 2022;12(4):e055679.

77. Sasangohar F, Dhala A, Zheng F, et al. Use of telecritical care for family visitation to ICU during the COVID-19 pandemic: an interview study and sentiment analysis. BMJ Qual Saf 2021;30(9):715–21.

78. Thomas KAS, O'Brien BF, Fryday AT, et al. Developing an innovative system of open and flexible, patient-family-centered, virtual visiting in ICU during the COVID-19 pandemic: a collaboration of staff, patients, families, and technology companies. J Intensive Care Med 2021;36(10):1130–40.

79. Kennedy NR, Steinberg A, Arnold RM, et al. Perspectives on telephone and video communication in the intensive care unit during COVID-19. Ann Am Thorac Soc 2021;18(5):838–47.

80. Hugelius K, Harada N, Marutani M. Consequences of visiting restrictions during the COVID-19 pandemic: an integrative review. Int J Nurs Stud 2021;121:104000.

81. Montauk TR, Kuhl EA. COVID-related family separation and trauma in the intensive care unit. Psychol Trauma Theory, Res Pract Policy 2020;12(S1):S96–7.

82. Bartoli D, Trotta F, Simeone S, et al. The lived experiences of family members of Covid-19 patients admitted to intensive care unit: a phenomenological study. Hear Lung 2021;50(6):926–32.

83. Antommaria AHM, Monhollen L, Schaffzin JK. An ethical analysis of hospital visitor restrictions and masking requirements during the COVID-19 pandemic. J Clin Ethics 2021;32(1):38–47.

84. Zeh RD, Santry HP, Monsour C, et al. Impact of visitor restriction rules on the postoperative experience of COVID-19 negative patients undergoing surgery. Surgery 2020;168(5):770–6.

85. Wakam GK, Montgomery JR, Biesterveld BE, et al. Not dying alone — modern compassionate care in the Covid-19 pandemic. N Engl J Med 2020; 382(24):e88.

86. Wendlandt B, Kime M, Carson S. The impact of family visitor restrictions on healthcare workers in the ICU during the COVID-19 pandemic. Intensive Crit Care Nurs 2022;68:103123.

87. Azad TD, Al-Kawaz MN, Turnbull AE, et al. Coronavirus disease 2019 policy restricting family presence may have delayed end-of-life decisions for critically ill patients. Crit Care Med 2021;49(10):e1037–9.

88. Teno JM, Fisher E, Hamel MB, et al. Decision-making and outcomes of prolonged ICU stays in seriously ill patients. J Am Geriatr Soc 2000;48(S1):S70–4.

89. LoGiudice JA, Bartos S. Experiences of nurses during the COVID-19 pandemic: a mixed-methods study. AACN Adv Crit Care 2021;32(1):14–26.

90. Diolaiuti F, Marazziti D, Beatino MF, et al. Impact and consequences of COVID-19 pandemic on complicated grief and persistent complex bereavement disorder. Psychiatry Res 2021;300:113916.

91. American nurses foundation, pulse on the nation's nurses COVID-19 survey series: family presence & visitation during COVID-19. Available at: https://www.nursing world.org/practice-policy/work-environment/health-safety/disaster-preparedness/ coronavirus/what-you-need-to-know/family-presence–visitation-during-covid-19- survey/. Accessed June 23, 2022.

92. Azoulay E, Cariou A, Bruneel F, et al. Symptoms of anxiety, depression, and peritraumatic dissociation in critical care clinicians managing patients with COVID-19. A cross-sectional study. Am J Respir Crit Care Med 2020;202(10):1388–98.

93. Wozniak H, Benzakour L, Moullec G, et al. Mental health outcomes of ICU and non-ICU healthcare workers during the COVID-19 outbreak: a cross-sectional study. Ann Intensive Care 2021;11(1):106.

94. Malliarou M, Nikolentzos A, Papadopoulos D, et al. ICU nurse's moral distress as an occupational hazard threatening professional quality of life in the time of pandemic COVID 19. Mater Socio Medica 2021;33(2):88.

95. States Pass Laws to Prevent Visitor Bans in Hospitals. Long-term care facilities. AJN, Am J Nurs 2022;122(7):16.

96. Hasenbeck, Pittman, Stark, et al. No Patient Left Alone Act. 2021.

97. Chapman DK, Collingridge DS, Mitchell LA, et al. Satisfaction with elimination of all visitation restrictions in a mixed-profile intensive care unit. Am J Crit Care 2016;25(1):46–50.

98. Strauss A. Corbin J. Basics of Qualitative Research. Sage; 1990.

99. General Assembly of North Carolina. The No Patient Left Alone Act; 2021.

100. Committee Substitute for Senate Bill No. 988. No Patient Left Alone Act; 2022.

101. Planetree International, American Nurses Foundation. Family Presence Policy Decision-Making Toolkit for Nurse Leaders. p. 1–17.

102. Fancott C, Yonadam A, Checkley J, et al. Advancing family presence policies and practices in the canadian health and care context: COVID-19 and beyond. Healthc Q 2021;24(1):14–21.

Development of the Modern Cardiothoracic Intensive Care Unit and Current Management

Ronald G. Pearl, MD, PhD, FCCM*, Sheela Pai Cole, MD, FASE, FASA

KEYWORDS

- Intensive care unit • Cardiac surgery • Mechanical circulatory support
- Echocardiography • Low cardiac output syndrome • Left ventricular failure
- Right ventricular failure • Postoperative complications

KEY POINTS

- The majority of preventable cardiac surgery complications occur in the postoperative period after cardiac surgery.
- The patient population in the cardiothoracic intensive care unit (CTICU) is now older, frailer, and has more advanced cardiac and noncardiac morbidities than in prior decades.
- Advances in cardiothoracic intensive care allows successful outcomes in both sicker patients and in patients undergoing more complex cardiac surgical procedures.
- The use of mechanical circulatory support such as ECMO and left and right ventricular assist devices now represents a significant portion of CTICU management.
- Optimum care in the CTICU involves collaboration between cardiac surgeons and intensivists with experience with multiple types of cardiac surgery patients and skills in hemodynamic management and echocardiography.

Over 400,000 patients undergo cardiac surgery in the United States each year and require postoperative care in the cardiothoracic intensive care unit (CTICU). The development of the modern CTICU has been the result of changes in three areas. One area is the development and expansion of the field of critical care medicine. As described elsewhere in this series, modern critical care began with the polio epidemics in the 1950s, requiring care of patients with respiratory insufficiency in specialized centers. Critical care science and technology then advanced in the 1960s and 1970s, including the establishment of the Society of Critical Care Medicine in 1971. The knowledge required to care for critically ill patients has continually increased over time, including

Department of Anesthesiology, Perioperative and Pain Medicine, Stanford University, Stanford University School of Medicine, 300 Pasteur Drive, Room H3589
* Corresponding author.
E-mail address: rgp@stanford.edu

Crit Care Clin 39 (2023) 559–576
https://doi.org/10.1016/j.ccc.2023.03.008
0749-0704/23/© 2023 Elsevier Inc. All rights reserved.

criticalcare.theclinics.com

advanced management of respiratory failure, hemodynamic instability, renal failure, liver failure, and neurologic disease. As a result, critical care fellowships expanded in the 1990s, and there are now over 150 programs in the United States accredited by the Accreditation Council for Graduate Medical Education, training over 1500 critical care fellows per year. As will be discussed in this article, the skills taught in such fellowships are necessary for optimum preoperative and postoperative care of the CTICU patient.[1,2]

The second major area has been advances in cardiology and the development of the modern coronary care unit (CCU). The original CCUs began in the 1960s with a focus on treating acute myocardial infarction and associated arrhythmias, including the use of external defibrillation for cardiac arrest. The use of continuous monitoring and intensive nursing care in the CCU resulted in improved outcomes and decreased mortality rates. Over time, the CCU patient population expanded, and CCUs now treat patients undergoing percutaneous coronary interventions (PCIs) for coronary artery disease, structural heart interventions for valvular disease, and patients with acute decompensated heart failure, including patients who require mechanical circulatory support (MCS) such as the use of an intra-aortic balloon pump or Impella RP (Abiomed, Danvers, MA), a catheter-based left ventricular (LV) heart pump. In the United States, there are now over one million PCI procedures performed per year. Because of the expansion of PCI, the number of coronary artery bypass grafting (CABG) procedures per year has dropped. The use of CABG peaked at slightly over 500,000 in 1997, but PCI procedures are now done at five times the rate of CABG procedures. Similarly, the number of transcatheter aortic valve replacement procedures per year is now triple the number of surgical aortic valve replacement procedures. The expansion of the CCU into management of sicker and more complex patients has resulted in the development of acute cardiovascular care as a potential subspecialty of cardiovascular medicine, often with dual fellowship-trained physicians and closed units.[3–10] As a result of the expansion of cardiology into areas that previously could only be treated surgically, the population of cardiac surgical patients is now older, has more noncardiac morbidities, and requires more complex procedures than before.

The third area responsible for the development of the modern CTICU has been technological advancements in cardiothoracic surgery and in cardiology. Open-heart surgery became a reality with the development of the cardiopulmonary bypass machine in the 1950s, allowing valve replacement. CABG surgery became practical in the 1960s. Refinements in the subsequent half-century have increased the safety of cardiac surgery, and advances in myocardial protection allow myocardial preservation despite prolonged aortic cross-clamp times. For routine cases, outcomes have markedly improved, and rates of blood transfusion have decreased. In addition, the expansion of cardiology into areas that previously could only be treated surgically has impacted not only the CCU population but also the population of cardiac surgical patients themselves, which is also now older, with more noncardiac morbidities, and requiring more complex procedures than before. The patient population in the CTICU has markedly shifted as a result of additional technological advances. The development of second and third-generation ventricular assist devices (VADs) has revolutionized the treatment of end-stage heart failure, both as bridge-to-transplant and as destination therapy. Advances in technology have resulted in rapid expansion of extracorporeal membrane oxygenation (ECMO) programs using venoarterial (VA) ECMO for circulatory support, veno-venous (VV) ECMO for acute respiratory failure, and combined techniques for complex patients. Advances in surgical techniques have increased survival in patients with aortic dissections and aneurysms, including the use of thoracic endovascular aortic repair. Patients who were not surgical candidates in the 20th century are now surgical candidates.

Most cardiac surgery patients now have a relatively uncomplicated postoperative course and are eligible for "fast-track" or "early recovery after cardiac surgery" programs that promote rapid extubation, removal of catheters, and transfer out of the CTICU.[11,12] However, other patients develop complications that can include low cardiac output syndrome due to LV, right ventricular, or biventricular dysfunction, hemorrhage, hypovolemia, vasoplegia, cardiac tamponade, arrhythmias, cardiac arrest, coronary air embolism, infection, pain, delirium, acute kidney injury, venous thromboembolism, LV outflow track obstruction (often due to systolic anterior motion of the mitral valve), and surgical issues such as kinked grafts after CABG or valvular dysfunction after repair. Low cardiac output syndrome is the most frequent major complication and results in decreased mental status, poor peripheral perfusion, decreased urine output, and lactic acidosis. The wide adoption of continuous cardiac output catheters has allowed earlier diagnosis of low cardiac output syndrome and confirmation of effective intervention. Respiratory failure with hypoxemia and/or hypercarbia is also common and may be due to pneumothorax, hemothorax, atelectasis, pneumonia, diaphragmatic dysfunction, and pulmonary embolism (PE).

As a result of the factors discussed above, care of patients in CTICUs has rapidly developed into its own subspecialty, requiring unique and highly specialized training.[2] In the 1970s and 1980s, intensive care management of cardiac surgery patients was primarily provided by cardiac surgeons without additional training in critical care. However, with the increased complexity of CTICU patients, including multiple noncardiac comorbidities, there has been a shift toward staffing the CTICU with critical care–trained physicians who also have expertise in the management of cardiothoracic patients. To illustrate the need for the specialized training and experience of CTICU providers, this article will discuss several types of cardiac surgery patients, common problems in the CTICU, and advanced techniques routinely used in the CTICU. Following this, we will discuss the ideal staffing of the CTICU.

CONTEMPORARY REASONS FOR CARDIOTHORACIC INTENSIVE CARE UNIT ADMISSION BEYOND STANDARD CARDIAC SURGERY
Heart Transplantation

In the United States, heart failure affects 6.2 million adults, which is predicted to increase. Approximately 10% to 15% of these patients will progress to end-stage heart disease. Even with modern guideline-directed medical therapy, median survival period with end-stage heart disease is only 5 years. Orthotopic heart transplantation is the most effective treatment for end-stage heart disease. Owing to the limited number of donors, the number of patients receiving heart transplants remains in the range of 3500 to 4000 per year. Although survival after heart transplantation varies based on patient factors, overall survival is approximately 88% at 1 year, 75% at 5 years, and 55% to 60% at 10 years, and most survivors have excellent quality of life. Patients who are potential candidates for heart transplantation may require critical care management because of acute decompensated heart failure, including MCS devices such as ECMO, Impella, TandemHeart (LivaNova, London, UK), or left ventircular assist device (LVAD) implantation. Critical care management immediately after heart transplantation can include management of primary graft dysfunction; right heart failure; hemorrhage; respiratory, kidney, or liver failure; neurologic dysfunction; or acute rejection.[13] Right heart failure frequently involves a combination of ischemia-reperfusion injury and elevated pulmonary vascular resistance. Management typically includes maintaining central venous pressure in the 10- to 12-mm Hg range, inotropic support, and pulmonary vasodilators, either intravenous inovasodilators such as milrinone or dobutamine, inhaled selective pulmonary vasodilators such as inhaled nitric oxide or inhaled epoprostenol, or oral vasodilators such as sildenafil. Finally, heart transplant patients may require ICU admission months or years after transplantation because of antibody or cellular rejection, accelerated atherosclerotic heart disease, or infectious complications from immunosuppression.

Lung Transplantation

In addition to the usual problems that may occur after a major cardiothoracic surgery such as hemorrhage and delirium, lung transplantation has additional specific concerns related to the transplant itself.[14] These include primary graft dysfunction, acute rejection, pulmonary vein stricture, bronchial anastomotic dehiscence, donor-associated pneumonia, phrenic nerve dysfunction, and severe deconditioning. Primary graft dysfunction manifests as altered gas exchange and associated pulmonary hypertension. Primary graft dysfunction is due to a combination of ischemia-reperfusion injury, pulmonary inflammation from bypass and blood transfusion, and altered anatomy from the transplant with factors such as loss of bronchial circulation and lymphatic drainage from the lungs. Primary graft dysfunction occurs in 20% to 30% of patients and increases short- and long-term mortality. Treatment of primary graft dysfunction is primarily supportive and may include the use of VV or VA ECMO. Critical care management of the patient after lung transplantation requires careful fluid optimization to prevent pulmonary edema while preserving renal function, adequate pain control such as regional anesthesia to promote early extubation and pulmonary toilet, and immunosuppression to prevent rejection. Patients who have severe deconditioning from chronic respiratory failure or prolonged ECMO support commonly require prolonged intubation and tracheostomy in the postoperative period. Patients may return to the ICU for respiratory failure due to deconditioning, pneumonia, systemic infection, rejection, or the development of bronchiolitis obliterans.

Combined Heart-Lung Transplantation

Combined heart-lung transplantation may be required in patients with both end-stage heart failure and end-stage lung disease. This combination generally involves patients with complex congenital heart disease with Eisenmenger's syndrome, patients with cardiomyopathy and severe pulmonary hypertension, patients with pulmonary hypertension and severe right ventricular failure (RVF), or patients with cystic fibrosis and pulmonary hypertension. Owing to the limited number of donors, the number of heart-lung transplants remains low at about 200 per year but has been progressively increasing. Many of these patients have prolonged ICU courses before and after transplantation, including the issues relevant to both heart transplantation and lung transplantation.

Thoracic Aortic Surgery

Thoracic aortic surgery is normally performed for an aortic aneurysm or dissection and may involve the ascending aorta, the aortic arch, or the descending thoracic aorta. Common etiologies are connective tissue disorders such as Marfan's syndrome, hypertension, and ascending aneurysms associated with a bicuspid aortic valve. Ascending aortic dissections may rupture or cause acute aortic regurgitation, cardiac tamponade, coronary artery dissection producing myocardial infarction, or innominate or carotid artery dissection producing stroke. In addition, ascending aortic dissections may extend into the descending aorta, causing malperfusion with hepatic, bowel, renal, or lower-extremity ischemia. Ascending (type A) aortic dissections have high mortality and, therefore, require emergency repair. Descending aortic aneurysms may be managed with open surgery, endovascular stenting, or medical therapy, depending on the evidence of malperfusion or progression. Ascending or arch aneurysms larger than specific diameters require elective open repair, and descending aneurysms that require intervention normally have endovascular stenting, with the exception of collagen vascular diseases that may require replacement of the entire aorta. Open repair of aneurysms or dissections that involve the aortic arch is normally done with deep hypothermic circulatory arrest (DHCA) and either antegrade or retrograde cerebral perfusion. Patients with thoracic aortic disease are treated with impulse therapy (control of heart rate and blood pressure) to prevent progression and rupture. Patients undergoing aortic surgery may require critical care management of ventricular dysfunction, spinal cord ischemia, bowel ischemia, coagulopathy, or pulmonary, neurologic, or renal failure.[15]

Congenital Heart Disease

Congenital heart disease may involve abnormalities of the atria, ventricles, valves, and aorta and pulmonary artery. Congenital heart disease occurs in approximately 1% of births, but many of these individuals do not require an intervention. Approximately one-quarter of babies born with congenital heart disease require surgery during the first year of life. With improved surgical techniques and medical therapy, patients with congenital heart disease are living longer lives, and approximately 90% of children born with congenital heart disease survive to adulthood. There are now one million adults with congenital heart disease in the United States, outnumbering children with congenital heart disease. Patients with congenital heart disease may require multiple surgeries throughout their lives and can develop end-stage heart disease or arrhythmias. As a result, the number of adults with congenital heart disease that require treatment in the adult CVICU has been progressively increasing. Treatment of these patients often requires a team that includes the intensivist, the cardiac surgeon, and a cardiologist who specializes in congenital heart disease.[16]

Extracorporeal Cardiopulmonary Resuscitation

Each year, there are over 500,000 cardiac arrests in the United States. Survival to hospital discharge is in the 10% range for out-of-hospital cardiac arrest and up to 25% for in-hospital cardiac arrest. However, many of these surviving patients have poor neurologic recovery. Successful resuscitation from a cardiac arrest using standard cardiopulmonary resuscitation becomes increasingly unlikely with longer resuscitation times. Extracorporeal cardiopulmonary resuscitation (ECPR) involves the use of ECMO in such patients. ECPR has two goals. The first is to maintain vital organ perfusion, especially perfusion to the brain and the heart. The second is to allow time for reversal of the underlying etiology of the cardiac arrest, such as PCI in the setting of acute coronary syndrome. Recent studies have been very mixed although some suggest improved survival, with good neurologic function, when ECPR is used in experienced centers.[17,18]

Cardiac Arrest After Cardiac Surgery

Although there is wide variation among published studies, the incidence of cardiac arrest after complex cardiac surgery is in the range of 5%, with good outcome in approximately half these patients. Rapid intervention is critical to good outcome. Management of the patient in cardiac arrest after cardiac surgery differs in several important ways compared to normal advanced cardiac life support (ACLS). Cardiac arrest after cardiac surgery may occur from hemorrhage, pericardial tamponade, intractable ventricular arrhythmias, cardiac failure, disconnection of vasopressor infusions or pacemaker leads, or surgical issues such as a malfunctioning graft or valve. The emphasis is on rapid correction of reversible conditions, opening the chest, open-heart massage, and institution of cardiac support.[19,20] In contrast to standard resuscitation, initial treatment of ventricular fibrillation or pulseless ventricular tachycardia begins with three attempts at immediate defibrillation rather than external chest compressions which can disrupt bypass grafts and cardiac surgical repair. If defibrillation is not successful or is not indicated, external cardiac compressions should begin, and plans for sternotomy should be initiated. Opening the chest may itself be therapeutic (relief of cardiac tamponade, kinked grafts, or right heart failure), may be diagnostic (hypovolemia, hemorrhage, graft disruption), allows direct placement of pacing wires, and provides more effective cardiac compression. Plans for institution of MCS should occur at the same time as the sternotomy. In contrast to normal ACLS, initial epinephrine administration in the patient with cardiac arrest after surgery is either avoided or used in significantly lower doses to avoid severe hypertension with return of spontaneous circulation, resulting in bleeding or disruption of surgical anastomoses.

COMMON PROBLEMS IN THE CARDIOTHORACIC INTENSIVE CARE UNIT
Bleeding

Bleeding after cardiac surgery has major implications and must be monitored closely. The definition of bleeding is challenging and has been represented by the number of red blood cell transfusions and by quantifying the amount of bleeding per hour. Conventional guidelines for re-exploration include more than 500 mL in the first hour, more than 800 mL at 2 hours, more than 900 mL at 3 hours, more than 1000 mL at 4 hours, or more than 1200 mL at 5 hours. Other descriptors such as chest tube output greater than 200 mL/h, greater than 2000 mL at any time point, and more than 1.5 mL/kg/h over 6 hours have also been used to define significant blood loss in the postoperative period.[21,22] Hemodynamically unstable hemorrhagic shock requires rapid mediastinal re-exploration at the bedside in the CTICU if transport to the operating room is deemed too risky or will require delay. The risk of reoperation after cardiac surgery is estimated at 2.2% to 4.3%, and the characteristics of patients at higher risk of bleeding and reoperation include older age, nonelective surgery, patients presenting for reoperation, need for greater than five bypass grafts, increased duration on cardiopulmonary bypass, and preoperative use of aspirin and clopidogrel.[23,24] Patients who require reoperation for bleeding have increased mortality as well as morbidity, including ventilator dependence, renal failure, circulatory failure, bowel ischemia, and multiorgan system failure.[24,25] Excessive bleeding may be due to coagulopathy and must be assessed by the CTICU team. In addition to traditional laboratory tests such as prothrombin time (PT), activated partial thromboplastin time (aPTT), platelet count, and fibrinogen, viscoelastic testing provides important real-time information about the integrity of the coagulation process. Thromboelastography (Haemonetics, Rosemont, IL, USA) and thromboelastometry (ROTEM; TEM Innovations, Munich, Germany) are currently available viscoelastic tests that inform the ICU team of abnormalities at various points in the coagulation cascade, including fibrin polymerization, fibrinolysis, platelet-fibrin interaction, and platelet function which is not adequately assessed with PT and aPTT testing alone.[26] Transfusion of fresh frozen plasma (FFP) and platelets form the mainstay of correction of coagulopathy in the cardiac surgical patient. Accelerated fibrinolysis after cardiopulmonary bypass and DHCA can be mitigated with the use of antifibrinolytics such as epsilon aminocaproic acid and tranexamic acid. Cryoprecipitate and fibrinogen concentrates are recommended for hypofibrinogenemia (normal levels 200–400 mg/L; treat for <150 mg/L). Following a period of widespread use of recombinant factor seven (rVII) concentrate in the United States, rVII is currently reserved for uncontrolled bleeding as its prothrombotic side effects in the arterial system can cause stroke and myocardial infarction.[27,28] Prothrombin complex concentrate (PCC) and activated PCC (factor eight inhibitor bypassing activity) are recommended for rapid reversal of vitamin K antagonist anticoagulants (warfarin) and also nonspecific reversal when bleeding is secondary to direct oral anticoagulants such as apixaban, rivaroxaban, and dabigatran. PCC requires low volumes, is rapidly available, and is more effective than traditional reversal with FFP transfusion.[26,29,30]

Pericardial Effusion, Tamponade, and Postpericardiotomy Syndrome

Pericardial complications such as effusions, tamponade, and postoperative pericardiotomy syndrome (PPS) occur with variable frequencies after cardiac surgery. Cardiac tamponade due to pericardial effusion and hematoma after cardiac surgery has an overall incidence of 0.1% to 0.6%.[31] Small pericardial effusions are common after cardiac surgery, occurring in about 84% of patients. These pericardial effusions gradually increase in size until 10 days after diagnosis and then resolve spontaneously. Twenty-five percent of asymptomatic pericardial effusions persist at day 20 and can cause pericardial tamponade in 1% to 2.6% of patients.[32] Early pericardial effusions are more common after CABG procedures, and late effusions are associated with valvular procedures.

Because most surgical procedures do not involve reapproximation of the pericardium, the classical hemodynamic and echocardiographic features of tamponade are not always adequate for assessment, especially as effusions and hematomas can be localized rather than circumferential. The presence of hemodynamic compromise, chamber compression, or evidence of low cardiac output syndrome with increasing filling pressures are reasons to perform a definitive intervention. The diagnosis of pericardial tamponade in the CVICU is made with a combination of hemodynamic collapse (low cardiac output and/or hypotension), escalating vasopressor requirements, and echocardiographic presence of fluid or clot in the pericardial space along with right atrial or right ventricular compression and an underfilled left ventricle. In this setting, urgent mediastinal re-exploration is warranted.

PPS, which develops in 15% of patients, is an immune-mediated inflammatory process. PPS can occur after pericardial trauma such as pericardial insult during surgery and bleeding into the pericardial sac. Late pericardial effusion is more likely to be associated with PPS.[33,34] Eighty percent of patients develop this syndrome within the first month after cardiac surgery and experience delayed recovery due to increased length of hospital stay and readmission. Diagnosis of PPS requires close surveillance in the postoperative period and is managed with anti-inflammatory therapies.[33]

Left Ventricular Failure

Low cardiac output syndrome secondary to LV dysfunction after cardiac surgery can be due to exacerbation of pre-existing LV dysfunction, inflammatory response from cardiopulmonary bypass, or new-onset coronary ischemia. New wall motion abnormalities on echocardiography can be due to a structural component such as a kinked coronary artery after valve repair or replacement. The incidence of coronary ostial stenosis is 1% to 5% after aortic valve replacement and can be due to the right coronary occlusion from the aortotomy suture, traumatic injury by sternal retractors, embolic debris from the aorta, and coronary spasm.[35–38] Similarly, with mitral valve repair or replacement, the left circumflex artery which lies in the left atrio-ventricular groove on the posterior aspect of the mitral valve can be injured. The incidence of injury is 0.5% to 2%. About 40% of the injuries are detected in the operating room during or immediately after separation from cardiopulmonary bypass, and the remaining have an urgent or delayed presentation up to 30 days after the procedure. In the ICU, these injuries should be suspected after mitral valve procedures when wall motion abnormalities or electrocardiogram changes are noted in the setting of low cardiac output syndrome. The mechanisms of injury include arterial entrapment, injury with a suture through the artery, endothelial laceration and thrombosis, external compression due to the annuloplasty ring, and coronary spasm.[39] In the ICU, persistent low cardiac output syndrome may require angiography to assess the coronary arteries. After coronary revascularization procedures, physical impediment to newly grafted coronary arteries can be due to hematoma, sternal reapproximation, or pressure from an ill-positioned chest tube.[40–42] Prompt identification of LV dysfunction is essential, and if inotropic escalation is ineffective, initiation of MCS is needed.

Right Ventricular Failure

RVF occurs after cardiopulmonary bypass due to some combination of pre-existing pulmonary hypertension, pulmonary inflammation from cardiopulmonary bypass and transfusion, pre-existing RV dysfunction, and ischemia-reperfusion injury during and after aortic cross-clamping. The incidence of RVF is approximately 3% after cardiac surgery and increases to 9% - 40% after LVAD implantation. RVF increases mortality and the length of ICU and hospital stay. Additionally, it increases the risk of respiratory failure, reintubation, mechanical ventilation, and stroke. In the ICU, diagnosis is made by a combination of clinical features such as systemic hypotension, increased pulmonary hypertension, decreased cardiac output, and specific echocardiographic features.

RVF is more frequent after mitral or tricuspid procedures or following orthotopic heart transplantation. RVF should be considered in patients requiring increased vasoactive support and increased central venous pressure (CVP) in the presence of either pulmonary hypertension or low pulmonary artery pulsatility index (calculated as the pulmonary artery pulse pressure divided by right atrial pressure). Refractory vasoplegia can be a manifestation of RVF. Additional diagnostic parameters include tricuspid annular plane systolic excursion (TAPSE) of less than 16 mm and tissue Doppler imaging with peak myocardial excursion at the lateral tricuspid annulus (S wave) less than 9.5 cm/s (in the absence of tricuspid procedures).[43]

RVF after LVAD implantation can be early or late based on occurrence within 14 days or more than 14 days after LVAD implantation. Characteristics associated with RVF after LVAD implantation include pre-existing RV dysfunction, pulmonary hypertension, mechanical ventilation, use of ECMO, and operative considerations such as loss of pericardial restraint and changes to tricuspid annular anatomy.[44,45] Blood transfusion and the presence of liver dysfunction increase the risk of vasoplegia and RV dysfunction.[45]

For patients with RVF and associated pulmonary hypertension, pulmonary vasodilators can be administered by inhalation or by intravenous infusion. Selective pulmonary vasodilation is achieved with continuous administration of inhaled nitric oxide (which increases cyclic guanosine monophosphate (GMP) and produces pulmonary vasodilation)[46] or aerosolized epoprostenol (a short-acting prostacyclin analog that increases cyclic adenosine monophosphate (AMP) and produces pulmonary vasodilation). Intermittent administration of aerosolized iloprost (a longer-acting prostacyclin analog) can be considered as an alternative.[47–50] Oral sildenafil can be used to transition from an inhaled pulmonary vasodilator. The use of inhaled milrinone and nitroglycerin has been reported in small studies, but data demonstrating benefit are limited.[51] Intravenous inovasodilators such as milrinone are first-line medications used to reduce pulmonary vascular resistance, alleviate right ventricular strain, and provide inotropic support. Levosimendan, a calcium-sensitizing agent, has inotropic and pulmonary vasodilator effects but is not approved for use in the United States. When inotropic support and pulmonary vasodilators are not sufficient to treat RV failure, temporary RV assist devices such as ProtekDuo (LivaNova, London, UK), the Impella, or even ECMO can be considered. Placement of these devices requires fluoroscopic and echocardiographic support and expertise and are described later in the article.

Heparin-Induced Thrombocytopenia

Heparin-induced thrombocytopenia (HIT) and its thrombotic version, heparin-induced thrombocytopenia with thrombosis (HITT), occur in 1.1% of patients after cardiac surgery.[52] HIT is a transient immune-mediated response to platelet and platelet-factor 4 complexes after heparin exposure (usually 5–10 days after exposure), resulting in platelet destruction, thrombotic response, and clotting in arterial and venous spaces.[53–56] The thrombotic version of this syndrome is HITT and can have devastating consequences. Cardiopulmonary bypass and inflammation from surgery cause platelet destruction and thrombocytopenia, so diagnosing HIT after cardiac surgery is challenging. The 4 Ts score (thrombocytopenia, timing, thrombosis, other cause of thrombocytopenia) is frequently used to determine when to obtain laboratory tests for HIT. In one study, patients who developed HIT after cardiac surgery had a mortality risk of 21.8% and a thromboembolic risk of 29.1% versus a non-HIT risk of 5.3% and 2.9% for mortality and thromboembolism, respectively.[52] Furthermore, for patients who develop HIT before a planned cardiac surgery, it is recommended to delay surgery until the patient is HIT negative if the clinical situation allows. There is no anamnestic response to HIT antigens so patients with prior HIT can be re-exposed to unfractionated heparin if there is no alternative for anticoagulation on cardiopulmonary bypass.[57]

Following confirmation of the diagnosis of HIT or HITT, the immediate first step in treatment is cessation of heparin administration and removal of all heparin-coated catheters, followed by anticoagulation with an alternative agent. Alternatives include intravenous direct thrombin inhibitors such as argatroban (metabolized by liver, so caution in patients with liver dysfunction is advised) and bivalirudin (a shorter-acting anticoagulant that is excreted by the kidneys). Oral anticoagulants such as warfarin, dabigatran, rivaroxaban, and apixaban are recommended after the platelet count has recovered. Warfarin requires close monitoring because of its low therapeutic index, whereas dabigatran, rivaroxaban, and apixaban have been shown to be superior to warfarin in stroke and embolism prevention but pose an increased risk of gastrointestinal bleeding.[58,59]

Respiratory Complications

Respiratory complications are common after cardiac surgery and include atelectasis in 50% to 80%,[60] pleural effusions in 10% to 40%,[61] adult respiratory distress syndrome (ARDS) in 0.4% to 20%,[62,63] pneumonia in 3.1% to 35%,[64,65] phrenic nerve injury in 10% to 21%,[66,67] pneumothorax in 0.7% to 1.7%,[61,67,68] and pulmonary embolism from deep vein thrombosis in 0.3% to 9.5%.[61,69,70] Radiographic atelectasis is seen in the early postoperative period because of lung deflation during cannulation for cardio-pulmonary bypass, internal mammary artery harvest, and manual compression of the lungs during heart exposure. This atelectasis normally responds to recruitment maneuvers during or after separation from cardiopulmonary bypass. In the ICU, symptomatic and radiographic atelectasis can occur due to impaired pain relief and chest wall splinting, impaired ciliary mobility and inspissation of secretions, gastric distension, and pleural effusions. Once the definitive cause is addressed, early postoperative mobility, chest physiotherapy, and pain control are important to maintain lung recruitment. Multimodal pain control including nonopioid medications and regional anesthesia with erector spinae plane or serratus anterior blocks can improve respiratory effort.

Postoperative hypoxia without major radiographic abnormalities is seen in 30% of patients after cardiac surgery and is associated with blood transfusions, inflammatory response generated by cardiopulmonary bypass, and aortic surgery.[61,67,71] Postoperative hypoxia usually resolves without intervention within 48 to 72 hours.

Patients with pre-existing chronic obstructive pulmonary disease and deconditioning are at increased risk of postoperative pneumonia. Furthermore, patients on prolonged mechanical ventilation (greater than 48 hours) are prone to develop ventilator-associated pneumonia.

Stroke, Delirium, and Atrial Fibrillation

Perioperative stroke can be categorized into early/intraoperative and delayed/postoperative after cardiac surgery. The mechanisms of stroke are primarily aortic manipulation in early stroke and atrial fibrillation, cerebrovascular disease, and cannulation and decannulation from ECMO in delayed stroke.[72] There is a 0.8% to 5.2% incidence of stroke after cardiac surgery, which is an important cause of death, prolonged hospitalization, and long-term disability.[73] Early awakening immediately after cardiac surgery is important to identify this devastating complication. Seizure prophylaxis, blood pressure augmentation, and early initiation of statin and aspirin therapy are important treatment considerations depending on the size and etiology of the postoperative stroke.

Delirium occurs in up to 50% of cardiac surgery patients and is associated with increased costs, length of stay in the ICU and hospital, long-term mortality, perioperative morbidity, and cognitive decline in a subset of patients experiencing delirium.[74–78] Perioperative factors predictive of delirium include older age, urgent surgery, hypertension, diabetes, preoperative cognitive decline or depression, carotid artery stenosis, New York Heart Association classification III or IV, increased length of stay in the ICU (possibly due to lack of sleep hygiene), and mechanical ventilation. Intraoperative findings such as low cerebral oximetry at baseline, low relative alpha waves and high theta waves on bispectral index raw data, and elevated cortisol and interleukin-6 levels appear to be associated with a higher incidence of delirium postoperatively.[79,80] Management of delirium includes a combination of supportive measures (restoring vision with glasses, dentures, sleep hygiene, addressing language barriers, etc.), minimizing benzodiazepine use, optimizing pain control with a multimodal approach, and early mobilization.[81] Recently, studies suggest that low-dose nocturnal dexmedetomidine may prevent delirium in some surgical and medically ill ICU patients in conjunction with reduction of other medications.[82–84]

New-onset atrial fibrillation occurs in up to 35% of cardiac surgery patients, versus 1% to 15% after noncardiac and nonthoracic surgery.[85] Inflammation, surgical trauma, presence of pericardial fluid, volume overload, electrolyte abnormalities, and cardiopulmonary bypass have been implicated in new-onset postoperative atrial fibrillation.[85] Furthermore, atrial fibrillation is an independent risk factor for adverse events postoperatively, associated with an increased risk of stroke, respiratory and renal failure, bleeding, and reoperation.

TECHNIQUES FREQUENTLY USED IN THE CARDIOTHORACIC INTENSIVE CARE UNIT
Ultrasonography and Echocardiography

Critical care ultrasonography and echocardiography (basic and advanced) may provide critical hemodynamic and therapeutic information in the intensive care setting.[86] In the CTICU, competence in ultrasonography and echocardiography is useful in inotropic decisions, initiation and weaning from mechanical support, need for reoperations, and deciding vascular access anatomy. Both transesophageal echocardiography (TEE) and transthoracic echocardiography (TTE) are important options for imaging in the cardiac surgery patient. The presence of thoracostomy tubes, postoperative dressings, and anatomic changes after cardiac surgery can make for difficult image acquisition with TTE; hence, TEE may be required. The use of TEE necessitates additional training expertise on the part of the intensivist. Complications can include endotracheal tube dislodgement (0.03%), laryngospasm and bronchospasm in nonintubated patients (0.06%–0.14%), and esophageal injury and perforation (0.01%–0.3%).[87,88]

Cannulation

Patients requiring ECMO require thoughtful venous and arterial cannulation after a complete assessment is made of vascular integrity. Presence of prior arterial or venous injury, thrombosis, presence of inferior vena cava filters, peripheral vascular disease, atheromatous aortic disease, and aortic dissection or aneurysm can aid in decision-making for arterial or venous cannulation. Echocardiography can assist in cannula insertion and positioning.

HEMODYNAMIC MONITORING

A pulmonary artery catheter (PAC) provides information above a central venous catheter, including filling pressures, cardiac output and indices, and mixed venous oxygen saturation. The use of a PAC has not resulted in improved mortality or morbidity after routine cardiac surgery.[89] PAC-based interventions may have a role in inotropic initiation and weaning in patients undergoing heart transplantation, VAD placement, multiple valvular procedures, and complex coronary and valve interventions. The lack of benefit in studies may have been due to inadequate training of providers. Continuous cardiac output PACs provide additional information including current cardiac output and mixed venous oxygen saturation.

Pulse wave analysis monitors are emerging to provide beat-to-beat cardiac output information using proprietary algorithms to analyze the arterial waveform. Noninvasive cardiac output monitor, FloTrac, and bioreactance monitors are examples of such devices. Some of these are able to generate a hypotension prediction index up to 15 minutes before occurrence by analyzing waveform patterns, amplitude, area, and segment slopes.[90]

Right ventricular ejection fraction (RVEF) catheters provide information regarding RV function. With the advent of echocardiography, RVEF and function can be estimated with TAPSE, RV fractional area change, RV strain measurements, and RV 3D measurements on both TTE and TEE.

Mechanical Circulatory Support

Patients with MCS are frequently managed in some CTICUs. MCS encompasses a spectrum of configurations for isolated cardiac, pulmonary, or combined cardiopulmonary support. MCS provides a bridge to definitive therapy or recovery, and clear discussion about its temporary nature should be conducted before the initiation of therapy.

Direct circulatory support is provided by VA ECMO and is reserved for patients in refractory cardiogenic shock on multiple vasoactive medications. Patients on VA ECMO require daily monitoring of machine-related factors including cannula position, adequacy of the oxygenator, measurement of flow, and end-organ perfusion and patient-related factors such as anticoagulation adequacy, degree of hemolysis, occurrence of bleeding and thrombosis, and end-organ function.

Indirect circulatory support is provided by VV ECMO and is used for refractory respiratory failure. Initiation of VV ECMO results in reduction in pulmonary vascular resistance and respiratory acidosis, which provides hemodynamic support and lung rest.[91]

Temporary assist devices are available for isolated left, right, or in combination for biventricular support. The Impella (family consisting of the Impella CP, 3.5, 5.5, and 5.0 LD that provide cardiac output from 3.5 L to 5.5 L) is inserted via the femoral or axillary artery for LV support. The Impella RP is placed into the pulmonary artery via the femoral vein for right ventricular support.[71] Similarly, the TandemHeart (LivaNova, London, UK) family consists of the Protek Solo device for LV support (transseptally placed 2 cannula approach) and the Protek Duo device (placed via the right internal jugular vein into the main pulmonary artery) for RV support. These devices are percutaneously placed and require either fluoroscopic or echocardiographic expertise for placement.

WHO SHOULD PROVIDE CARE IN THE CARDIOTHORACIC INTENSIVE CARE UNIT?

As discussed in this article, the CTICU physician needs to understand cardiopulmonary physiology and have experience dealing with all the patient types, surgical procedures, postoperative complications, and techniques discussed. In addition, the provider should have fellowship-level training in critical care medicine for two reasons. First, advanced management of many postoperative problems such as septic shock and ARDS are routinely managed in critical care medicine. While less common in the CTICU, they are nonetheless complications that may occur. Second, there has been a shift toward surgery in patients with more complex cardiac disease with worse ventricular function, more pulmonary hypertension, more comorbidities, increased frailty, and older age. As a result, patients are more likely to have complications of hemorrhage, poor LV function, poor right ventricular function, prolonged intubation, postoperative renal failure, and altered mental status. The best care of the CTICU patient is provided by a multidisciplinary collaboration that includes the critical care physician; the cardiac surgeon; providers with relevant expertise such as the heart failure cardiologist, the lung transplant pulmonologist, the infectious disease expert, and the neurologist; as well as allied health professionals such as a respiratory therapist, pharmacist, nutritionist, and physical therapist.

Anesthesiologists have had leadership roles in critical care medicine since the earliest days of the specialty. Anesthesiologists, especially cardiac anesthesiologists, have had increasing roles in CTICUs throughout the past half-century. One advantage of dual-fellowship-trained anesthesiologists (cardiac anesthesia and critical care medicine) is their advanced echocardiography skills that include both TTE and TEE. Cardiac anesthesiologists who work in both the operating room and the CTICU collaborate with cardiac surgeons in both arenas, have a deep understanding of MCS, and recognize how decisions made in the operating room affect the postoperative course in the CTICU as, in many respects, postoperative care of the cardiac surgery patient is an extension of intraoperative anesthetic management. Dual-trained cardiac anesthesiologists add value in being able to immediately take a patient from the CTICU to the operating room in an emergency situation. Cardiac anesthesiologists without critical care fellowship training have many of the skills of the dual-trained anesthesiologists. Although they have not completed critical care fellowship, they frequently have had extensive critical care and CTICU experience during anesthesia residency and cardiac anesthesia fellowship and have worked extensively with the cardiac surgeons in the operating room.

As discussed at the beginning of this article, there is a growing specialty of critical care cardiology.[7] Some data demonstrate improved survival with cardiology providers with expertise in critical care medicine practicing in closed CCUs. Although the focus of these units has primarily been on nonsurgical patients, critical care cardiologists have relevant training and experience for CTICU patient management, either as a primary physician or as a consultant.

Physicians with training in internal medicine or emergency medicine who have also completed critical care medicine fellowship are increasingly involved in CTICU. Although they have outstanding critical care skills, their training normally does not include TEE, advanced MCS, or experience in the cardiac operating room. Therefore, these providers often gain additional experience with a "mini-fellowship" in CTICU before becoming independent CTICU providers.

SUMMARY

Cardiopulmonary bypass was first used clinically 70 years ago. Since then, cardiac surgery and the postoperative care of the cardiac surgery patient have markedly advanced. As a result, we can now successfully operate on patients who are older, have more complex and advanced cardiac disease, and have more noncardiac comorbidities such as renal, respiratory, and neurologic dysfunction. Successful outcomes can require advanced techniques such as TEE, viscoelastic testing, and MCS. However, success in the care of the postoperative cardiac surgery has also depended on the development of CTICU providers with expertise in cardiac physiology and in critical care medicine. In the future, CTICU may develop into its own specialty, combining the skills and expertise from the different specialties involved in care of the CTICU patient.

CLINICS CARE POINTS

- Low cardiac output syndrome following cardiac surgery can be due to multiple etiologies, including left ventricular failure, right ventricular failure, biventricular failure, and cardiac tamponade.

- Echocardiography (transthoracic or transesophageal) can help identify the etiology of low cardiac output syndrome following cardiac surgery.

- Surgical complications such as coronary artery injury should be considered when patients have low cardiac output or excessive bleeding after cardiac surgery.

- Excessive bleeding after cardiac surgery requires aggressive diagnosis and treatment and may require re-sternotomy if not responsive to transfusion of blood and blood products.

- The management of cardiac arrest after cardiac surgery differs from standard ACLS and should include rapid re-sternotomy and preparation for mechanical circulatory support if return of spontaneous circulation does not rapidly occur.

DISCLOSURE

The authors have nothing to disclose.

REFERENCES

1. Stephens RS, Whitman GJ. Postoperative critical care of the adult cardiac surgical patient: Part II: Procedure-specific considerations, management of complications, and quality improvement. Crit Care Med 2015;43:1995–2014.
2. Kopanczyk R, Kumar N, Bhatt AM. A brief history of cardiothoracic surgical critical care medicine in the United States. Medicina (Kaunas) 2022;58:1856.
3. Miller PE, Chouairi F, Thomas A, et al. Transition from an open to closed staffing model in the cardiac Intensive Care Unit improves clinical outcomes. J Am Heart Assoc 2021;10:e018182.
4. O'Malley RG, Olenchock B, Bohula-May E, et al. Organization and staffing practices in US cardiac intensive care units: a survey on behalf of the American heart association Writing Group on the Evolution of critical care cardiology. Eur Heart J Acute Cardiovasc Care 2013;2:3–8.
5. Brusca SB, Barnett C, Barnhart BJ, et al. Role of critical care medicine training in the cardiovascular Intensive Care Unit: survey responses from dual certified critical care cardiologists. J Am Heart Assoc 2019;8:e011721.
6. Lüsebrink E, Kellnar A, Scherer C, et al. New challenges in cardiac intensive care units. Clin Res Cardiol 2021;110:1369–79.
7. Morrow DA, Fang JC, Fintel DJ, et al. Evolution of critical care cardiology: transformation of the cardiovascular intensive care unit and the emerging need for new medical staffing and training models: a scientific statement from the American Heart Association. Circulation 2012;126:1408–28.
8. Bonnefoy-Cudraz E, Bueno H, Casella G, et al. Editor's Choice - acute cardiovascular care association position paper on Intensive Cardiovascular Care Units: an update on their definition, structure, organisation and function. Eur Heart J Acute Cardiovasc Care 2018;7:80–95.
9. Katz JN, Minder M, Olenchock B, et al. The genesis, maturation, and future of critical care cardiology. J Am Coll Cardiol 2016;68:67–79.
10. Gross CR, Adams DH, Patel P, et al. Failure to Rescue: a quality metric for cardiac surgery and cardiovascular critical care. Can J Cardiol 2023;39:487–96. S0828-282X(23)00003-X.
11. Charlesworth M, Klein A. Enhanced recovery after cardiac surgery. Anesthesiol Clin 2022;40:143–55.
12. Stephens RS, Whitman GJ. Postoperative critical care of the adult cardiac surgical patient. Part I: routine postoperative care. Crit Care Med 2015;43:1477–97.
13. Freundt M, Lavanga E, Brehm C. Optimal, early postoperative management of cardiac transplant and durable left ventricular assist recipients. Curr Cardiol Rep 2022;2023–9.
14. Di Nardo M, Tikkanen J, Husain S, et al. Postoperative management of lung transplant recipients in the Intensive Care Unit. Anesthesiology 2022;136:482–99.
15. De Paulis S, Arlotta G, Calabrese M, et al. Postoperative intensive care management of aortic repair. J Pers Med 2022;12:1351.
16. Kratzert WB, Boyd EK, Schwarzenberger JC. Management of the critically ill adult with congenital heart disease. J Cardiothorac Vasc Anesth 2018;32:1682–700.
17. Kim C, Vigneshwar M, Nicolato P. Extracorporeal cardiopulmonary resuscitation: is it futile? Curr Opin Anaesthesiol 2022;35:190–4.

18. Abrams D, MacLaren G, Lorusso R, et al. Extracorporeal cardiopulmonary resuscitation in adults: evidence and implications. Intensive Care Med 2022;4:1–15.

19. Brand J, McDonald A, Dunning J. Management of cardiac arrest following cardiac surgery. BJA Educ 2018f;18:16–22.

20. Rus IA, Kudela M, Suffredini G, et al. Implementing change in the care of the complex cardiac patient. Curr Opin Anaesthesiol 2023;36:57–60.

21. Colson PH, Gaudard P, Fellahi JL, et al. Active bleeding after cardiac surgery: a prospective observational multicenter study. PLoS One 2016;11:e0162396.

22. Elassal AA, Al-Ebrahim KE, Debis RS, et al. Re-exploration for bleeding after cardiac surgery: revaluation of urgency and factors promoting low rate. J Cardiothorac Surg 2021;16:166.

23. Karthik S, Grayson AD, McCarron EE, et al. Reexploration for bleeding after coronary artery bypass surgery: risk factors, outcomes, and the effect of time delay. Ann Thorac Surg 2004;78:527–34.

24. Kristensen KL, Rauer LJ, Mortensen PE, et al. Reoperation for bleeding in cardiac surgery. Interact Cardiov Th 2012;14:709–13.

25. Hall TS, Brevetti GR, Skoultchi AJ, et al. Re-exploration for hemorrhage following open heart surgery differentiation on the causes of bleeding and the impact on patient outcomes. Ann Thorac Cardiovasc Surg Official J Assoc Thorac Cardiovasc Surg Asia 2001;7:352–7.

26. Bolliger D, Tanaka KA. Coagulation management strategies in cardiac surgery. Curr Anesthesiol Reports 2017;7:265–72.

27. Gill R, Herbertson M, Vuylsteke A, et al. Safety and efficacy of recombinant activated factor VII. Circulation 2009;120:21–7.

28. Levi M, Levy JH, Andersen HF, et al. Safety of recombinant activated factor VII in randomized clinical trials. New Engl J Med 2010;363:1791–800.

29. Siegal DM, Garcia DA, Crowther MA. How I treat target-specific oral anticoagulant–associated bleeding. Blood 2014;123:1152–8.

30. Raleigh L, Cole SP. Con: factor concentrate usage in cardiac surgery—a paucity of data limits their universal adoption. J Cardiothor Vasc An 2018;32:1068–71.

31. Leiva EH, Carreño M, Bucheli FR, et al. Factors associated with delayed cardiac tamponade after cardiac surgery. Ann Cardiac Anaesth 2018;21:158–66.

32. Khan NK, Järvelä KM, Loisa EL, et al. Incidence, presentation and risk factors of late postoperative pericardial effusions requiring invasive treatment after cardiac surgery. Interact Cardiovasc Thorac Surg 2017;24:835–40.

33. Maranta F, Cianfanelli L, Grippo R, et al. Post-pericardiotomy syndrome: insights into neglected postoperative issues. Eur J Cardiothorac 2021;61:505–14.

34. Imazio M. The post-pericardiotomy syndrome. Curr Opin Pulm Med 2012;18:366–74.

35. Turillazzi E, Giammarco GD, Neri M, et al. Coronary ostia obstruction after replacement of aortic valve prosthesis. Diagn Pathol 2011;6:72.

36. Santini F, Pentiricci S, Messina A, et al. Coronary ostial enlargement to prevent stenosis after prosthetic aortic valve replacement. Ann Thorac Surg 2004;77:1854–6.

37. Pillai JB, Pillay TM, Ahmad J. Coronary ostial stenosis after aortic valve replacement, revisited. Ann Thorac Surg 2004;78:2169–71.

38. Thomopoulou S, Sfirakis P, Spargias K. Angioplasty, stenting and thrombectomy to correct left main coronary stem obstruction by a bioprosthetic aortic valve. J Invasive Cardiol 2008;20:E124–5.

39. Hiltrop N, Bennett J, Desmet W. Circumflex coronary artery injury after mitral valve surgery: a report of four cases and comprehensive review of the literature. Cathet Cardiovasc Intervent 2017;89:78–92.

40. Svedjeholm R, Håkanson E. Postoperative myocardial ischemia caused by chest tube compression of vein graft. Ann Thorac Surg 1997;64:1806–8.

41. Sulimovic S, Noyez L. Postoperative myocardial ischemia caused by compression of a coronary artery by chest tube. J Cardiovasc Surg 2006;47:371–2.

42. Kwiatt M, Tarbox A, Seamon MJ, et al. Thoracostomy tubes: a comprehensive review of complications and related topics. Int J Critical Illn Inj Sci 2014;4:143–55.

43. Levy D, Laghlam D, Estagnasie P, et al. Post-operative right ventricular failure after cardiac surgery: a cohort study. Frontiers Cardiovasc Medicine 2021;8:667328.

44. Estep JD, Stainback RF, Little SH, et al. The role of echocardiography and other imaging modalities in patients with left ventricular assist devices. Jacc Cardiovasc Imaging 2010;3:1049–64.

45. Stainback RF, Estep JD, Agler DA, et al. Echocardiography in the management of patients with left ventricular assist devices: Recommendations from the American Society of Echocardiography. J Am Soc Echocardiog 2015;28:853–909.

46. Ichinose FJDR, Zapol WM. Inhaled nitric oxide. Circulation 2004;109:3106–11.

47. Kallet RH. Expanding the use of inhaled vasodilators in managing right ventricular dysfunction in the emergency and critical care setting: should we broaden our vision? Respir Care 2019;64:864–5.

48. Enomoto TM, Treggiari MM, Yanez ND, et al. Inhaled iloprost versus epoprostenol in heart transplant recipients. Respir Care 2019;64:743–51.

49. McGinn K, Reichert M. A Comparison of inhaled nitric oxide versus inhaled epoprostenol for acute pulmonary hypertension following cardiac surgery. Ann Pharmacother 2016;50:22–6.

50. Krug S, Sablotzki A, Hammerschmidt S, et al. Inhaled iloprost for the control of pulmonary hypertension. Vasc Heal Risk Management 2009;5:465–74.

51. Thunberg CA, Morozowich ST, Ramakrishna H. Inhaled therapy for the management of perioperative pulmonary hypertension. Ann Cardiac Anaesth 2015;18:394–402.

52. Brown JA, Aranda-Michel E, Kilic A, et al. Outcomes with heparin-induced thrombocytopenia after cardiac surgery. Ann Thorac Surg 2021;112:487–93.

53. Pishko AM, Cuker A. Heparin-induced thrombocytopenia and cardiovascular surgery. Hematology 2021;2021:536–44.

54. Pishko A, Cuker A. Heparin-induced thrombocytopenia in cardiac surgery patients. Semin Thromb Hemost 2017;43:691–8.

55. Holmes-Ghosh E. Heparin-induced thrombocytopenia and thrombosis syndrome after cardiopulmonary bypass. Am J Critical Care 2000;9:276–8.

56. Szokol JW. Heparin-induced thrombocytopenia. Seminars Cardiothorac Vasc Anesthesia 2010;14:73–4.

57. Warkentin TE, Greinacher A. Heparin-induced thrombocytopenia and cardiac surgery. Ann Thorac Surg 2003;76:2121–31.

58. Ho PJ, Siordia JA. Dabigatran approaching the realm of heparin-induced thrombocytopenia. Blood Res 2016;51:77–87.

59. Lauffenburger JC, Farley JF, Gehi AK, et al. Effectiveness and safety of dabigatran and warfarin in real-world us patients with non-valvular atrial fibrillation: a retrospective cohort study. J Am Heart Assoc 2015;4:e001798.

60. Szelkowski LA, Puri NK, Singh R, et al. Current trends in preoperative, intraoperative, and postoperative care of the adult cardiac surgery patient. Curr Prob Surg 2015;52:531–69.
61. Weissman C. Pulmonary complications after cardiac surgery. Seminars Cardiothorac Vasc Anesthesia 2004;8:185–211.
62. Asimakopoulos G, Taylor KM, Smith PL, et al. Prevalence of acute respiratory distress syndrome after cardiac surgery. J Thorac Cardiovasc Surg 1999;117:620–1.
63. Kor DJ, Lingineni RK, Gajic O, et al. Predicting risk of postoperative lung injury in high-risk surgical patients. Anesthesiology 2014;120:1168–81.
64. Allou N, Bronchard R, Guglielminotti J, et al. Risk factors for postoperative pneumonia after cardiac surgery and development of a preoperative risk score. Crit Care Med 2014;42:1150–6.
65. He S, Chen B, Li W, et al. Ventilator-associated pneumonia after cardiac surgery: a meta-analysis and systematic review. J Thorac Cardiovasc Surg 2014;148:3148–55.
66. Canbaz S, Turgut N, Halici U, et al. Electrophysiological evaluation of phrenic nerve injury during cardiac surgery – a prospective, controlled, clinical study. BMC Surg 2004;4:2.
67. Tanner TG, Colvin MO. Pulmonary complications of cardiac surgery. Lung 2020;198:889896.
68. Urschel JD, Parrott JC, Horan TA, et al. Pneumothorax complicating cardiac surgery. J Cardiovasc Surg 1992;33:492–5.
69. Josa M, Siouffi SY, Silverman AB, et al. Pulmonary embolism after cardiac surgery. J Am Coll Cardiol 1993;21:990–6.
70. Ho KM, Bham E, Pavey W. Incidence of venous thromboembolism and benefits and risks of thromboprophylaxis after cardiac surgery: a systematic review and meta-analysis. J Am Heart Assoc 2015;4:e002652.
71. Rong LQ, Franco AD, Gaudino M. Acute respiratory distress syndrome after cardiac surgery. J Thorac Dis 2016;8:E1177–86.
72. Gaudino M, Rahouma M, Mauro MD, et al. Early versus delayed stroke after cardiac surgery: a systematic review and meta-analysis. J Am Heart Assoc 2019;8:e012447.
73. Sun LY, Tu JV, Lee DS, et al. Disability–free survival after coronary artery bypass grafting in women and men with heart failure. Open Hear 2018;5:e000911.
74. Rudolph JL, Inouye SK, Jones RN, et al. Delirium: an independent predictor of functional decline after cardiac surgery. J Am Geriatr Soc 2010;58:643–9.
75. Gottesman RF, Grega MA, Bailey MM, et al. Delirium after coronary artery bypass graft surgery and late mortality. Ann Neurol 2010;67:338–44.
76. Martin BJ, Buth KJ, Arora RC, et al. Delirium as a predictor of sepsis in post-coronary artery bypass grafting patients: a retrospective cohort study. Crit Care 2010;14:R171.
77. Brown CH, Probert J, Healy R, et al. Cognitive decline after delirium in patients undergoing cardiac surgery. Anesthesiology 2018;129:406–16.
78. Brown CH. Delirium in the cardiac surgical ICU. Curr Opin Anaesthesiol 2014;27:117–22.
79. Schoen J, Meyerrose J, Paarmann H, et al. Preoperative regional cerebral oxygen saturation is a predictor of postoperative delirium in on-pump cardiac surgery patients: a prospective observational trial. Crit Care 2011;15:R218.

80. Plaschke K, Fichtenkamm P, Schramm C, et al. Early postoperative delirium after open-heart cardiac surgery is associated with decreased bispectral EEG and increased cortisol and interleukin-6. Intensive Care Med 2010;36:2081–9.

81. Barr J, Kishman CP, Jaeschke R. The methodological approach used to develop the 2013 Pain, Agitation, and Delirium Clinical Practice Guidelines for adult ICU patients. Crit Care Med 2013;41:S1–15.

82. Su X, Meng ZT, Wu XH, et al. Dexmedetomidine for prevention of delirium in elderly patients after non-cardiac surgery: a randomised, double-blind, placebo-controlled trial. Lancet 2016;388:1893–902.

83. Skrobik Y, Duprey MS, Hill NS, et al. Low-dose nocturnal dexmedetomidine prevents ICU delirium. A randomized, placebo-controlled trial. Am J Resp Crit Care 2018;197:1147–56.

84. Nuzzo E, Girard TD. The sandman in the ICU: a novel use of dexmedetomidine? Am J Resp Crit Care 2018;197:1098–9.

85. Greenberg JW, Lancaster TS, Schuessler RB, et al. Postoperative atrial fibrillation following cardiac surgery: a persistent complication. Eur J Cardio Thorac Surg 2017;52:665–72.

86. Mayo PH, Beaulieu Y, Doelken P, et al. American College of chest physicians/La Société de Réanimation de Langue Française statement on competence in critical care ultrasonography. Chest 2009;135:1050–60.

87. Hahn RT, Abraham T, Adams MS, et al. Guidelines for performing a comprehensive transesophageal echocardiographic examination: Recommendations from the American Society of echocardiography and the Society of cardiovascular anesthesiologists. J Am Soc Echocardiog 2013;26:921–64.

88. Nicoara A, Skubas N, Ad N, et al. Guidelines for the use of transesophageal echocardiography to assist with surgical decision-making in the operating room: a surgery-based approach from the American Society of Echocardiography in collaboration with the Society of Cardiovascular Anesthesiologists and the Society of Thoracic Surgeons. J Am Soc Echocardiog 2020;33:692–734.

89. Brown JA, Aranda-Michel E, Kilic A, et al. The impact of pulmonary artery catheter use in cardiac surgery. J Thorac Cardiovasc Surg 2022;164:1965–73.

90. Maheshwari K, Shimada T, Fang J, et al. Hypotension Prediction Index software for management of hypotension during moderate- to high-risk noncardiac surgery: protocol for a randomized trial. Trials 2019;20:255.

91. Cole SP, Martinez-Acero N, Peterson A, et al. Imaging for temporary mechanical circulatory support devices. J Cardiothorac Vasc Anesth 2022;36:2114–23.

Four Decades of Intensive Care Unit Design Evolution and Thoughts for the Future

Neil A. Halpern, MD, MCCM, FCCP, FACP[a,b,]*,
Elizabeth Scruth, PhD, MPH, RN, CNS, CCRN-K, CCNS, FCCM, FCNS, CPHQ[c],
Michelle Rausen, MS, RRT, RRT-NPS[d], Diana Anderson, MD, MArch[e]

KEYWORDS

- Intensive care unit • Critical care unit • Design • Evolution • Informatics
- Future-proofing

KEY POINTS

- The design of adult intensive care units (ICUs) in the United States has evolved significantly over four decades from the mid-1980s until 2022.
- ICUs have transformed from beds in open spaces to single-bed patient rooms with associated enhancements in patient privacy, safety, infection control, aesthetics, and experiences for patients, visitors, and staff.
- Hospitals and ICUs have shifted from paper-based medical records to electronic health records; this change guides the design to support advanced computers and displays.
- As medical device technologies evolve, standalone devices (ie, physiologic monitors, mechanical ventilators, infusion pumps and ICU beds) are now health care informatics platforms.
- Connectivity, interoperability, and association of the patient with all technologies and caregivers, data management and alarm distribution are now integral to ICU design.

INTRODUCTION

Over the past four decades intensive care unit (ICU) design has evolved. Herein, we explore the design changes that have occurred primarily in adult ICUs in the United States. Our discussion is predicated on our combined ICU design writings,[1–4] work

[a] Critical Care Center, Department of Anesthesiology and Critical Care, Memorial Sloan Kettering Cancer Center, 1275 York Avenue, C-1179, New York, NY 10065, USA; [b] Department of Anesthesiology, Weill Cornell Medical College, New York, NY, USA; [c] Kaiser Permanente, NCAL Quality, Safety, Risk Department, 1950 Franklin Street, 14th Floor Quality Department, Oakland, CA 94612-1950, USA; [d] Respiratory Therapy, Department of Anesthesiology and Critical Care, Memorial Sloan Kettering Cancer Center, 1275 York Avenue, C-1176A, New York, NY 10065, USA; [e] VA Boston Healthcare System, 150 S Huntington Avenue, Room 12C-34C, Boston, MA 02130, USA
* Corresponding author.
E-mail address: halpernn@mskcc.org

Crit Care Clin 39 (2023) 577–602
https://doi.org/10.1016/j.ccc.2023.01.008
0749-0704/23/© 2023 Elsevier Inc. All rights reserved.

experiences, visits to many ICUs, participation in decades of the ICU design award process of the Society of Critical Care Medicine (SCCM),[5] reviews of ICU design guidelines from the SCCM,[6,7] International Health Facility Guidelines (iHFG),[8] US Department of Health and Humans Services (DHHS) Guidelines,[9] Facility Guideline Institute (FGI)[10] and long-term ICU design architectural analyses.[11–14] We also compare the 1983-1984 and 2022 FGI design guidelines and briefly address "future-proofing," namely, anticipating the future design needs for ICUs.

Background Intensive Care Unit Data

It is difficult to accurately determine the number of ICUs in US hospitals. Using 2020 American Hospital Association (AHA) data, there were approximately 3000 acute care hospitals (nonfederal short-term general and other special) with ICUs.[15] Assuming an average of 2 to 3 adult ICUs per hospital, there are approximately 6000 to 9000 ICUs in the United States with an estimated 83,000 adult ICU beds. Larger hospitals have multiple ICUs that are more specialized than ICUs in smaller hospitals. To the best of our knowledge, it is not possible to approximate the number of ICUs that have been renovated or newly built over time.

In the past, smaller units (8 to 14 beds/ICU) dominated and were built where space was available. Current ICUs, especially in newly constructed acute care towers (pavilions), seem to be large units (ie, $\geq$20 beds/ICU) that are co-located (ie, either on the same floor or stacked one on top of another) to take advantage of economies of scale (**Fig. 1**). In theory, the modern ICU-centric environment allows for pharmacy, imaging, respiratory therapy, supply chain, and critical care office space to support all the ICUs. This scenario may optimize staff requirements and transit times for devices, supplies, and imaging equipment. In addition, these towers may co-locate operating rooms and interventional radiology (IR) procedural suites near the ICUs as well.

Evolution of Intensive Care Unit Design

ICU design began in the 1950s to 1960s.[16,17] However, in the early days of ICU design, there was a dearth of available information to inform the design process, and often general wards or other hospital spaces were adapted for use as an ICU. Currently, there are outstanding award-winning ICU designs and family-centered ICU care innovation strategies available for study through the SCCM website,[5] ICU design publications, and evidence-based design studies.[18–20] ICU design writings now include strategic thinking[21,22] and capacity modeling[23,24] to address the optimal number of ICU beds and ICU locations. This process has also expanded to include ICUs within Emergency Departments[25–28] and placement of Stepdown Units as standalone or co-located within ICUs.[29,30]

Local hospital administrative and clinical organizational culture guide ICU design development.[1,31] For decades the design planning process relied on physical drawings and mockups.[2] Currently design engagement has shifted to dynamic, three-dimensional electronic displays and virtual reality imaging that are provided by both vendors and architects.[20] Finally, ICU design articles traditionally addressed ICU design as the process to build a new ICU. However, today, ICU design has expanded to include "re"design within functioning ICUs as hospitals refurbish existing ICUs.[32,33] Such evolution in busy ICUs operating under exigent circumstances was highlighted by acute ICU redesign during the recent coronavirus disease-2019 (COVID-19) pandemic.[34]

Anecdotally, there has been a swinging pendulum in the makeup of ICU design teams. Initially, these teams were composed primarily of hospital administrators

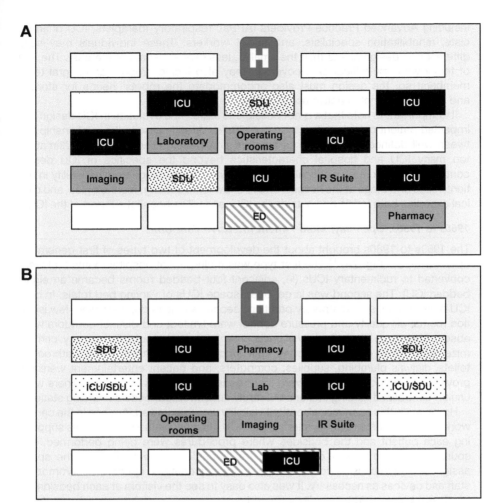

Fig. 1. Location of ICU within a hospital. ICUs are positioned randomly in a hospital with no relation to SDUs, the ED or other core hospital services (*A*). Today, in inpatient acute care towers, ICUs and SDUs are purposefully located taking advantage of core facilities (*B*). In B, SDUs are either combined with an ICU or located next to an ICU. In addition, an ICU is incorporated within an ED. SDU-Step-Down Unit. ED-Emergency Department. IR-Interventional Radiology.

and architects with minimal input from providers of critical care medicine (CCM). As time passed, broad-based and in-depth participation by ICU clinical leaders and the ancillary staff was sought to create a more inclusive design team that incorporated expert advice of end users.[1,35] However, more recently, with the building of large inpatient hospital pavilions, we have seen a transition back to administrators and architects with minimal CCM involvement as universal acuity-adaptable inpatient room design with minor customization for ICU-level care has returned to the fore.[36–39]

Another element that should be considered in the design process is the evolution of ICU staffing. There has been a shift in all types of medical centers from an ICU team made up of only physicians and nurses to much larger multidisciplinary teams including Advanced Practice Providers (APPs), respiratory therapists, ICU pharmacists, rehabilitation specialists, and social workers. These individuals may have different ICU design needs than the smaller, less diverse teams of the past. The ICU of today with tele-critical care coverage may also include robots as integral team members; so, the design must also accommodate the robots' needs for storage and power when not in active use.[40]

It is important to note that it is not possible to state if the evolution in ICU design has impacted patient outcomes because few studies directly assess the relationship between well-defined ICU design parameters and patient outcomes.[41–43] Ultimately, too many ICU and hospital characteristics beyond the specifics of ICU design contribute to outcomes of critically ill ICU patients. These range from variability in patient intake and triage at the hospital and ICU levels, to staffing, technologies, and clinical expertise both inside and outside the ICU, as well as hospital support of the ICUs.

1960s to 1980s: Open Bay, Multi-Patient Intensive Care Units

The 1960s to 1980s brought about the development of two types of first-generation open bay ICUs (**Fig. 2**A).[17] The first type was multi-patient hospital rooms that were converted to rudimentary ICUs (ie, adjacent four-bedded rooms became an eight-bedded ICU). The second was large, open-space ICUs of varying bed totals. In both ICU types, curtains, or temporary partitions separated the beds; there were few isolation rooms; air quality and pressure control were limited; and distinct corridors were absent. There was little in the way of environmental control to establish privacy, or minimize transmission of infection, sound, light, smoke, or fire. Similarly, sinks, bathrooms, toilets, dialysis plumbing, supplies, computers, and patient entertainment were not provided at each bedside. Nor were there bedside amenities for visitors. There were usually centralized nursing stations but rarely decentralized, bedside nursing stations.

However, in this open model, patient visibility was maximized. Anyone in the central work area could visualize the entirety of the ICU, the associated technologies supporting each patient and the bedsides where procedures were being performed. Resources could be rapidly deployed to the bedside. In the open ICU, the space assigned to each bedside could "stretch" to the adjacent bed space to accommodate staff and devices as necessary. It was also easy to see the visitors at each bedside, so family meetings could be readily arranged.

1980s Going Forward: Development of Single Patient Rooms

The major transformative ICU design change in the United States was the evolution from an open space to ICUs with single (private) patient rooms.[9] This shift happened gradually and variably across the United States, first with walls (glass or opaque) constructed between the beds and curtains for privacy in front of the room (**Fig. 2**B) followed by metal framed doors with glass panels (ie, single doors that open and close or multi-door configurations with doors that both slide or break away) that replaced the curtains (**Fig. 2**C). The shift to single-bed rooms offered many improvements in terms of patient privacy, and control of infection, room temperature, sound, light, smoke, and fire. Also, private rooms allowed for air pressure control, logistical support, visitor amenities, and opportunities for visitors to stay at the bedside and not interfere with the care of other patients. Single rooms also are thought to potentially decrease the incidence of delirium.[44,45]

The major disadvantage of the single-patient ICU room is the elimination of direct visibility of all ICU patients that existed in open bay ICUs, as each bedside can no longer be readily observed.[42] Thus, nurses and other caregivers (ie, respiratory therapists) must rely upon electronic surveillance solutions such as split screen physiologic

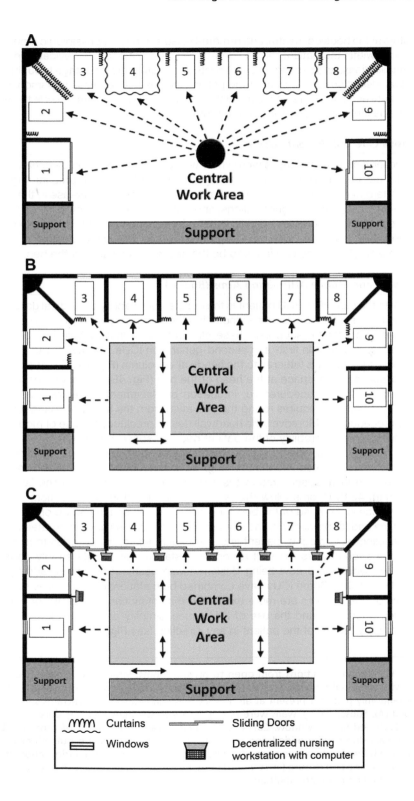

monitors at the bedside, central and remote-based stations for physiologic monitoring, webcams within the patient rooms, web-based views of bedside devices, electronic communications, and secondary alarm systems. Another disadvantage brought about by privacy solutions at the front of the patient room is the decrease in personal interaction between the ICU teams commonly rounding in the corridors outside the rooms and the patients and visitors inside the rooms.

Intensive Care Unit Patient Rooms

First-generation patient spaces were small with a minimal focus on designated locations for devices or visitors; windows may or may not have been present (**Fig. 3**A).[9] Recent iterations of the FGI guidelines have recommended an increase in the square footage of the ICU room, higher ceilings, and windows in each room.[10,12,46] The larger room footprint incorporates dedicated zones for nursing work, patient care and visitors (**Fig. 3**B). However, even with larger ICU rooms, the actual patient, caregiver, and procedural interface continues to be the space directly around the bed.

Headwalls and Mobile Articulating Arms (Booms)

Integral to the care of the ICU patient is the constant availability of medical gasses (oxygen and air), suction, power, data, mounting for physiologic monitors, and other devices, and baskets for supplies. These elements were initially built into stationary headwalls or columns in first- and second-generation ICUs. However, with a stationary model, the patient is tethered to the headwall or column (**Fig. 4**A). This design limits the available physical space at the head of the bed (**Fig. 4**B). Although possible, it is difficult to perform procedures (ie, intubation or placement of central lines) at the head of the bed and requires rolling the bed away from the headwall to create space for the proceduralist. Moreover, the headwall design precludes the use of mobile head scanners as maneuverability of the patient bed and space is limited.

As time progressed, operating room technologies such as mobile articulating arms, or booms, were adopted into the ICU (**Fig. 4**A1). The mobile nature of booms greatly expanded the local space around the patient, taking advantage of the larger ICU rooms (**Fig. 4**B1). Booms allow the patient to be turned in any direction; staff can not only access the head of the bed for procedures but space can be opened up all around the bed for procedures and visitors. Recently, booms have integrated safe patient handling technologies (patient lifts), procedure lights, accessories to hang infusion pumps, computers, as well as docking stations for mobile supply carts and ventilators. Booms are now being designed with aesthetics in mind, adding color and calming lights. Some ICUs have combined both stationary and mobile solutions. In terms of cost, booms are more expensive than stationary headwalls or columns. However, booms expand the use of ICU space, simplify access to the patient and allow for easy turning of the patient in any direction (see **Fig. 4**B1).

Fig. 2. ICU design transitions from open to private rooms. Initially, ICU spaces were wide open with few isolation beds. Most patients were easily visible from a central area. Windows were randomly placed if present at all. Privacy was enabled through curtains surrounding the bed (A). Subsequently, walls were put up between the beds and corridors were developed. Each bed had a window. Curtains provided privacy in the front of room (B). Later, sliding glass doors were added and local nursing workstations were put either at each room or in between every two rooms (C). Sliding doors have multiple configuration options for door opening and closure (ie, standard push and push, electronic powered by buttons or sensors), smoke rating, and multiple privacy options.

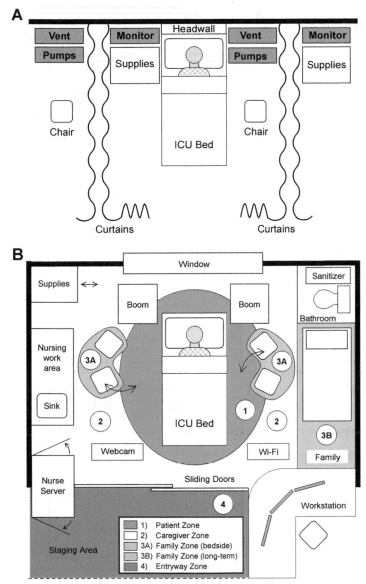

Fig. 3. Open space ICU rooms to zone-based ICU rooms. Initially, the open ICU rooms had no defined zones for work or family (*A*). With time and the installation of walls between beds came the development of zone-based ICU rooms (*B*). In 3B, we see a patient zone, caregiver zone, family zones, and an entryway zone (staging area). The rooms themselves also became larger.

Privacy options

Privacy options that are deployed at the patient rooms' "front door," the interface between the room and the corridor, have evolved over the years. ICU designers can select from curtains alone, glass doors and curtains, glass doors with built-in electronic or manual blinds, or glass doors with integrated electronic glass. ICU doors are rarely opaque. However, visibility of the patient through the front door is also dependent on

Headwall

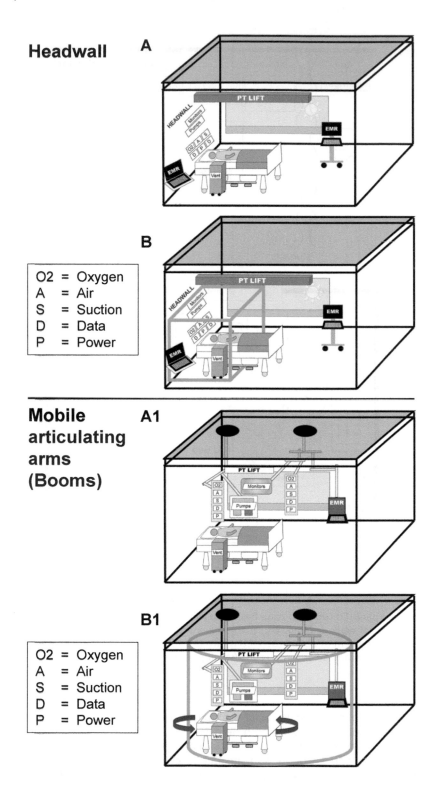

bed positioning and the height and width of the transparency approach deployed within the front door. Thus, the patient may be fully or partially visible or not visible at all. In addition, ICUs have transitioned the walls in between ICU rooms from see-through glass to solid materials. Patients and families value their privacy and designs are now optimized to ensure that the preferences of these individuals are readily addressed.[47]

Bedside Devices

The core devices of an ICU room, over the decades, are relatively unchanged and include an ICU bed, physiologic monitor, mechanical ventilator, and infusion pumps. These devices, however, have evolved from simple devices into advanced informatics platforms that incorporate many of the standalone devices of the past (ie, pulse oximeters and cardiac output devices into the physiologic monitor and a scale into the bed) (**Fig. 5**A, B). With this consolidation of standalone devices, space is freed up in the ICU room. In addition, space previously needed for storage of standalone devices in equipment supply rooms is also liberated. Moreover, the challenges of triage, distribution, and cleaning of standalone devices are minimized.

However, an evolutionary cycle may occur as prior standalone devices are incorporated into core ICU platforms, new technologies (ie, sonography devices, hemodynamic systems, mobility units) will take their place in the ICU (see **Fig. 5**C). Thus, the same issues of space constraints at the bedside and supply rooms, and the associated device triage, distribution, cleaning and cost will continue to exist until these newer technologies are also ultimately consolidated into core ICU platforms and replaced through further device development.

Intensive Care Unit Rooms Within the Context of Flexibility Adaptability Rooms

Today there is a renewed interest in building rooms described as having "flexible adaptability," otherwise known as the "acuity adaptable model" or "universal design rooms." This concept was introduced over two decades ago to purportedly address nursing shortages, achieve cost-effective care, decrease patient movement during a hospital stay, and increase "customer" satisfaction.[48] Its application requires a transformable room larger than the typical inpatient room and includes critical care technologies.[38] This approach was initially applied to specialized patient groups (ie, maternity, cardiac surgical). However, there were many challenges in its widespread adoption including operationalizing the concept, achieving defined goals, and performing data-driven studies to support the model.[37,39,49,50] Despite these barriers, we have recently observed that flexible adaptability rooms are being built in large acute care inpatient towers.

In this model, administrators primarily control the design process without much CCM clinician input. All adult inpatient rooms are similarly configured with stationary headwalls to handle both medical-surgical patients as well as ICU patients. Some units are simply named ICUs with a modicum of ICU-type technologies (ie, physiologic monitors, device integrators, patient lifts) added to the room. In theory, patient acuity can flex up or down in exactly the same room and patient movement throughout the continuum of inpatient care is minimized. In practice, highly acute critically ill patients may be co-located with much lower acuity patients. ICU nurses are handling both

Fig. 4. Headwalls and mobile articulating arms (booms). Stationary headwalls are on the top (A and B) and mobile articulating arms (booms) are on the bottom (A1 and B1). The active care spaces as related to the headwall are represented by a cube (B) and by a circle with booms (B1). Importantly, the space of the cube is very restricted; in contrast, the circle with the patient in the middle is much larger and can rotate as the bed and booms rotate.

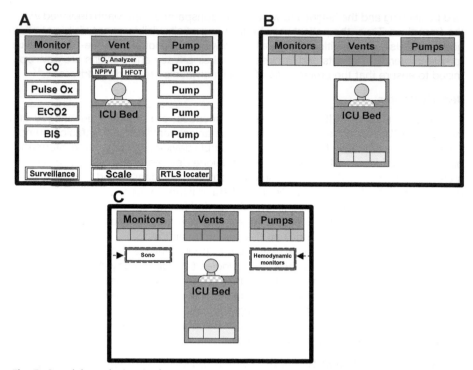

Fig. 5. Standalone devices in the ICU patient room versus integrated components. Standalone devices (*A*) (that is, cardiac output [CO], pulse oximeter [pulse Ox], End-tidal CO2 [EtCO2], bispectral index [BIS], O2 analyzer, noninvasive positive pressure ventilator [NPPV] and high-flow oxygen therapy [HFOT], scale, surveillance for patient fall system, Real-Time Locating System [RTLS] and infusion pumps) were common decades ago. Currently these stand-alone monitors or devices are directly integrated into physiologic monitors; mechanical ventilator; and ICU beds *(B)*. Infusion pump channels or independent infusion pumps are integrated together around a core brain or attached to one another, respectively *(B)*. As new technologies are introduced into the ICU, a new generation of standalone devices will appear at the patient bedside as they did in the past (ie, Sono device, hemodynamic monitors) *(C)*.

critically and non-critically ill patients and their ICU skillsets are diluted. The same is true for ICU pharmacists, respiratory therapists, and other providers.

Flexible adaptability patient rooms are not designed and dedicated specifically to ICU care. Mobile articulating arms (booms) are eliminated; a shift in our opinion, that although decreases initial construction costs, represents a devolution in the design of well-configured and dedicated ICU rooms. However, we do believe that flexible adaptability in inpatient medical-surgical rooms has a place within the hospital construct for specific populations including step-down patients. Moreover, the availability of such rooms and wards enables the hospital to rapidly stand-up ICU-type rooms in disaster circumstances (ie, acute replacement of an ICU that cannot be used due to smoke, fire, or electrical failure or for acute surge capacity).[51]

Bedside Laboratory Diagnostics and Imaging

In past decades, blood specimens were transported to the central hospital laboratory or to a STAT laboratory, possibly located within the central laboratory or near the ICU. Point of Care Lab Testing (POCT) has evolved and now offers bedside or local ICU whole blood gas and electrolyte testing as well as coagulation examinations. Whole blood analyzers were historically large and complicated, requiring dedicated laboratory staff to maintain them; however, the more recent generations of POCT devices (handheld or cartridge driven) are much smaller, more durable, and are easy to use and maintain. Moreover, the cartridge-based POCT devices are equipped with automated quality control (Auto-QC), and all POCT devices have connectivity to Laboratory Information Systems and electronic health records (EHRs).

Today, with increased sonographic training in bedside Point of Care Ultrasound Skills (POCUS), bedside imaging, and procedural teams, are part of typical diagnostic and therapeutic processes. However, patients are still commonly transported to centrally based computed tomography (CT) and MRI scanners. This process is resource, time, and staff intense. However, in the last decade, an unknown, but probably small, number of ICUs have incorporated permanent or mobile scanners to avoid long-distance transports. The mobile CT or MRI scanners bring highly advanced and safe imaging to the ICU bedside.[52] The new generation of CT scanners does not scatter x-rays and likewise the new generation of MRIs does not pull metal into the MRI core. Thus, these mobile devices offer an entirely new perspective to the ICU design as their incorporation mitigates the transport of ICU patients. "Garage space" must, however, be dedicated in the ICU to house and provide power and safe calibration areas for these large mobile imaging devices and the ICU floors must be capable of supporting the weight-load.

Intensive care unit environment: aesthetics, time, ergonomics, safety, and sustainability

In the early decades there was minimal attention to ICU aesthetics, ergonomics, safety, and sustainability. The rooms felt cold and sterile. This inattention to environmental conditions was thought to lead to sleep deprivation or fragmentation, and therefore impair recovery.[53] Today we focus on enhancing the ICU physical environment[54] using artistic and coordinated designs with comfortable flooring, aesthetically pleasing wall and window finishings, and contemporary and electronic art on walls and ceilings.[35] Similarly, there is an emphasis on sound control and computerized lighting to minimize disruption of circadian regulation.[55,56] Patient rooms themselves may feel less crowded with fewer built-in drawers and more mobile supply carts. Attention paid to these details may also help lessen stress for providers working in these conditions which in turn may lessen errors in human performance.[57] Family-oriented spaces and comfortable seating options are now provided because improving the ICU environment has been shown to increase patient and family satisfaction while reducing the duration of delirium.[58]

ICUs have also evolved in the way they keep time. Standalone battery-operated clocks are replaced with synchronized clock systems that unify timekeeping across health care facilities through a wired or wireless network by leveraging Network Time Protocol (NTP) acquired time. These systems eliminate the need to locally change the time twice a year on each clock and also notify hospital engineers when the clocks fail or batteries need replacement.

Concomitantly, there has been a recognition that ergonomic design plays a major role in preserving the physical well-being and safety of staff by protecting staff from injury and facilitating patient mobilization. Lastly, today as opposed to decades ago, there is a major thrust to consider sustainability, energy and ecological efficiency, and environmental concerns when designing, building, and addressing disposable supplies, electrical utilization, and waste management.[11,59–63]

Patient Engagement

In the first-generation open ICU model, the patient space was not designed for a positive patient engagement nor was it practical or prioritized to monitor or control the environment (ie, sound light, temperature, and airflow). Presently, patient engagement is heavily considered and feasible, especially in the private room construct.[27,47] Within this context, each patient room has a window; environmental parameters can be monitored; temperature control is local; shades on outside windows are electrically powered. In select ICUs, computerized lighting may be coordinated with circadian rhythms. These individual systems can be integrated electronically with environmental control assigned to the bedside nurse and/or the patient using remote controls.

Patient entertainment has evolved from televisions attached to the walls, ceilings, or bedrails to large flat-screen displays embedded in the rooms' walls. These displays feature hotel-like user menus that may include options for patient education and food selections. Bluetooth-enabled speakers also permit the patient to link their own mobile devices.

Infection control

Historically only a minority of available ICU rooms in first-generation ICUs were capable of negative or positive pressure. The number of these types of rooms may have been based on local Department of Health regulations (ie, one negative pressure room to every 10 ICU beds). The recommendations as well as the descriptive terminology of these rooms have evolved over time. According to the CDC,[64] negative pressure rooms are now referred to as airborne infection isolation (AII) rooms. In AII rooms, the heating, ventilation, and air conditioning (HVAC) exhaust value exceeds the supply value making the room negatively pressured. Negative pressure confines room based pathogens to the room itself preventing outward dissemination. Current ICU design now includes negative pressure in most ICU rooms. An enclosed anteroom was the norm in the past for negative pressure rooms; however, today such enclosed spaces may or may not be present in front of AII rooms. Commonly anteroom spaces, whether enclosed or open, are used to don and doff personal protective equipment (PPE) (see **Fig. 3**B).

Conversely, positive pressure rooms or protective isolation rooms as they are sometimes referred to, have HVAC systems where the supply value exceeds the exhaust value making the room positively pressured to the area outside the room. In many cases, the air supply into these rooms is also HEPA filtered in the room's ceiling diffuser providing additional protection to the patient. The positive pressure provides a constant level of fresh highly filtered air into the room and keeps contaminants and pathogens out.

Infection control processes in the ICU have improved. In early ICUs there were few sinks, today, there are sinks inside and outside each room. Moreover, the culture emphasizing the importance of handwashing in reducing infections has improved with sink availability, as well as the use of gloves and gowns and the emphasis of sterility while performing bedside procedures.

ICUs are now being designed with passive systems that continuously or periodically disinfect the room (ie, self-disinfecting copper or silver coated surfaces,[65] special light fixtures, disposable bed-rail covers) while the room is occupied.[66] Other more active methods of room disinfection have been used including ultraviolet (UV) light devices and hydrogen peroxide systems.[67] Not only do these active systems require mobile devices and trained operators, but they are limited to use only when rooms are vacant.

Plumbing and Preventative Maintenance

Similarly, older ICU rooms did not have the necessary plumbing to support hemodialysis or continuous renal replacement therapy (CRRT) devices. Today, especially after

COVID-19, in our opinion, all ICU rooms should be capable of plumbing to support renal therapeutics. With all room advances comes the need for ongoing preventive maintenance (ie, air filters, headwalls and booms, and sliding doors).[59] The control panels for room based systems used to be incorporated within the patient room itself, limiting their accessibility when the room was occupied; we recommend locating control panels outside each room.

Mobilizing the patient

In the past, ICU patients were commonly heavily sedated and remained in bed for prolonged periods of time. Patients are now minimally sedated and are mobilized much more quickly out of bed. Concomitant with the evolution in the care model has come enhancements in bedside mobility technologies. Thus, current room ceilings incorporate patient lift devices to help mobilize the patient and ICU beds now have features to assist the patient in getting out of bed. ICU patients are encouraged to walk around the ICU corridors even if they are tethered to physiologic monitors (wired or wireless) and mechanical ventilators.

Waste Disposal

Patient bathrooms were rare in the early-generation ICUs. Human waste products were carried by staff to dirty utility rooms. Subsequently, toilets were built into the room's millwork, however, as bedpans were dumped into them, the room sometimes became contaminated through splashes and these toilets also leaked. The FGI guidelines now mandate bathrooms for new ICU rooms.[10]

Corridors

Accompanying the conversion from open ICUs to the single patient room model (see **Fig. 2A–C**), came well-defined corridors. These corridors, when thoughtfully located and designed, have the potential to organizationally integrate separate ICU pods especially in large ICU platforms (**Fig. 6**). Furthermore, from a practical perspective, patient visibility and wayfinding were not problems in open ICUs. With the development of large ICUs, patient visibility and wayfinding have become more challenging (see **Fig. 2A–C**).

ICU layout typologies are commonly integrated into hospital floorplates and may include a linear configuration, a racetrack configuration (ie, rectangle, square, oval, circle, or triangle with service in the center and patient beds on the perimeter with a loop corridor space in between), or a pod arrangement (often done for ease of patient monitoring and decreased walking distances by staff). Sometimes an "X" shape is used; this design integrates four pods at the periphery of the X and usually does not follow the hospital floorplate. In a study of award-winning ICU designs, layout typologies varied from unit to unit, but racetrack was the most frequently used.[12,68,69] Large ICU complexes may include characteristics of multiple layout types. No single ICU geometry has ever been noted to be superior.

Clearly delineated wayfinding instructions and bed numbers are especially needed in large ICUs with long corridors. Moreover, ICU corridors serve as peripheral and central pathways for internal navigation and usually include "cut throughs" from one area to another to minimize transit time across large ICU platforms (see **Fig. 6**). In these environments, patient rooms, placed along the periphery to obtain window views, or along the interior core, may not be visible from central working areas that cannot be constructed along the entirety of the ICU corridors.

Corridors serve many purposes. Well-appointed corridors offer the opportunity to set an environmental tone that was not available in an open space ICU. Thus light,

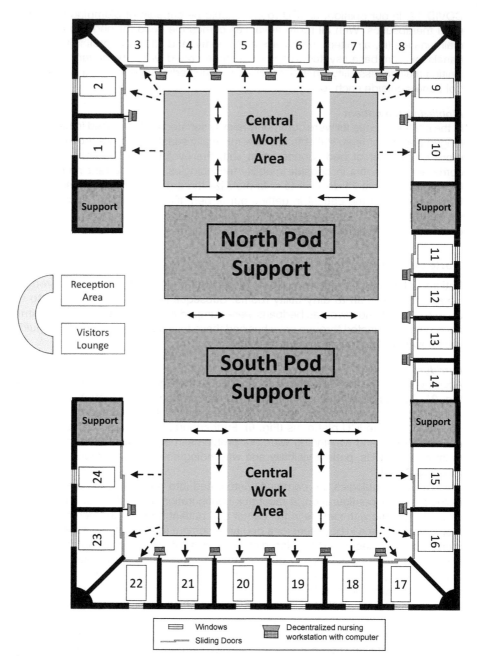

Fig. 6. Large rectangular 24-bed ICU. This ICU has 12-beds in both the North and South pods. Patient rooms are located on the periphery so that each room has a window. Of note, ICU Beds 11 to 14 are not directly visible from the Central Work Areas, an unfortunate feature not uncommon in very large ICUs. Remote visibility (and audio) may be achieved by installing webcams in each room.

sound, and art with day and night rhythms can now be integrated. Corridors are used as meeting spaces for rounding teams, and simultaneously for mobilization of critically ill patients. Logistically the corridors are integrated into the hospital supply chain with entries to large supply and device storage rooms and with the placement of alcoves for local cart-based storage. Supply chains may use a combination of formal centralized supply rooms and storage located near or inside the patient rooms including bidirectional storage with nurse servers (accessible from the corridor and inside the room).

Supply chain

Supply chain and ICU device and supply storage have evolved. Today, there are fewer built-in supply cabinets with drawers along the inside walls of the ICU room. Many ICUs use mobile supply carts, some with their own electronic access and supply tracking controls. Similarly, the maintenance of standardized minimum and maximum ICU supply par (periodic automatic replenishment) levels performed manually in the past is now handled by computerized (ie, bar code) approaches to inventory control. In addition, supplies can be electronically associated (tagged) with the patient for tracking and billing purposes.

Another major change is the shift from reusable supplies that required cleaning (ie, in the ICU or in a sterilization area) to predominantly single-patient-use disposable supplies. This change may require increased local supply storage and waste receptacles. Environmental concerns may be factored into the ICU supply chain equation as a portion of the single-use supplies may be sent to third-party vendors that re-process them for future use.

Central work areas

Over the decades ICUs have been built with central work areas which have been described by many terms (ie, central nursing or staffing stations) (see **Fig. 6**). They are commonly labeled by letter or location and are associated with pods or groups of ICU beds (See **Fig. 6**, Central Work Area - North Pod - covers ICU beds 1 to 12). Historically, these spaces were used for charting, congregating, consulting, and communicating among both ICU and non-ICU staff. However, with modernity and the EHR, the configurations of the central spaces have changed. Carts and cubbies for storage of paper-based charts have been minimized and replaced with computers and printers. Whiteboards with markers and magnets to illustrate patient names and bed numbers have transitioned to electronic bed boards linked to the EHR or other hospital patient tracking systems. However, central physiologic monitor displays of all ICU beds remain. Design adjustments in these central areas may now include adjacent offices, conference rooms, pharmacy, and automated medication dispensing cabinets, and supply storage spaces.

Central versus decentralized nursing (staff) spaces

With the transition to private rooms came the option to shift nursing charting from centralized staffing or nursing stations to room based, or decentralized, nursing stations. These decentralized stations can be permanently built both inside and outside the patient rooms. Alternatively, permanently built decentralized stations can be avoided with the deployment of mobile computers outside the rooms or with computers mounted on headboards or permanent columns or attached to mobile articulating arms within the patient rooms.[70]

These choices opened an important debate about preferences for central versus decentralized stations.[71] Supporting decentralization are studies that focus on the decreased distance for bedside located staff to respond to patient-related alarms and reach requisite medications, equipment, and supplies.[72] However, due to the lack of ICU nurses, many ICUs cannot even achieve a 1:2 much less a 1:1 nurse-to-patient ratio that permits bed-based staffing. Also, eliminating or minimizing central workspaces may have many unintended ramifications for all the other functions (ie, ICU and non-ICU staff communicating, charting, consulting, reviewing images, and ultimately building an ICU community) that routinely occur at central work areas. Decentralization may also lead to the social isolation of the nurses.[68] Therefore, our belief is that a hybrid approach with both central and decentralized spaces (including directly outside the bedside and within the patient room) is best (see **Figs. 2**C, **3**B, and **6**).

Intensive Care Unit-Based Respite and Sleeping Accommodations

Spaces for nurses to relax continues to be a vital element of the ICU design.[2] Over the years, these lounge areas have been improved aesthetically and ergonomically. At the same time, the need for the multi-bed on-call suites for house staff diminished with the imposition of work-hour limitations for physician trainees. However, as ICU night staffing now includes night Intensivists, Hospitalists and APPs, the need for similar respite areas returned.

Visitor Lounges

Visitor lounges, formerly known as waiting rooms, provide a space for patient visitors to relax before, or after, visiting their loved ones in the ICU. These spaces continue to be positioned adjacent to the ICU. Historically, the visitor lounges were not aesthetically pleasing and provided just simple chairs and tables. Over the decades, the décor has been upgraded, televisions and Wi-Fi added, and vending machines installed. Some ICUs have also provided sleeping accommodations.[73]

Before COVID restrictions, family participation in the care of the ICU patient was encouraged, with a focus on improving the ICU visitor experience with visitor zones and amenities[19](see **Fig. 3**B). However, with COVID visitor restrictions, came a decrease in the use of the visitor lounges and even visitor spaces within patient rooms. Only time will tell if such spaces will again accommodate the large number of visitors as in the past. Currently, the FGI prescribes a certain ratio of waiting room chairs to ICU beds.[10]

Step-down units

Step-down units and step-down beds were introduced as care concepts in the 1960s.[29] It is important to recognize that many step-down models exist.[30] For example, hospitals may have step-down units as independent entities or co-located within ICU complexes or scattered among hospital wards (see **Fig. 1**). To further confuse this discussion, many terms have been used to describe step-down units or beds (ie, Progressive care, Intermediate care, Transitional care) and diverse formulations of location, ICU integration, staffing, patient triage, and care patterns exist. A detailed discussion of step-down units is beyond the scope of this review; however, new ICU design should account for the evolving models of step-down units and beds.

Informatics: pre- and post-electronic health records eras

A clear distinction must be recognized between the pre- and post-EHR eras. In the 1980s to 1990s, paper charts were the norm (**Fig. 7**A). Flowsheets and daily notes were completed by hand. Laboratory data were delivered to the ICU on paper. In this paper-based environment, the ICU had to maintain large cabinets or mobile carts for storage of paper-based charts as well as desk space to place and read the charts. Staff members were commonly competing to engage with the paper charts. ICUs also had to maintain large x-ray viewing devices to store and look at film-based x-rays and

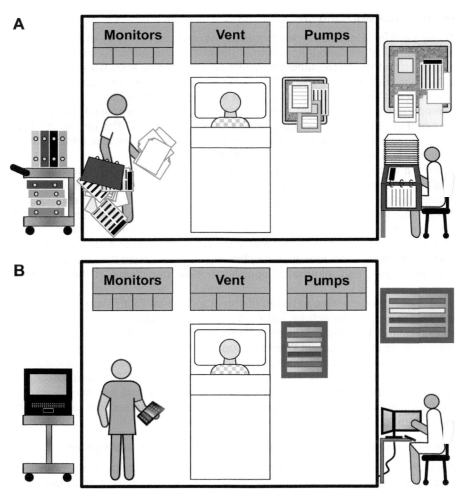

Fig. 7. Paper vs EHR. The ICU of the past was managed with paper for charting and reading diagnostic or therapeutic reports (A). Charts were stored in central areas in rolling carts that were brought to the bedside for rounds. Bedside charting was performed at bedside tables. Papers were posted on bulletin boards both inside and outside the patient room. With time, the paper record system was mostly replaced by the EHR. Associated with this transition were mobile and handheld computers, computers at bedside locations, and electronic displays (B).

keep track of the films and coordinate their return to the Radiology File Room. Today, imaging data is housed within the EHR and viewed online (**Fig. 7**B). This paradigm shift to the EHR is associated with many benefits as information is consolidated and simultaneously available for all staff to both view and edit.

However, the EHR comes with its own costs to the ICU environment. The ICU must maintain many computers and displays centrally, at the bedside, in offices, and conference spaces. Similarly, the ICU must house a large cadre of workstations on wheels and provide parking spaces with electrical outlets to charge them.[70] A fast and secure network (wired and wireless) must be functional and updated as necessary for the computers and EHR to be efficiently used. Interestingly, paper has not fully disappeared in the EHR era; thus, many ICUs still have to maintain paper and printers.

Health Care Device Platforms

Today's evolution in health care informatics has changed the nature of infusion pumps and mechanical ventilators from simple devices to sophisticated health care informatics platforms. These platforms require an entirely new knowledge base to evaluate, pilot, deploy, integrate, maintain and finance.[3,74] The older devices were not electronically associated with the patient or caregiver and lacked connectivity and interoperability, and could not transmit data or alarms, or integrate into the EHR continuum (**Fig. 8**A). Older devices simply required a warranty. The new technologies must be broadly integrated into the hospital's and ICU's informatics infrastructure in a manner that advances patient and staff focused care.[75]

From a technical standpoint, successfully integrating smart technologies into a health care informatics platform requires the placement of bar code readers or permanent device integrators into each ICU room (**Fig. 8**B). Their implementation in the design process requires simulation laboratories that address connectivity with the EHR, data flow, information security, and fail-safe server architecture. Modern health care platforms also require an entirely new system of ongoing support (ie, software and hardware licenses, and upgrade planning) and cost projections. Thus, biomedical engineering and informatics specialists must participate in the ICU design process.

Devices from decades ago posed no threat to hospital information security simply due to their lack of connectivity. There was no need for ICU designers or informaticists to understand the core informatics elements of devices at the bedside. Current devices however, pose great threats through their integration into hospital networks; hospital information security teams must perform deep dives into each vendors' technologies to mitigate the risk of hospital network compromise. The need for such vigilance at the design level will only expand as ICU device data are incorporated into continuously evolving artificial intelligence, clinical decision support tools, and machine learning platforms.[76]

Intensive Care Unit Design Drives Data, Alarm Distribution, and Storage

Another major change in ICU design is the need to address data generated within each ICU room. In the past, manual entry of data to flowsheets was the primary goal. Physiologic monitor alarms were sent to central stations and unfiltered ventilator alarms were transmitted through nurse call systems or annunciators. Otherwise, alarms were mostly confined to the patient's room. In contrast, today we deal with staggering quantities of electronic data that are captured, filtered, validated, and transmitted to the EHR and distributed as secondary alarms to other middleware and receiving systems. Concomitantly, there is an ongoing focus on reducing alarm fatigue by transmitting or creating alarms that are meaningful, actionable, and useful for real-time clinical decision-making including the use of early warning systems and artificial intelligence middleware.[77] In addition, hospitals and ICUs have shifted the storage of data from local or remote physical servers to cloud-based support. Thus, the ICU informatics design must be integral to the entire ICU design process and developed with the hospital's informatics and information security specialists.

Remote monitoring and management (control)

The 2020 COVID-19 pandemic highlighted the need for remote monitoring and care of ICU patients.[34] This included visualizing bedside monitors remotely or placing duplicate monitoring displays outside the patient rooms. Moreover, remote management was also advanced as bedside physiologic monitors were remotely controlled using wired remotes; infusion pumps were placed outside the rooms, monitored and controlled; and ventilators were either placed outside the room or remotely controlled.[78] In terms of ICU design, the remote placement of devices outside the patient rooms requires power, connectivity, and possibly conduits (for ventilator circuits and IV tubings) in the front of each ICU patient room. Most ICUs did not have such support outside each room and had to improvise these elements.

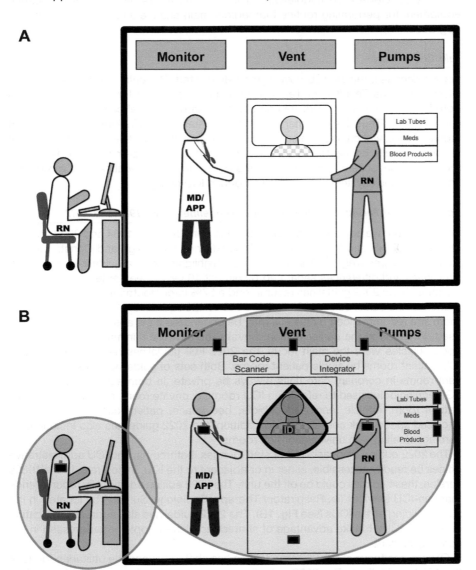

Fig. 8. Association of staff, devices, and samples with the patient. Initially, devices, staff, medications, laboratory samples, and blood products were only associated, if at all, with the patient through manual means in the paper medical record because there were no electronic association (linkage) capabilities (A). Currently, by using ICU patient rooms as digital locations, in conjunction with room based or mobile barcode scanners and device integrators, the patient, medical devices, staff members as well as medications, laboratory samples, and blood products, each with their own unique identifiers (ie, Bar code) are associated electronically with the patient (B).

Real-Time Locating Systems

Locating mobile devices or staff assigned to an ICU was very challenging in the past. The use of Real-Time Locating Systems (RTLS) technologies has transformed the ICU environment permitting tagged devices, staff, patients and visitors to be tracked using RTLS web-based middleware. These systems are also helpful in locating equipment for performing routine biomedical maintenance and delivering software upgrades.

Tele-Critical Care

In past decades, remote ICU coverage rarely existed. Currently, remote coverage of ICUs, known as Tele-ICU or Tele-Critical Care, is available for hospitals and ICUs both large and small.[79,80] Private companies or large medical centers often provide such services. Thus, the designers of new ICUs may need to include remote enabling technology (ie, webcams and alerting for a tele-intensivist). The tele-critical care bunker (a room virtually connected to patient rooms where the tele-critical care team can round) may be located anywhere; thus the design for the tele-critical care monitoring space is a specialty item not usually included in ICU design.

Comparison of Facility Guideline Institute Guidelines: 1983-1984 and 2022

In this section, we compare the ICU guidelines from the 1983-1984 and 2022 editions of the US DHHS and the US-based FGI Guidelines for Design and Construction of Hospitals, respectively.[9,10] This comparison highlights, from a guideline standpoint, similarities and differences separated by almost 40 years (see **Table 1**).

Although the 2022 guidelines recommend a 67% larger footprint for the ICU patient room than the earlier edition (200 sq ft in 2022 vs 120 sq ft in 1983), both stress that the room size recommended by the FGI may be undersized if the absolute minimums are used. Whereas in the earlier edition, private rooms were minimally mentioned and open cubicles were the main focus, the 2022 FGI guidelines recommends that all ICU patient rooms be single patient rooms. Both sets of guidelines endorse that patient rooms in coronary care units always be private. In both editions, the multiple FGI terminologies used to refer to an ICU room (ie, private room, patient room, single patient room, cubicle, enclosed cubicle, bed space, patient care station, private enclosed space) lack consistency. In addition, the 2022 guidelines also include brief verbiage dealing with universal or flex rooms.

The 2022 edition emphasizes that staff lounges, bathrooms, and ICU administrative offices be readily accessible, either in or adjacent to the ICU. In contrast, in the 1980s version, these spaces could be off the unit. The 2022 edition additionally recommends that non-ICU services (ie, Respiratory Therapy, Radiology, Surgery) be located in the same building as the ICUs (see **Fig. 1**B). The 2022 guidelines also address co-location of multiple ICUs to take advantage of shared facilities—a topic not addressed in the earlier guidelines.

Of note, the focus of the 2022 guidelines has shifted beyond the utilitarian focus of the 1980s guidelines. The 2022 guidelines now recognize the stress and complexities of care and the environment experienced by staff and families and highlight the need for improved aesthetics, privacy, ambience, comfort, safety, visitor seating in each ICU room, and corridor separation for patient transport. In addition, the 2022 guidelines emphasize the need for providing and correctly sizing spaces that incorporate privacy for staff to concentrate during data review. The 2022 guidelines also include an infection control section mandating handwashing sinks at each bedside as well as direct access for toilets and for waste disposal in each patient room.

Table 1 Major foci of intensive care unit design evolutionary changes	
Mid 1980s	**Present**
Small ICUs located anywhere	Large, purposefully located ICUs and SDUs
Open space for patient	Single dedicated room
Central work/staffing spaces	Central and/or decentralized spaces
No corridors	Corridors
Stationary support (headwalls or columns)	Stationary and mobile articulating arms (booms)
Minimal concerns for ICU environment	Focus on aesthetically pleasing, warm environment, and design encouraging positive engagement for staff, patients, and visitors
Paper health record	Electronic health records (EHR)
Standalone medical devices	Integrated health care informatics platforms
No informatics	Informatics with connectivity, interoperability, and association
Care monitored and rendered locally	Care monitored and rendered locally and remotely
No thought for the future	Future-proofing integral to design

Abbreviations: ICU, intensive care unit; SDU, step down unit.

We would like to highlight two additional differences between the two guidelines. The first addresses the positioning of nursing staff (see **Figs. 2** and **6**). In the early edition, a central work area (central nursing station) with visibility to all ICU beds was the main focus; in contrast, the 2022 edition discusses both central and decentralized (near the bedside) work areas. Although the 2022 edition continues to emphasize direct vision of all beds from central stations, there is now mention of remote visibility. The second difference is with regard to informatics. In the 1980s, informatics was not a major component of the ICU, but the 2022 guidelines address the presence of automated information systems and the need for space for computers and printers to support informatics.

Future-Proofing

Future-proofing is loosely defined as designing a space or technology so that its usefulness will be long term, continuing even if the situations that existed at the time of the original design change. In the past, this concept was not addressed. Thus, although ICUs may have been meant to last for decades, there was not much thought to actualizing this intent.

ICU future-proofing requires several steps. First, scalable power and connectivity across ICU platforms should be included to address future needs.[3,74] Caring for patients during COVID-19 highlighted the absence of available ICU power and connectivity both inside and outside the patient rooms[4] necessary to incorporate additional health care informatics platforms and changes in practice patterns.[34,51,81] Second, future-proofing requires the inclusion of both sufficient heights between floors and weight density capacity to accommodate new technologies (eg, a mobile CT scanner). Third, we suggest that ICU design include negative pressure (AII rooms) in a majority of ICU rooms regardless of minimalist state or FGI recommendations.

SUMMARY

Concepts of ICU design have changed dramatically since the mid-1980s until 2022. However, it is not possible to precisely target the timing, speed, and incorporation of the multiple, dynamic and concomitant evolutionary processes that occurred. Our impression is that evolution in ICU design will certainly continue and those designs that both address the current state of ICU affairs and look to the future will successfully create long-lasting ICUs.

CLINICS CARE POINTS

- ICU design publications now include strategic thinking and capacity modeling to optimize ICU bed locations and numbers.
- It is not possible to state if the evolution in ICU design has impacted patient outcomes because few studies directly assess well-defined ICU design parameters and patient outcomes.
- Improving the ICU environment has been shown to increase patient, family, and staff satisfaction.
- The adoption of Electronic Health Records (EHR) and the incorporation of medical devices that are all healthcare informatics platforms has strongly influenced the design of the ICU and advanced the need to address data management and cybersecurity.
- Optimally, ICUs should include both centralized and decentralized staff and nursing stations to address the specific needs of staff and patient care at different locales.
- With the recent building of large inpatient hospital pavilions, we have seen a shift to universal acuity-adaptable inpatient room design with minor customization for ICU-level care; a possible economic advance associated with a devolution in ICU design.
- The 2020 COVID-19 pandemic highlighted the need for enhanced remote monitoring and remote management of ICU patients.

FUNDING

This work was supported in part by the MSK Cancer Center Support Grant/Core grant (P30 CA008748) and the Department of Anesthesiology and Critical Care Medicine.

ACKNOWLEDGMENTS

The authors thank Elaine Ciccaroni for her development of the figures.

REFERENCES

1. Halpern NA. Innovative designs for the smart ICU: part 1: from initial thoughts to occupancy. Chest 2014;145(2):399–403.
2. Halpern NA. Innovative designs for the smart ICU: Part 2: the ICU. Chest 2014; 145(3):646–58.
3. Halpern NA. Innovative designs for the smart ICU: Part 3: advanced ICU informatics. Chest 2014;145(4):903–12.
4. Halpern NA, Anderson DC, Kesecioglu J. ICU design in 2050: looking into the crystal ball! Intensive Care Med 2017;43(5):690–2.
5. Award SCCM. Winning ICU designs. 2021 [cited 2022 11/17/2022]. Available from: https://store.sccm.org/SearchResults.aspx?searchterm=icu+design&search option=ALL.
6. Guidelines for intensive care unit design. Guidelines/practice parameters committee of the American college of critical care medicine, society of critical care medicine. Crit Care Med 1995;23(3):582–8.

7. Thompson DR, Hamilton DK, Cadenhead CD, et al. Guidelines for intensive care unit design. Crit Care Med 2012;40(5):1586–600.
8. iHG. International health facility guidelines. Available from: http://www.health facilityguidelines.com/.
9. DHHS. Guidelines for construction and equipment of hospital and medical facilities. 1983-1984. Publication No. (HRS-M-HF) 84-1: [cited 2022 10/23/2022].Available at: https://fgiguidelines.org/guidelines/earlier-editions/.
10. FGI. Guidelines for design and construction of hospitals. St. Louis: The Facilities Guidelines Institute; 2022.
11. Verderber S, Gray S, Suresh-Kumar S, et al. Intensive care unit built environments: a comprehensive literature review (2005-2020). HERD 2021;14(4): 368–415.
12. Rashid M. Two decades (1993-2012) of adult intensive care unit design: a comparative study of the physical design features of the best practice examples. Crit Care Nurs Q 2014;37(1):3–32.
13. Vincent JL. Critical care–where have we been and where are we going? Crit Care 2013;17(Suppl 1):S2.
14. Hamilton DK, Shepley MM. Design for critical care: an evidence-based approach. Oxford, UK: Architectural Press; 2010.
15. AHA. Fast facts on U.S. Hospitals, 2022. American hospital association 2022 january 2022 [cited 2022 10/23/2022]. Available from: https://www.aha.org/statistics/fast-facts-us-hospitals#: ∼ :text=Fast%20Facts%20on%20U.S.%20Hospitals%2C%202022%201%201.,4%204.%20Medical-surgical%20intensive%20care.%20.%20More%20items.
16. Thompson JD. Short-stay and long-stay: study of two recovery rooms offers clues to intensive care unit design. Hospitals 1958;32(21):35.
17. Rourke AJ, Peters DA, Kronebusch DD. Details are critical; in intensive care unit design. Hospitals 1966;40(9):81–6.
18. Bingham E, Whitaker D, Christofferson J, et al. Evidence-based design in hospital renovation projects: a study of design implementation for user controls. HERD 2020;13(2):133–42.
19. Sundberg F, Fridh I, Lindahl B, et al. Visitor's experiences of an evidence-based designed health care environment in an intensive care unit. Herd 2021;14(2): 178–91.
20. Shultz J, Jha R. Using virtual reality (VR) mock-ups for evidence-based health care facility design decisions. Int J Environ Res Public Health 2021;18(21):11250.
21. Gooch RA, Kahn JM. ICU bed supply, utilization, and health care spending: an example of demand elasticity. JAMA 2014;311(6):567–8.
22. Barbash IJ, Wallace DJ, Kahn JM. Effects of changes in ICU bed supply on ICU utilization. Med Care 2019;57(7):544–50.
23. McManus ML, Long MC, Cooper A, et al. Queuing theory accurately models the need for critical care resources. Anesthesiology 2004;100(5):1271–6.
24. Mathews KS, Long EF. A conceptual framework for improving critical care patient flow and bed use. Ann Am Thorac Soc 2015;12(6):886–94.
25. Gunnerson KJ, Bassin BS, Havey RA, et al. Association of an emergency department-based intensive care unit with survival and inpatient intensive care unit admissions. JAMA Netw Open 2019;2(7):e197584.
26. Jeong H, Jung YS, Suh GJ, et al. Emergency physician-based intensive care unit for critically ill patients visiting emergency department. Am J Emerg Med 2020; 38(11):2277–82.

27. Du J, Gunnerson KJ, Bassin BS, et al. Effect of an emergency department intensive care unit on medical intensive unit admissions and care: a retrospective cohort study. Am J Emerg Med 2021;46:27–33.

28. Jayaprakash N, Pflaum-Carlson J, Gardner-Gray J, et al. Critical care delivery solutions in the emergency department: evolving models in caring for ICU boarders. Ann Emerg Med 2020;76(6):709–16.

29. Prin M, Wunsch H. The role of stepdown beds in hospital care. Am J Respir Crit Care Med 2014;190(11):1210–6.

30. Plate JDJ, Leenen LPH, Houwert M, et al. Utilisation of intermediate care units: a systematic review. Crit Care Res Pract 2017;2017:8038460.

31. Kesecioglu J, Schneider MM, van der Kooi AW, et al. Structure and function: planning a new ICU to optimize patient care. Curr Opin Crit Care 2012;18(6):688–92.

32. Halpern NA, Anderson DC. Keeping a 2009 design award-winning intensive care unit current: a 13-year case study. HERD 2020;13(4):190–209.

33. Lin FF, Foster M, Chaboyer W, et al. Relocating an intensive care unit: an exploratory qualitative study. Aust Crit Care 2016;29(2):55–60.

34. Halpern NA, Kaplan LJ, Rausen M, et al. *Configuring ICUs in the COVID-19 era.* COVID-19 rapid resource center. Society of Critical Care Medicine; 2020. June 15, 2020; Available from: https://www.sccm.org/COVID19RapidResources/Resources/Configuring-ICUs-in-the-COVID-19-Era-A-Collection.

35. Ferri M, Zygun DA, Harrison A, et al. Evidence-based design in an intensive care unit: end-user perceptions. BMC Anesthesiol 2015;15:57.

36. Bonuel N, Cesario S. Review of the literature: acuity-adaptable patient room. Crit Care Nurs Q 2013;36(2):251–71.

37. Venditti A. Patient-centered care: impacting quality with the acuity adaptable model. Nurs Manage 2015;46(7):36–42.

38. Bonuel N, Cesario S, Cabading AD. The need for critical care nursing skills in an acuity-adaptable care delivery system. Crit Care Nurs Q 2010;33(4):356–60.

39. Kwan MA. Acuity-adaptable nursing care: exploring its place in designing the future patient room. HERD 2011;5(1):77–93.

40. Alnobani O, Zakaria N, Temsah MH, et al. Knowledge, attitude, and perception of health care personnel working in intensive care units of mass gatherings toward the application of telemedicine robotic remote-presence technology: a cross-sectional multicenter study. Telemed J e Health 2021;27(12):1423–32.

41. Saha S, Noble H, Xyrichis A, et al. Mapping the impact of ICU design on patients, families and the ICU team: a scoping review. J Crit Care 2022;67:3–13.

42. Lu Y, Ossmann MM, Leaf DE, et al. Patient visibility and ICU mortality: a conceptual replication. HERD 2014;7(2):92–103.

43. Ferri M, Zygun DA, Harrison A, et al. A study protocol for performance evaluation of a new academic intensive care unit facility: impact on patient care. BMJ Open 2013;3(7):e003134.

44. Caruso P, Guardian L, Tiengo T, et al. ICU architectural design affects the delirium prevalence: a comparison between single-bed and multibed rooms*. Crit Care Med 2014;42(10):2204–10.

45. Lee HJ, Bae E, Lee HY, et al. Association of natural light exposure and delirium according to the presence or absence of windows in the intensive care unit. Acute and Critical Care 2021;36(4):332–41.

46. Rashid M. Space allocation in the award-winning adult ICUs of the last two decades (1993-2012): an exploratory study. HERD 2014;7(2):29–56.

47. Andersson M, Fridh I, Lindahl B. Is it possible to feel at home in a patient room in an intensive care unit? Reflections on environmental aspects in technology-dense environments. Nurs Inq 2019;26(4):e12301.
48. Gallant D, Lanning K. Streamlining patient care processes through flexible room and equipment design. Crit Care Nurs Q 2001;24(3):59–76.
49. HCD GA. Beyond the universal patient room. Health care Design 2005 4/30/2005 [cited 2022 10/23/2022]. Available from: https://healthcaredesignmagazine.com/architecture/beyond-universal-patient-room/.
50. Bonuel N, Degracia A, Cesario S. Acuity-adaptable patient room improves length of stay and cost of patients undergoing renal transplant: a pilot study. Crit Care Nurs Q 2013;36(2):181–94.
51. Hidalgo J, Baez AA. Natural disasters. Crit Care Clin 2019;35(4):591–607.
52. Maury E, Arrive L, Mayo PH. Intensive Care Medicine in 2050: the future of medical imaging. Intensive Care Med 2017;43(8):1135–7.
53. Meyer TJ, Eveloff SE, Bauer MS, et al. Adverse environmental conditions in the respiratory and medical ICU settings. Chest 1994;105(4):1211–6.
54. Shepley MM, Gerbi RP, Watson AF, et al. The impact of daylight and views on ICU patients and staff. HERD 2012;5(2):46–60.
55. Voigt LP, Reynolds K, Mehryar M, et al. Monitoring sound and light continuously in an intensive care unit patient room: a pilot study. J Crit Care 2017;39:36–9.
56. Fan EP, Abbott SM, Reid KJ, et al. Abnormal environmental light exposure in the intensive care environment. J Crit Care 2017;40:11–4.
57. Donchin Y, Seagull FJ. The hostile environment of the intensive care unit. Curr Opin Crit Care 2002;8(4):316–20.
58. Kesecioglu J. Improving the patient's environment: the ideal intensive care unit. Reanimation 2015;24(2):341–3.
59. Huffling K, Schenk E. Environmental sustainability in the intensive care unit: challenges and solutions. Crit Care Nurs Q 2014;37(3):235–50.
60. McGain F, Muret J, Lawson C, et al. Environmental sustainability in anaesthesia and critical care. Br J Anaesth 2020;125(5):680–92.
61. Yu A, Baharmand I. Environmental sustainability in Canadian critical care: a nationwide survey study on medical waste management. Healthc Q 2021; 23(4):39–45.
62. Pollard AS, Paddle JJ, Taylor TJ, et al. The carbon footprint of acute care: how energy intensive is critical care? Publ Health 2014;128(9):771–6.
63. Chapman M, Chapman A. Greening critical care. Crit Care 2011;15(2):302.
64. Airborne CDC. Infections isolations (AII) room. Interactive core curriculum on tuberculosis 2005 [cited 2022 11/10/2022]. Available from: https://www.cdc.gov/tb/webcourses/course/chapter7/7_infection_control_7_infection_control_program_airborne_infection_isolation_aii_room.html.
65. Boyce JM. Modern technologies for improving cleaning and disinfection of environmental surfaces in hospitals. Antimicrob Resist Infect Control 2016;5:10.
66. Esolen LM, Thakur L, Layon AJ, et al. The efficacy of self-disinfecting bedrail covers in an intensive care unit. Am J Infect Control 2018;46(4):417–9.
67. Weber DJ, Rutala WA, Sickbert-Bennett EE, et al. Continuous room decontamination technologies. Am J Infect Control 2019;47S:A72–8.
68. Hamilton DK, Swoboda SM, Lee JT, et al. Decentralization: the corridor is the problem, not the alcove. Crit Care Nurs Q 2018;41(1):3–9.
69. Hadi K, Zimring C. Design to improve visibility: impact of corridor width and unit shape. HERD 2016;9(4):35–49.

70. Halpern NA, Burnett G, Morgan S, et al. Remote communication from a mobile terminal: an adjunct for a computerized intensive care unit order management system. Crit Care Med 1995;23(12):2054–7.
71. Fay L, Cai H, Real K. A systematic literature review of empirical studies on decentralized nursing stations. HERD 2019;12(1):44–68.
72. Silvis J. Unit design is secret to successful patient room. Health care design 2014 11/7/2014 [cited 2022 11/11/2022]. Available from: https://healthcaredesignmagazine.com/trends/interior-design/unit-design-secret-successful-patient-room/.
73. Peterson MJ, Woerhle T, Harry M, et al. Family satisfaction in a neuro trauma ICU. Nurs Crit Care 2020;27(3):334–40.
74. Anderson DC, Jackson AA, Halpern NA. Informatics for the modern intensive care unit. Crit Care Nurs Q 2018;41(1):60–7.
75. Meissen H, Gong MN, Wong AI, et al. The future of critical care: optimizing technologies and a learning health care system to potentiate a more humanistic approach to critical care. Crit Care Explor 2022;4(3):e0659.
76. Vellido A, Ribas V, Morales C, et al. Machine learning in critical care: state-of-the-art and a sepsis case study. Biomed Eng Online 2018;17(Suppl 1):135.
77. Lewandowska K, Weisbrot M, Cieloszyk A, et al. Impact of alarm fatigue on the work of nurses in an intensive care environment-A systematic review. Int J Environ Res Public Health 2020;17(22).
78. Rausen MS, Nahass TA, Halpern NA. Novel technology deployed for remote ventilator management by respiratory therapists during the COVID-19 pandemic: lessons learned. J Intensive Care Med 2022;37(12):1662–6.
79. Guinemer C, Boeker M, Furstenau D, et al. Telemedicine in intensive care units: scoping review. J Med Internet Res 2021;23(11):e32264.
80. Khurrum M, Asmar S, Joseph B. Telemedicine in the ICU: innovation in the critical care process. J Intensive Care Med 2021;36(12):1377–84.
81. Drumheller BC, Mareiniss DP, Overberger RC, et al. Design and implementation of a temporary emergency department-intensive care unit patient care model during the COVID-19 pandemic surge. Journal of the American College of Emergency Physicians open 2020;1(6):1255–60.

Critical Care 1950 to 2022
Evolution of Medicine, Nursing, Technology, and Design

D. Kirk Hamilton, BArch, MSOD, PhD[a],*, Jeanne Kisacky, MArch, PhD[b], Frank Zilm, DArch[c]

KEYWORDS

- ICU • Regulations • Technology • Acuity-adaptable • Intensivist

KEY POINTS

- Critical care and ICU design has been influenced by advances in medicine and technology, and training of clinicians, along with economic and regulatory factors.
- Early ICUs were modeled on surgical recovery rooms and military field hospitals where vulnerable patients were under high levels of observation. These units serving the most critically ill patients have evolved to provide more space for equipment, patient care, and greater privacy.
- The challenge of COVID-19 has resulted in a re-examination of design concepts for ICUs that include: amount of dedicated isolation rooms, ability to manage equipment from outside the room, video and telemedicine patient monitoring, communication technologies, design for high levels of visualization, and consideration of increased corridor widths.

INTRODUCTION

The idea of today's critical care units (referred to as ICUs in this article)—spaces designed for concentrated and specialized care of critically ill patients—developed out of multiple parallel advances in medical, surgical, as well as nursing techniques and training which took advantage of new therapeutic technologies. These advances supported the development of innovative and successful strategies to prolong life in the face of critical illness. Extensive regulatory requirements and national health care policy impacted ICU design and practice throughout that development.

THE EARLIEST ANTECEDENTS

Advancements in anesthesia in the mid-1800s and its adoption for surgery allowed for new surgical techniques and permitted operations of greater length. As a result, new

[a] Department of Architecture, College Station, TX 77843, USA; [b] Independent Historian, 111 Brandon Place, Ithaca, NY 14850, USA; [c] Institute for Health & Wellness Design, University of Kansas, Lawrence, KS 66045, USA
* Corresponding author. Department of Architecture, Texas A&M University, College Station, Texas 77843-3137, USA.
E-mail address: khamilton@tamu.edu

Crit Care Clin 39 (2023) 603–625
https://doi.org/10.1016/j.ccc.2023.01.002
0749-0704/23/© 2023 Elsevier Inc. All rights reserved.

higher risk types of surgeries were introduced, which led some surgeons to create recovery rooms for the immediate postoperative period as patients came out from anesthesia. In spite of the growing professionalism of nursing, following Florence Nightingale's reforms to give nurses roles beyond hygiene, delivery of medications, nutrition, and custodial care, the experienced surgeons and surgical nurses were most qualified to look after these postsurgical cases.

A few surgeons in the United Kingdom introduced spaces for immediate postsurgical care, and the concept appeared in the literature as early as 1847,[1] only one year after ether was demonstrated in an operation at the Massachusetts General Hospital. In the United States, recovery rooms, such as the surgical recovery space at Charity Hospital in New Orleans created for Dr Alton Ochsner, were appearing in hospitals by the 1890s. These early recovery spaces—located adjacent to the surgical suites which were frequently located at the top levels of hospitals to access the best possible lighting[2]—were precursors of today's postanesthesia care units and intensive care units.

EVOLUTION OF PATIENT CARE AFTER WORLD WAR II (WWII) AND KOREAN WAR (1950S)

Doctors and nurses who worked in military field hospitals during WWII and Korea treated large numbers of casualties suffering from major trauma and gained extensive experience in caring for patients requiring intensive life-saving medical and surgical interventions. To deal with the challenges of having limited experienced clinical staff available, field hospital structures not optimally arranged for care, and high rates of postoperative complications, the military medical staff developed specialized recovery rooms. These were large, open, multi-bed spaces offering high-intensity observation during the critical postanesthesia recovery period. Postwar physicians and nurses carried their wartime experiences home and advocated for the inclusion of recovery rooms (for short-term care of immediately postoperative patients) either as additions to existing hospitals or as an essential component in the hundreds of hospitals built under the new Hill–Burton program. This program was Congress' way to expand hospitals beyond America's large cities by funding hospital construction in underserved rural and small-town communities.

After WWII, as medical practice and medical education promoted increasing specialization, civilian hospitals offered newer, more extreme, and often highly specialized surgical treatments. Advances in surgery and anesthesia enabled these longer, more complex procedures but also left postoperative patients extremely vulnerable, increasing the risk of complications. The difficulties of caring for these vulnerable postoperative patients remained a problem, particularly in multi-story, sprawling hospital structures with surgical suites distant from nursing units and with limited medical technologies available on these nursing units.[3] By concentrating critically ill patients, special groups of nurses, and medical technologies into one space, these recovery rooms and ICUs fostered critical care specialization and led to the development of new life-saving procedures and practices[4] (Fig. 1).

EARLY GENERATIONS OF CRITICAL CARE (MID-1950S TO 1960S)

Modern ICUs developed in the mid-1950s, driven by experience providing care to postsurgical patients, polio patients, and later, coronary patients. Many of the first ICUs developed by providing a recovery room's high level of observation and specialized nursing and then expanding the patient base to include any critically ill person whether medical or surgical. Unlike the recovery room which closed at the end of the day, these ICUs offered care around the clock with the continuous presence of a nurse.[5] The earliest of these ICUs used portable equipment, including oxygen tanks,

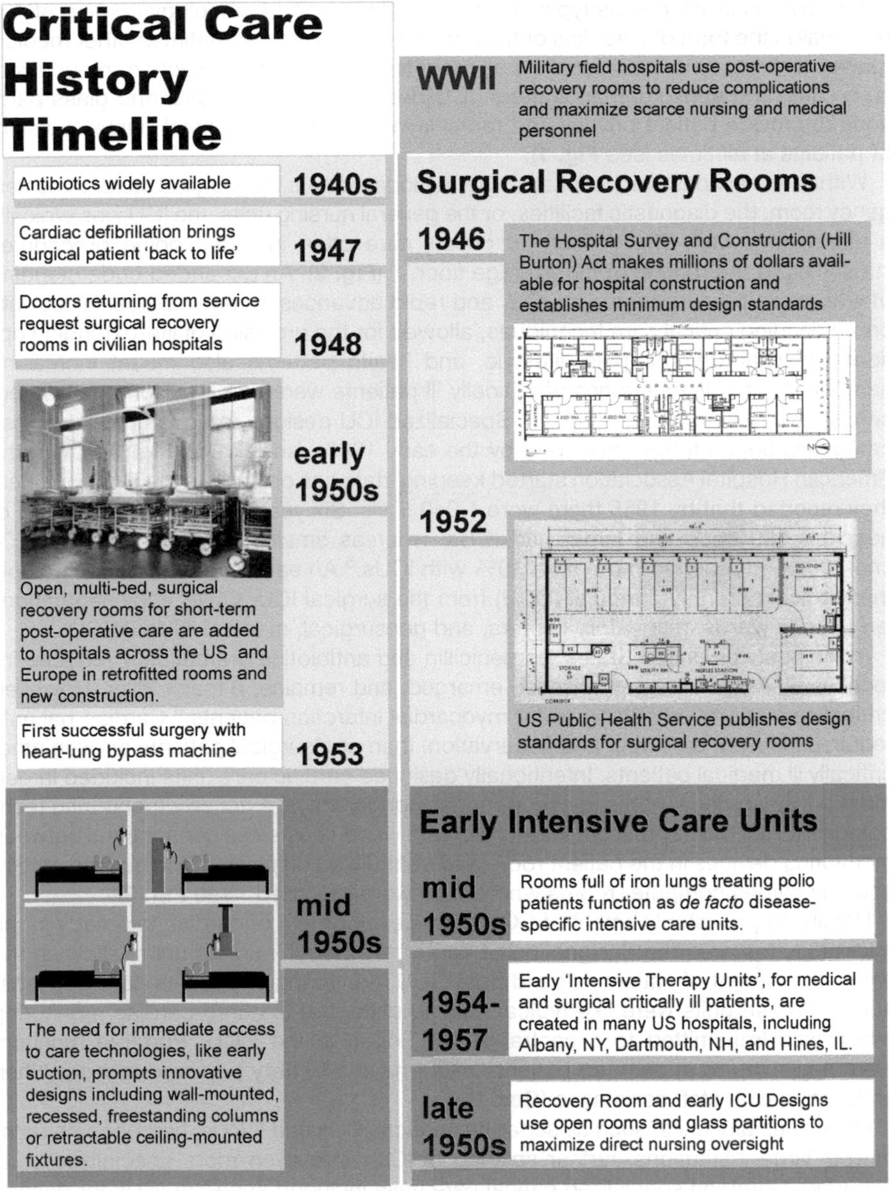
Critical Care History Timeline
Antibiotics widely available
1940s
Cardiac defibrillation brings surgical patient 'back to life'
1947
Doctors returning from service request surgical recovery rooms in civilian hospitals
1948
early 1950s
Open, multi-bed, surgical recovery rooms for short-term post-operative care are added to hospitals across the US and Europe in retrofitted rooms and new construction.
First successful surgery with heart-lung bypass machine
1953
mid 1950s
The need for immediate access to care technologies, like early suction, prompts innovative designs including wall-mounted, recessed, freestanding columns or retractable ceiling-mounted fixtures.
WWII
Military field hospitals use post-operative recovery rooms to reduce complications and maximize scarce nursing and medical personnel
Surgical Recovery Rooms
1946
The Hospital Survey and Construction (Hill Burton) Act makes millions of dollars available for hospital construction and establishes minimum design standards
CORRIDOR
1952
ISOLATION
STORAGE
UTILITY RM
NURSES STATION
CORRIDOR
US Public Health Service publishes design standards for surgical recovery rooms
Early Intensive Care Units
mid 1950s
Rooms full of iron lungs treating polio patients function as de facto disease-specific intensive care units.
1954-1957
Early 'Intensive Therapy Units', for medical and surgical critically ill patients, are created in many US hospitals, including Albany, NY, Dartmouth, NH, and Hines, IL.
late 1950s
Recovery Room and early ICU Designs use open rooms and glass partitions to maximize direct nursing oversight

Fig. 1. Critical care historical timeline: recovery rooms to early ICUs. (*Adapted from* US Public Health Service, "Elements of the General Hospital," Hospitals 20:5 (May 1946) p. 70; US Public Health Service "Recovery Rooms", Hospitals 26:11 (Nov 1952) p. 74; F.T. Crossling and John Hutchison, "Special Series on Hospital Planning. V. Experience in the use of a recovery room during the past four years," 6:7(July 1961) p. 329; Diagram of suction mounting options by author, with permissions.)

but newly constructed units typically featured life-support technology coming off the headwall in the form of electrical outlets, piped oxygen, and sometimes other medical gasses, lighting, and occasionally wall mounted equipment like suction, blood pressure cuffs, and sphygmomanometers. ICU designers used curtains and glass partitions to provide patient privacy and radial layouts to maintain direct nurse oversight of patients at all times (see **Fig. 1**).

Within the new postwar hospitals, whether located near the surgical suite, the emergency room, the diagnostic facilities, or the general nursing units, the ICU was typically a stand-alone unit. The delivery of critical care often included doing procedures "upsetting to the routine of the average floor."[3] (**Fig. 2**). An expanded understanding of who could be cared for in an ICU, and rapid advances in medical specialties with corresponding critical care techniques, allowed for the provision of life-extending options. Postwar demographic, lifestyle, and health patterns also meant increasing numbers of unique categories of critically ill patients were admitted to hospitals (eg, coronary, pediatric, burn, surgical). Specialized ICU designs to accommodate these categories began to be developed by the early 1960s (see **Fig. 2**; **Fig. 3**). Once the American Hospital Association started keeping statistics on ICUs in the United States, they reported that by 1965 there were 1,040 ICUs. Six years later more than 90% of hospitals 500 beds and larger had ICUs, whereas smaller hospitals between 100 and 200 beds reported more than 30% with ICUs.[5] An early separation of ICUs split the medical coronary care unit (CCU) from the surgical ICU. Other early separations led to polio wards, respiratory centers, and nonsurgical, medical ICUs (MICU).

In the postwar United States, as penicillin and antibiotics dramatically reduced infectious diseases, coronary disease emerged, and remains, a major killer. However, critical care improved outcomes for myocardial infarction patients.[6] Cardiac patients required different care (rest and observation) than postsurgical patients or even other critically ill medical patients. Intentionally designed cardiac care units included larger, more private, patient rooms to accommodate longer stays, extensive monitoring technologies (EKG, blood pressure, heart rate) with wired or wireless connections between monitoring devices in the patient room and centralized displays at the nursing station and sometimes computer rooms where data were recorded[7] (see **Fig. 3**).

Parallel to the establishment of CCUs, the development of cardiac telemetry in the mid-1960s fostered the designation of acute "telemetry" nursing units, allowing the early assessment of patient risk and post-CCU monitoring of patients during rehabilitation.[8] These units were like typical nursing units, but featured cardiac monitoring which was transmitted to a central station, often in the CCU. Portable monitors were beginning to appear, so patients might have a battery powered monitor when ambulating with staff assistance (**Box 1**).

Once specialty units, such as separate surgical ICUs and CCUs, had become common in large institutions, further splitting of ICUs into even more specialized units occurred. Common specialized critical care units included separate ICUs for general surgical and cardiovascular patients (Surgical ICU [SICU], Cardiovascular ICU [CVICU]) and for medical and coronary care patients (MICU, CCU). Such specialty ICUs for multiple services began to appear at teaching hospitals as demand in such centers could be justified. Medical education favored specialization and physician specialists made the case for other specialized ICUs such as burn, trauma, respiratory, neurosurgery, nephrology, pediatrics, and others.

Second Generation of Critical Care (1970–1995)

By the end of the 1960s, nearly every hospital had at least one ICU and many also had an additional specialized unit. ICU growth was explosive (see **Fig. 3**). As the 1970s

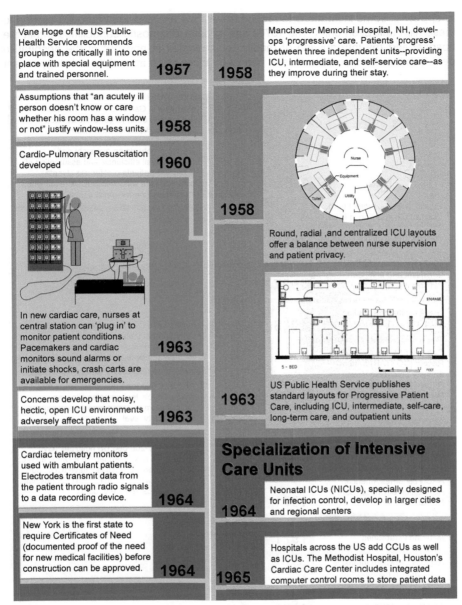

1957 Vane Hoge of the US Public Health Service recommends grouping the critically ill into one place with special equipment and trained personnel.

1958 Manchester Memorial Hospital, NH, develops 'progressive' care. Patients 'progress' between three independent units--providing ICU, intermediate, and self-service care--as they improve during their stay.

1958 Assumptions that "an acutely ill person doesn't know or care whether his room has a window or not" justify window-less units.

1960 Cardio-Pulmonary Resuscitation developed

1958 Round, radial ,and centralized ICU layouts offer a balance between nurse supervision and patient privacy.

1963 In new cardiac care, nurses at central station can 'plug in' to monitor patient conditions. Pacemakers and cardiac monitors sound alarms or initiate shocks, crash carts are available for emergencies.

1963 Concerns develop that noisy, hectic, open ICU environments adversely affect patients

1963 US Public Health Service publishes standard layouts for Progressive Patient Care, including ICU, intermediate, self-care, long-term care, and outpatient units

Specialization of Intensive Care Units

1964 Cardiac telemetry monitors used with ambulant patients. Electrodes transmit data from the patient through radio signals to a data recording device.

1964 Neonatal ICUs (NICUs), specially designed for infection control, develop in larger cities and regional centers

1964 New York is the first state to require Certificates of Need (documented proof of the need for new medical facilities) before construction can be approved.

1965 Hospitals across the US add CCUs as well as ICUs. The Methodist Hospital, Houston's Cardiac Care Center includes integrated computer control rooms to store patient data

Fig. 2. Critical care historical timeline: early ICUs to specialization of intensive care units. (*Adapted from* Plan diagram of radial ICU layout by author; Diagram of cardiac care with central nurse station and bedside unit; US Public Health Service, Elements of Progressive Care, US Govt Printing Office: Washington, DC, 1963, p. 77; with permissions.)

began, larger hospitals began to group multiple specialized ICUs into "Critical Care Complexes" on single floors, wings, or towers[9] (**Fig. 4**). A project at the Medical College of Virginia in Richmond had seven specialized ICUs on a single floor. Clustering ICUs near one another provided advantages for support functions such as pharmacy and laboratory medicine. Satellite pharmacy and laboratory locations near ICUs began to appear at some institutions to reduce travel time and provide improved service to these high utilization units. The 1970s saw greater diagnostic capabilities within the hospital and the introduction of mobile technologies in and out of the hospital to deal with the rising complexities of care. Advances such as mobile radiology meant

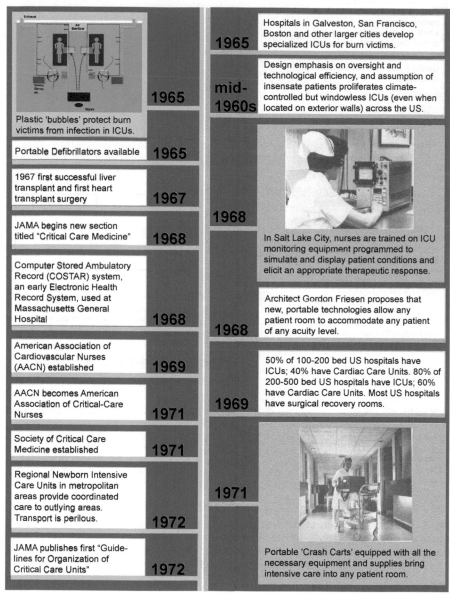

Fig. 3. Critical care historical timeline of specialization of intensive care units. (*Adapted from* Plan diagram of bubble isolation enclosures around patients in burn unit by author; Homer R. Warner, Alberto Budkin "A 'link trainer' for the coronary care unit," Computers and Biomedical Research 2:2 (Oct 1968) p. 137; Richard A. Fairchild and Howard N. Allen "Monitoring Systems for Intensive Care," Medical Clinics of North America 55:5 (Sept 1971) p. 1122; with permission.)

Box 1
Evolution of ICU Privacy

Although recovery room designers had presumed an unconscious patient, insensible to and thus not in need of any patient amenities such as privacy, visitor accommodations, or ambulation space, the longer stay of the ICU patient prompted designs for increased patient privacy, usually by partitions while maintaining direct lines of nurse oversight. Whether or not a critical patient space required an outside window remained a matter of debate. Suspecting that "an acutely ill patient doesn't know or care whether his room has a window or not," the designers of an experimental ICU at the Rochester Methodist Hospital in Minnesota provided one of the cubicles in the radial unit "with an illuminated scene in place of a window" to gauge the effect on the patient.[36] Numerous early ICUs were designed and built with windowless patient rooms. Awareness of the negative effect of these early ICU environments on patient recovery appeared as early as 1963.

---

vulnerable and unstable patients could be x-rayed in their ICU bed without a disruptive trip to another department, often on another floor.

As significant numbers of patients experienced ICU treatment, new patterns and designs emerged. The awareness of ICU delirium prompted many efforts to ameliorate ICU noise and lighting. Marker boards indicating the date and providing names of assigned staff members were installed to better coordinate care and visiting. As early ambulation for categories of critically ill patients proved impactful on patient outcomes, ICU designs with corridors or other walkable spaces increased, sometimes at the expense of nurse oversight. These patterns and the widespread usage of ICUs led to increasingly focused studies by researchers. One study, *Planning for Cardiac Care* led by Clipson and Wehrer at the University of Michigan, documented analysis of existing units, functional needs for patient care, full scale mock-ups of patient rooms used in clinical scenarios, simulation model outputs for bed need, and recommendations regarding unit design such as increased room size and the use of commode chairs for toileting to reduce patient stress and avoid disconnecting the heart monitor[10] (see **Fig. 4**). In 2006, David Allison at Clemson University and Kirk Hamilton at Texas A&M produced a study of hospital departmental square footage allocations, which included critical care units[11] (**Box 2**).

ICUs had often been large open bays divided only by curtains; this was, after all, the model learned from wartime, surgical recovery rooms, and polio wards. Private rooms were initially only for private-pay patients, disruptive, or infectious cases. The 1980s and 1990s began to see a shift toward increased numbers of private rooms in hospitals, in part to attract insured, middle-class patients.[5] The first justifications were for privacy and dignity, and there was usually a pay differential. Some institutions elected to change their acute care units to all private rooms so there would be no pay difference for a multi-bed room. Hospitals that made the change to all private rooms for financial and patient satisfaction reasons sometimes also made the change in their ICUs. Although some raised concerns about reduced ability to observe patients and increased isolation of staff members, the trend continued (**Figs. 5** and **6**).

During the 1990s, the rationale for private rooms changed. Studies of infection indicated transmission was facilitated by multi-bed settings. Given the immunocompromised condition of the most vulnerable critical care patients, infection control became a compelling new argument for a shift to private rooms throughout the hospital, including in critical care.[12] ICUs featuring private rooms were inevitably larger than open bays, as the square footage per bed increased. The need to accommodate increasing medical technologies associated with care of the highest acuity cases provided a further impetus for larger rooms (see **Fig. 5**).

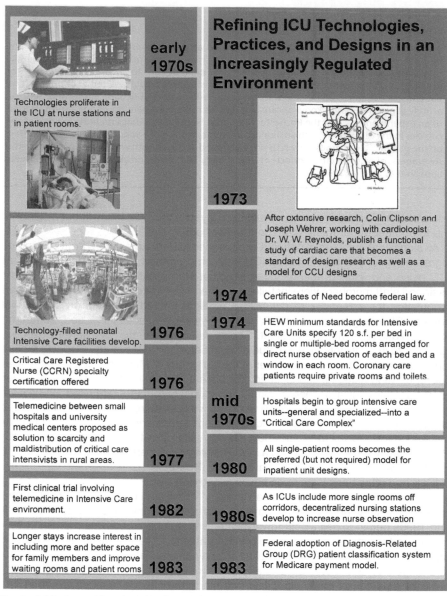

Fig. 4. Critical care historical timeline: refining ICU technologies, practices, and designs in an increasingly regulated environment. (*Adapted from* Richard A. Fairchild and Howard N. Allen "Monitoring Systems for Intensive Care," Medical Clinics of North America 55:5 (Sept 1971) p. 1108; D.E.M. Taylor "Problems of patients in an intensive care unit: The prevention of the intensive care syndrome," International Journal of Nursing Studies 8:1 (Feb 1971) between pp. 52 and 53; Richard S. Baum "The Large Private Hospital and Neonatal Intensive Care," Clinics in Perinatology 3:2 (Sep 1976) p. 308; Drawing by Frank Zilm, adapted from Clipson CW; Wehrer JJ, Planning for cardiac care; a guide to the planning and design of cardiac care facilities. Ann Arbor: Ann Arbor Health Administration Press; 1973; with permissions.)

Box 2
Clipson & Wehrer's *Planning for Cardiac Care*

One of the earliest comprehensive research studies of critical care unit design was initiated in the early 1970s through a Kellogg Foundation grant as part of the Michigan Comprehensive Coronary Care Project. Directed by the cardiologist Dr E.W. Reynolds, the design research was led by the University School of Architecture professors Colin Clipson and Joseph J. Wehrer. The resulting 300-page publication, *Planning for Cardiac Care*, documented a detailed analysis of existing units, the functional needs for patient care, full-scale mock-ups of patient rooms, simulation model output to determine bed needs, and overall recommendations regarding unit design.[10] Medical and nursing staff were recruited to participate in critical care scenarios in the mock-up spaces, which were video recorded for detailed analysis. The resulting recommendations regarding patient room sizes range from a standard room of 150 net square feet (nsf) to larger "expanded" rooms of 180 nsf and procedure rooms of 280 nsf. This research mock-up approach was subsequently used to analyze the proposed patient room configurations for the University of Michigan replacement hospital.[37] While not widely disseminated in the health care architecture community, the study was awarded the first Progressive Architecture Design Research Award (see **Fig. 4**).

The ICU fostered the development of specially trained physicians, known as intensivists, who had no practice other than in critical care. Similarly, advanced practice nurses received specialty training to serve in critical care. These specialized clinicians provided 24-hour care, supporting admitting physicians who often came only twice a day at early morning and late evening to protect their routine daily private practice obligations. By the 1990s, specialized critical care medicine, nursing, and technology could save patients who, a decade earlier, might not have survived. High-acuity critical care populations filled units with increasingly vulnerable, unstable, and high-risk cases. To accommodate the increasing patient volume, hospital administrators investigated units called stepdown or intermediate care that were intended to treat patients whose acuity fell between the ICU and a typical nursing unit.

Advances in specialized treatments—open heart surgery, transplants, trauma, neurosurgery, microsurgery, and other demanding specialties—fueled a parallel development of critical nursing skills and training. ICU nurses' work was increasingly challenged by the growing numbers of physiologically frail and unstable patients who needed a great deal of individual care. The American Association of Cardiovascular Nurses was founded in 1969 for specialized nurses, changing its name to the American Association of Critical-Care Nurses and retaining the AACN acronym in 1971.[5] These nurses developed training and certification for critical care specialization as they developed new ways of organizing their increasingly complex work. At the same time, the Society of Critical Care Medicine (SCCM) was founded in 1971, with a multidiscipline membership that includes physicians, nurses, pharmacists, respiratory personnel, and even a few architects. Critical Care Registered Nurse (CCRN) certification began in 1976 (see **Figs. 3** and **4**). These organizations pioneered recognition, training, and certification of specialized clinicians in multiple disciplines, including intensivists and advanced practice nurses.

Third Generation of Mature Critical Care (1995–2019)

In the mature phase of critical care development,[13,14] life-support systems were further developed. No longer simple interventions with a few utilities on the headwall behind the bed, ICU room designs proliferated to include the ability to deliver more gasses, uninterruptible power, examination lighting, and physiologic monitors capable of multiple parameters. IV pumps were usually hung on rolling poles or bed-mounted

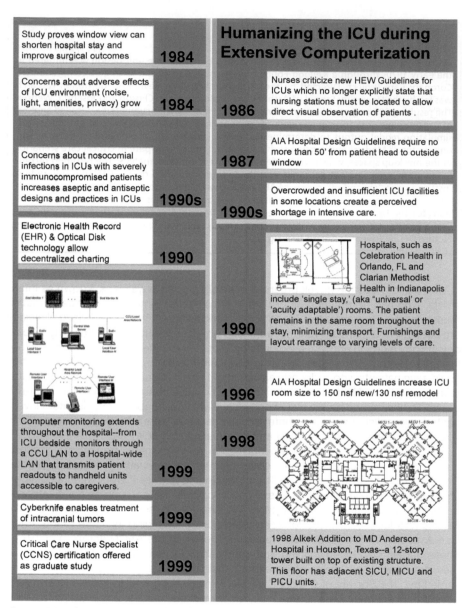

Fig. 5. Critical care historical timeline: humanizing the ICU during extensive computerization. (*Adapted from* Jastremski CA, ICU Bedside Environment: A Nursing Perspective, Critical Care Clinics, Volume 16, Issue 4, (October 2000), p. 728; Courtesy of HKS Architects.)

poles. In some cases, IV poles hung from ceiling tracks running parallel to each side of the bed. Although most of the ICU rooms featured headwall designs and continue to do so today, variations were innovated to remove the bed from the headwall; after all, in a crisis or code situation, the bed must be pulled away from the wall and someone must carefully step over the many connected utility umbilicals to stand at the patient's head and assure the airway remains open.

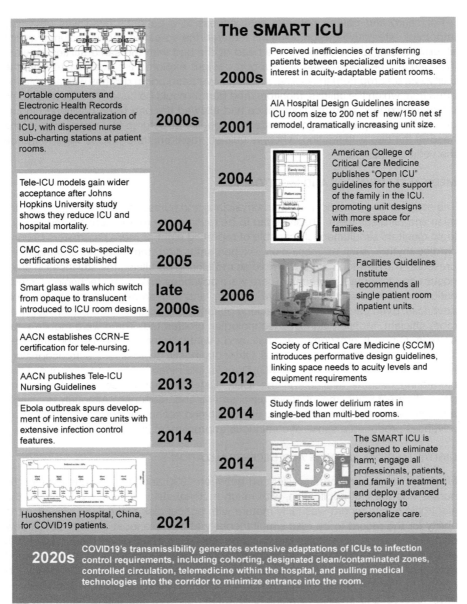

The SMART ICU

2000s Perceived inefficiencies of transferring patients between specialized units increases interest in acuity-adaptable patient rooms.

2001 AIA Hospital Design Guidelines increase ICU room size to 200 net sf new/150 net sf remodel, dramatically increasing unit size.

2004 American College of Critical Care Medicine publishes "Open ICU" guidelines for the support of the family in the ICU. promoting unit designs with more space for families.

2006 Facilities Guidelines Institute recommends all single patient room inpatient units.

2012 Society of Critical Care Medicine (SCCM) introduces performative design guidelines, linking space needs to acuity levels and equipment requirements

2014 Study finds lower delirium rates in single-bed than multi-bed rooms.

2014 The SMART ICU is designed to eliminate harm; engage all professionals, patients, and family in treatment; and deploy advanced technology to personalize care.

2000s Portable computers and Electronic Health Records encourage decentralization of ICU, with dispersed nurse sub-charting stations at patient rooms.

2004 Tele-ICU models gain wider acceptance after Johns Hopkins University study shows they reduce ICU and hospital mortality.

2005 CMC and CSC sub-specialty certifications established

late 2000s Smart glass walls which switch from opaque to translucent introduced to ICU room designs.

2011 AACN establishes CCRN-E certification for tele-nursing.

2013 AACN publishes Tele-ICU Nursing Guidelines

2014 Ebola outbreak spurs development of intensive care units with extensive infection control features.

2021 Huoshenshen Hospital, China, for COVID19 patients.

2020s COVID19's transmissibility generates extensive adaptations of ICUs to infection control requirements, including cohorting, designated clean/contaminated zones, controlled circulation, telemedicine within the hospital, and pulling medical technologies into the corridor to minimize entrance into the room.

Fig. 6. Critical care historical timeline: the smart ICU and coronavirus (COVID-19. (*Adapted from* Virginia Commonwealth University Hospital, (Courtesy of Frank Zilm, D.Arch, Lawrence, KS); Fakhry M, and Mohammed WE, "Impact of Family Presence on Healthcare Outcomes and Patients' Wards Design." Alexandria Engineering Journal 61:12 (2022): 10713-26; Magdzinski A, Marte A, Boitor M, Raboy-Thaw J, Paré B, and Gélinas C. "Transition to a Newly Constructed Single Patient Room Adult Intensive Care Unit - Clinicians' Preparation and Work Experience," Journal of Critical Care 48 (2018/12/01/ 2018): 426-32, page 428; Halpern NA. "Innovative Designs for the Smart ICU: Part 2: The ICU." CHEST 145:3 (2014): 646-58, Page 650; and Chen Y, Lei J, Li J, Zhang Z, Yu Z, and Du C. "Design Characteristics on the Indoor and Outdoor Air Environments of the Covid-19 Emergency Hospital." Journal of Building Engineering 45 (01/01/2022): 103246, Page 4; with permissions.)

For neuro and trauma patients, easy access to a patient's head was obviously important; alternative design solutions featured the so-called "power column" which stood vertically at the corner of the head of the bed with the same utilities as were included in a headwall. Other life support designs explored the potential to have the utility system drop from the ceiling, including overhead boom designs with articulating arms from which the utilities, monitors, and pumps could be hung.[15] These adjustable overhead fixtures freed the floor space and allowed the bed to be positioned in any orientation. European designs included bridge-like structures that spanned over the head of the bed with lighting, whereas utilities, monitors, and pumps were found on the vertical columns.

MEDICAL TECHNOLOGY AND MONITORING

The early cardiac monitors permitted physicians and nurses to rapidly identify arrhythmias and cardiac stress. These began to be replaced by more sophisticated physiologic monitors simultaneously capable of reporting eight or more parameters beyond cardiac rhythm, such as respiration, oxygen saturation, temperature, or intracranial pressure. The development of physiologic monitoring paralleled the advances in diagnostics and treatment protocols. There were advances in IV pump technology, medication administration, point-of-care testing, and research-based pharmaceutical advances. Even barcoding made tracking patients, medications, and billable supplies more efficient. Mobile diagnostic technologies proliferated. There were mobile x-ray devices, C-arm fluoroscopy machines, and eventually even a mobile Computerized Tomography (CT) for imaging in place. Other diagnostic devices for Electroncephalography (EEG), Electromyography (EMG), Doppler examination of extremities, or glucose monitoring became available in the ICUs. Satellite pharmacies, laboratories, and point-of-care testing meant rapid assessment and response. Although no single advance represented a watershed, the combined technical, surgical, and medical advances produced a sense of continuous improvement in critical care.

DIGITAL MEDICAL RECORDS AND DECENTRALIZATION

Electronic medical records proliferated between 1990 and 2000. Documentation by nurses was the first application, with much material still in hard copy. By 2000, the electronic health record was fairly mature with optical disk technology providing the ability for the record to be read simultaneously at multiple locations. Almost all new diagnostic images were digital and could be made part of the digital record. Hospitals struggled with the cost of transitioning older film files to digital media, but reclaimed silver that had been used to develop the x-ray images helped offset the huge investment. The 2014 Accountable Care Act mandated electronic records. The ability to have records and images at multiple locations allowed the first experiments with decentralized charting, moving documentation closer to the bedside in units with all private rooms that had become quite large (see **Fig. 5**).

The shift in medical records from a single hard copy binder that had to be kept at a central station to portable electronic records allowed experimentation with decentralized critical care unit designs. The fundamental concept is to move the responsible nurse closer to the patient's bedside, whether in the room, just outside the room, or just across the corridor from the room. A typical ICU nurse must assess and document each of their patient's conditions every 1, 2, or 4 hours, depending on acuity, so moving electronic documentation and charting closer to the patient can greatly reduce nurse travel distance. Decentralized nurse stations could also include other helpful elements, such as observation windows, medications, supplies, telephones, seating, bookshelves, personal storage (sweaters, purses, lunches), and more (see **Figs. 5** and **6**). Problems cropped up in decentralized units that completely eliminated their central stations and for less experienced nurses who lost some of the mentoring advantages associated with central stations.

Decentralized design variations are numerous. A literature survey by Fay and colleagues[16] provided examples of the most prominent variations in configuration along with some of the arguments for and against models of decentralization. Ultimately, a rough consensus in the industry has gathered around the concept of combining the advantages of decentralization with the advantages of centralization, resulting in an effective hybrid model that spreads some activities (such as charting and medication administration) but concentrates others (such as a unit clerk, telephone answering, pneumatic tubes, and copy machines) into "collaboration" or team areas.

One justification for decentralization was the increasing size of critical care units. As units included more patients and housed them in large private rooms, the size increased beyond the ability to observe every room and patient from a central position. Decentralized charting allowed some to imagine there might no longer be a need for a central station, and decentralization suggested that the corridor could be straight instead of concentric or radial. If this was true, ICUs could be placed within the same structural footprint as a typical patient unit, and many examples were built along this model.[17] Unfortunately, straight corridors and private rooms drastically reduced the observation of patients and many nurses felt a lack of colleague support as they could no longer see each other and each other's patients. When observation and contact are reduced, nurses fear sentinel events can occur in one room while they are in another, and no one else is responsible for watching their patients. As a result, some have proposed returning to designs that offer increased visualization of staff and patients.[18]

THE ROLE OF CODES AND STANDARDS

Hospitals are one of the most highly regulated organizations in the United States, with multiple laws and organizations monitoring care, including the spaces where care is provided. Licensure of nonfederal hospitals is established by the state laws and regulations. In addition to state requirements, federal agencies providing reimbursement for the cost of care for selected patients, and voluntary compliance review commissions, have mandated conformity with national building codes as a requirement for payment.

A key evolution in the design of hospitals was the enactment of the Hill–Burton program, initiated in 1946 to stimulate construction of needed hospital capacity in the United States, particularly in rural areas. It quickly became apparent that some proposed projects lacked experienced health care design architects. In 1947, the Public Health Service published rules and regulations regarding the components of hospitals. Included in the initial regulation were requirements regarding the maximum nursing unit size (30 beds), the mix of single, double, and four-bed patient rooms, and the minimum size of those rooms: 125 net square feet (nsf) of usable floor area in a room for single rooms and 80 nsf per bed for multi-patient rooms. They listed isolation room requirements and guidance for other building components.

Hill–Burton standards led to the proliferation of nursing unit designs with multiple small rooms off a central double-loaded corridor, which made nurse oversight of patients more difficult.[5] The prevalence of these nursing unit layouts in postwar hospital designs, in which critical care was difficult to provide, contributed to the rapid adoption of separate, smaller, ICUs where observation could be increased.

As with many care components, the response to space needs of critical care units lagged the initial implementation of new care protocols. In 1964, the federal agency for Health, Education, and Welfare (HEW) through the Public Health Service published *Coronary Care Unit*, including the description, and illustrations, of a prototype unit. In 1965, this was expanded to *A Facility Design for Coronary Care*.[19,20] The suggested size of this unit for a community hospital was 4 to 5 beds, with the individual area per bed 11 feet by 11 feet (121 nsf). An addendum to this publication pointed out that the layout illustrations did not indicate windows in the unit, which were required at the time by the General Guidelines for construction.

Over time three key organizations have been instrumental in establishing space guidelines for critical care in the United States: HEW, the American Institute of Architects (AIA), and the Facilities Guidelines Institute (FGI). **Table 1** documents the evolution of two components: room size and isolation room requirements. Early guidelines did not specify requirements for critical care units. The base area requirement was 100 nsf for single bedrooms and 80 nsf per bed for multiple occupancy. The first mention of critical care beds was in the 1974 HEW Minimum Standards, requiring single patient rooms, with a toilet, for coronary care patients. Since that period, the area required for single bedrooms in new construction has grown from 150 to 200 nsf, with leniency for remodeling plans. Access to windows with outdoor views has also been modified, with early requirements allowing up to 50 feet from the head of a patient to an outside window, to the current requirement of a window at each patient bed. Toileting requirements have also changed, particularly with recent studies of potential self-contamination of patients through aerosols associated with flushing toilets.[21] Patient toilet rooms are now required in all critical care patient rooms and cannot be shared.

Although these guidelines were proposed as minimum standards, pressure to reduce health care costs and the costs of construction resulted in many cases where interpretation of the standards were instead used as maximum allowable. The use of these guidelines should not be a substitute for the functional and space programming of these units on a case-by-case basis.

ICU DESIGN GUIDELINES ARE TRANSFORMED

The SCCM task force produced design guidelines in 2012 which introduced performance (not prescriptive) guidelines.[22] Minimum sizes for patient rooms in prior guidelines from the Public Health Service, HEW, AIA, or FGI were not suited to the significant differences between ICUs found in smaller rural facilities, community hospitals, or large tertiary medical centers. Performance guidelines identified space needs according to acuity levels and equipment requirements. Since the 1980s, there has been an increased emphasis on evidence-based design as a parallel to evidence-based medicine.[12,23]

FINANCIAL INCENTIVES AND DISINCENTIVES

On January 4, 1975, the US Congress enacted Public Law 93-641 in an effort to control health care costs. Rising costs brought public attention and concern, and ICUs were among the most expensive services in the hospital. Among the provisions of the law was the creation of a regional and state-level Certificate-of-Need (CON) process to assure that capital investments were filling needs and not duplicative of existing services. The federal government funded the creation of regional Health Systems

Table 1
ICU patient room design guidelines and regulations 1947 to 2022

| | Year | Guidelines/Standard | Organization | Minimum Room Size (Net Square Feet) and Requirements | | | |
				Single	Multiple (per Bed)	Isolation Rooms	Comments
1940–1970	1947	Hill–Burton (Appendix A)	PHS	125	80	1	No specific critical care standards
	1955	Hill–Burton (Appendix A)	PHS	100	80	1 per hospital	No specific critical care standards
	1960	Minimum Requirements of Construction	HEW	100	80		No specific criteria for critical care beds
	1962	General Standards for Construction and Equipment of Hospitals	HEW	100	80		No specific criteria for critical care beds
	1967	General Standards for Construction and Equipment of Hospitals	HEW	100	80	1 for every 30 beds	No specific criteria for critical care beds anteroom required for isolation. Toilets for every patient room.
	1969	General Standards for Construction and Equipment of Hospitals	HEW	100	80	1 for every 30 beds	No specific criteria for critical care beds anteroom required for isolation. Toilets for every patient room.
1970–1990	1974	Minimum Requirements of Construction	HEW	120	120	At least 1 private room per unit	Private rooms, with toilet, for cardiac windows required in each patient room
	1975	Minimum Requirements of Construction	HEW	120	120	At least 1 private room per unit	Private rooms, with toilet, for cardiac windows required in each patient room
	1984	Guidelines for Construction and Equipment of Hospital and Medical Facilities	HHS	120	100		Private rooms, with toilet, for cardiac windows required in each patient room

(continued on next page)

Table 1
(continued)

	Year	Guidelines/Standard	Organization	Minimum Room Size (Net Square Feet) and Requirements			
				Single	Multiple (per Bed)	Isolation Rooms	Comments
1990–2000	1996	Guidelines for the Design and Construction of Hospitals	AIA	150 for New 130 remodel	Same as Single room	No minimum	At least one outside window per room
	1987	Guidelines for Construction and Equipment of Hospital and Medical Facilities	AIA	200 New 150 Remodel	Same as Single room	At least 1	50 foot maximum distance from patient head to outside window
	1993	Guidelines for Construction and Equipment of Hospital and Medical Facilities	AIA	200 New 150 Remodel	150 per bed	No minimum identified. Anteroom required	50 foot maximum distance from patient head to outside window
	1997	Guidelines for Construction and Equipment of Hospital and Medical Facilities	AIA	200 New 150 Remodel	Same as Single room	At least 1	50 foot maximum distance from patient head to outside window
2000–2022	2001	Guidelines for Construction and Equipment of Hospital and Medical Facilities	AIA	200 New 150 Remodel	Same as Single room	At least 1	50 foot maximum distance from patient head to outside window. Toilet required in coronary care
	2006	Guidelines for Construction and Equipment of Hospital and Medical Facilities	AIA	200 New150 Remodel	Same as Single room	At least 1	Patient window required per each bed. If combined ICU/CCU 50% private rooms. Toilets in CCU rooms
	2010	Guidelines for the Design and Construction of Health Care Facilities	FGI	200 New 150 Remodel	150 per bed	At least 1	Patient window required per each bed. Direct access to an enclosed toilet
	2014	Guidelines for the Design and Construction of Health Care Facilities	FGI	200 New 150 Remodel	Same as single room	At least 1	13-foot minimum headwall width. Window required; 50-foot maximum distance from patient bed, where bays or cubicles are

Year	Document					
						provided, no more than one intervening patient care station between any patient bed and window. Direct access to an enclosed toilet or human waste disposal room.
2018	Guidelines for the Design and Construction of Health Care Facilities	FGI	200 New 150 Remodel	Same as single room	At least 1	13-foot minimum headwall width. Window required; 50-foot maximum distance from patient bed, where cubicles are provided, no more than one intervening patient care station between any patient bed and window. Direct access to an enclosed toilet or human waste disposal room.
2020	Guidelines for the Design and Construction of Health Care Facilities	FGI	200 New 150 Remodel	Same as single room	At least 1	Patient window required per each bed. Patient toilet required in each room.

Abbreviations: AIA, The American Institute of Architects; FGI, Facilities Guidelines Institute; HEW, Department of Health, Education and Welfare; HHS, Department of Health and Human Services; PHS, Public Health Service.

Agencies (HSAs) charged with assessing regional health care needs, the resulting facility priorities, and to approve applications for major construction, new services, and major capital equipment purchases. A frequently referenced theory influencing this approach was called the "Roemer effect," based on the research presented by Dr Milton Roemer that a built bed was a filled bed (regardless of medical need).[24]

Each state has authority to develop a review process and guidelines for project reviews. Some states developed the target ratios of acute hospital beds per 1,000 population. The development of space guidelines regarding room sizes, shell space, and other building characteristics was also established on a state-by-state basis. One of the unintended consequences of this approach was a rush to get approval of a bed project, potentially locking out competing hospitals from expansion. This included critical care beds, which provided higher reimbursements for each day of care than acute care beds. Centers for Medicare & Medicaid Services (CMS) policies during the early 1980s requiring the separate physical designation of "stepdown" intermediate acute care units delayed the development of intermediate levels of care, resulting in many critical care units providing patient days of care which fell below their target acuity standards.[25]

In 1983, Congress allowed CMS to implement a prospective payment model for hospitals based on diagnostic-related groups (DRGs) to identify the patient case mix, using statistical modeling initially developed by Robert Fetter and John Thompson at Yale University in the 1970s. This reversed some of the financial incentives for extended ICU days, resulting in a shift of some ICU days into "stepdown" beds, particularly for coronary care.[26]

In 1986, Congress passed legislation ending this health planning law, leaving the continuation of CON reviews up to each state. Currently, 35 states maintain some form of CON reviews. Few states have continued the original HSAs. As health care finance shifted from reimbursement to capitated care models, the decisions regarding capital expenditures have shifted, with critical care bed needs aligned more closely with actual anticipated demand.

In the 1980s and 1990s, hospitals and health systems found themselves in competitive situations. The organizations with the strongest market shares, especially in high-cost services such as surgery, imaging, emergency, and critical care, had an advantage. During this period, hospitals made every effort to gain regulatory permission for expansions, renovations, or replacements of these high-dollar services. Hospitals engaged in aggressive marketing of these services. As a result, this period saw many critical care facilities constructed.

UNIVERSAL ROOM AND ACUITY-ADAPTABLE ROOM EXPERIMENTS

Universal confusion. The preferred model for inpatient unit design shifted to all single bedrooms in the 1980s, and the move to all single-patient rooms was accelerated when the FGI established this model as the recommended standard in 2006. As state licensing agencies adopted the FGI Guidelines as their minimum space standards, the strategies of matching patient care and staffing generated concepts incorporating terms including universal patient rooms, universal patient care, stepdown units, intermediate care, and acuity-adaptable rooms. Application of these terms has been inconsistent and often confusing.

One concept tested in the 90s was the "single stay" patient room, which was called a universal, or acuity-adaptable, room concept. The key concept was that patients would be admitted and stay in one patient room. Two examples are Celebration Health in Orlando, Florida, and Clarian (Methodist) Health in Indianapolis (see **Figs. 5** and **6**).

The Methodist hospital design of two 28-bed Cardiac Comprehensive Critical Care units was based on data showing that transfers of patients between critical care and acute care nursing units were associated with a risk of medication errors, higher costs, and potential longer lengths of stay.[27] "Technologically, the rooms are state of the art. All equipment and supplies required for the medical needs of critical care patients are easily accessible, including transforming (acuity-adaptable) headwalls and advanced computer technology..."[27]

Post-occupancy studies of the unit reported a 90% reduction in patient transports and a 70% reduction in medication errors.[27] Reports from other units indicated similar positive results, including pediatric cardiac care,[28] cardiothoracic units,[29,30] and kidney transplant units.[31]

Despite these care improvements, this acuity-adaptable strategy has not been generally adopted. Ann Hendrich, who developed Clarian's unit, believed that the acuity-adaptable room should only be used within a single service line and only for ICU and stepdown patients. Massachusetts General Hospital's universal room experiment promoted by manufacturers was intended to cover every room in the hospital so it could flex up or down as needed. It proved to be too expensive and was abandoned. Melissa Kwan reported in 2007 that several issues have limited the success of these approaches[32]: she identified specific issues, including the need to train all nursing staff on the units to provide care for high-risk patients, the maintenance of the required unit-wide nurse to patient ratios, high initial turnover of staff not comfortable with a new organizational model, complications with state licensure agencies and insurers, and physician discomfort with the mix of patients. At the time of the Kwan article, only a dozen sites were identified as acuity-adaptable units. She reported that at least three had abandoned the concept, including Clarian Methodist and Celebration Health.

What has since emerged from these early models is a redefinition of acuity-adaptable and universal care. The ability to flex-up to support higher acuity patients or to flex-down to move critical care patients safely into acute units has been developed to complement the traditional ICU. As the net square footage of acute patient rooms has evolved, and the width of the typical nursing unit room has approximated critical care rooms, many units are being labeled "universal" patient rooms, meaning they could be configured to accommodate critical care patients.

With aging of the US population, pressure to shift lower acuity patients out of inpatient beds, and implementation of patient rooms designed to accommodate all levels of care, revisiting the single-bed universal concept may occur.

SAME-HANDED ROOMS AND ERROR REDUCTION

A critical care issue which originated from typical nursing unit design has been the question of whether so-called same-handed rooms would reduce error. Same-handed rooms mean rooms that are literally identical in orientation and location of objects and services, as opposed to the more frequent back-to-back room designs.[33] Same-handed rooms are intended to enforce standardization as one might find in an aircraft cockpit or at a nuclear installation where error is unacceptable. The concept was proposed by John Reiling, administrator at a small hospital in West Bend, Wisconsin, based on the study of failsafe organizations.[34] A successful example of a larger ICU featuring same-handed rooms is Cedars Sinai in Los Angeles where the bed faces the corridor. Nurses generally scoff at the idea that orienting in only one way is sensible, as patients can have conditions at many locations on the body, and it remains to be seen whether research data will support reductions in error. Although many organizations have adopted the concept, no study has yet been published to demonstrate improved outcomes.

COVID-19 PANDEMIC EXPERIENCE AND LESSONS (2019-TODAY)

The world of critical care has been significantly disrupted by the COVID-19 pandemic. The global crisis has impacted the two most challenging room types: ICU rooms and infectious disease isolation rooms with anterooms. Many hospitals and health systems discovered that they were woefully ill prepared for huge numbers of highly contagious patients. The lessons of COVID will inevitably change the way hospitals and critical care units are designed in the future.

In Ontario, where planners remember the deadly Severe Acute Respiratory Syndrome (SARS) epidemic, current hospital plans recognize the importance of increasing isolation capacity so they plan for entire "cohort" isolation *units*, not just isolation rooms. The anteroom concept for entire units means dedicated space for donning and doffing of protective gear, perhaps in space that converts when the need arises. They are planning for 100% filtered outside air, exhausted directly with no recirculation. The lack of viable tests for new epidemic agents may limit the initial ability to implement cohort quarantine strategies, resulting in increased demand for isolation rooms.

Other examples included rapid conversion of nonclinical space to create improvised COVID units with donning and doffing capabilities. Will this mean some large spaces need to be prepared with medical gasses and electrical capacity in spaces that might be converted? Some institutions drilled holes in corridor walls to create technology ports so monitors, pumps, and medical equipment could be managed without entering the patient room. Will this mean future nursing unit corridors should be wider? An example from Israel used a telemedicine model for an expert "control room" outside the direct "hot zone" for work in the patient rooms.[35] Separating some of the staff to minimize exposure is an effective strategy and may become a more common approach when infection control is a priority.

SUMMARY

It should be clear that critical care and ICUs developed as a result of parallel advances in medicine and surgery, along with advances in nurse education and training, while benefiting from a constant introduction of new technology to support critical care. All of this occurred while being significantly impacted by changes in regulatory requirements, national health policy, and financial limitations. It is an astonishing story based on a rich mix of influences and a steady advancement of the healing arts. The story cannot be told without reference to the contributions of multiple actors from many disciplines. More patients than ever before now survive major illness and trauma and go on to have full lives. The complex world of critical care is indeed something close to the elusive "medical miracle."

The authors believe that future ICUs will be ever more important for patient care, more prevalent in hospitals, and will continue to evolve and change in positive ways as new procedures and technologies contribute to our post-COVID world. With the continuing shift of lower acuity care to outpatient settings, the aging of the US population, and increasingly sophisticated medical procedures, it is reasonable to project the continued growth and importance of critical care and acuity-adaptable stepdown care. Knowing how critical care emerged, how it progressed, and the problems that have been solved or created along the way, offers a greater ability to assess where design for critical care is (and perhaps should be) as it evolves in the future. Planners are advised to use evidence-based design concepts and performance criteria as they develop superior critical care environments of the future to flexibly serve increasingly high-acuity patients, their families, and their committed cadre of expert caregivers.

CLINICS CARE POINTS

- Surgical recovery rooms including examples from military field hospitals were models adapted for the earliest ICUs.
- Early ICUs (1950s and 1960s) were in large open bays with a central nursing station.
- High levels of observation and support from colleagues are crucial to quality care.
- Codes, standards, and government regulations profoundly influenced ICU designs in the United States.
- The development of cardiac monitors led to specialized coronary care units supported by cardiologists and specially trained nurses.
- ICUs supporting additional specialties were created at large or teaching hospitals.
- Advances in medical and diagnostic technologies that permitted the survival of increasingly vulnerable and acute patients influenced caregiving and design.
- As ICUs cared for higher acuity patients, the development of stepdown or intermediate care units with telemetry monitoring allowed for a level of care between the ICU and the acute nursing unit which reduced pressure on numbers of ICU beds.
- Attempts to reduce capital expenditures for hospital facilities at the national and state levels in the United States were not successful in blocking ICU development.
- As patient room size increased and more single-patient rooms were planned, unit size increased, creating problems with travel distance, support from colleagues, and contributed to experimentation with decentralization.
- Electronic health records accessed from multiple locations reduced dependence on a single paper medical record and made decentralization possible.
- The introduction of intensivists and advanced practice nurses provided more consistent care around the clock.
- Experience with COVID provided new appreciation for the importance of isolation and staff protection. This experience has shown the need to provide appropriate staff support spaces to help reduce the stress of patient care.

REFERENCES

1. Zuck D. Anaesthetic and postoperative recovery rooms. Anaesthesia 1995;50(5): 435–8.
2. Rustow I. Empire of the scalpel. New York, NY: Scribner; 2022.
3. Sadove MS, Cross J, Higgins HG, et al. The recovery room expands its service. Mod Hosp 1954;83(6):65–75.
4. Dunn FE, Shupp MG. The recovery room: a wartime economy. Am J Nurs 1943; 43(3):279–81.
5. Fairman J, Lynaugh J. Critical care nursing: a history. Philadelphia, PA: University of Pennsylvania Press; 1998.
6. Lockward HJ, Lundberg J, George AF, et al. Effect of intensive care on mortality rate of patients with myocardial infarcts. Public Health Rep 1963;78(8):655–61.
7. Sadove MS, Albrecht RF, Schumer W. Monitoring in the intensive care unit and the recovery room. Surg Clin 1968;48(1):9–15.
8. Rowe G. Cardiac telemetry and monitoring. JAMA 1964;187(5):31–2.

9. Cioppa FJ. The critical care complex. JAMA 1971;216(5):886.

10. Clipson C. Planning for cardiac care; a guide to the planning and design of cardiac care facilities. Ann Arbor, MI: Health Administration Press; 1973.

11. Allison D, Hamilton D. Area calculations for major hospital departments. Washington, DC: AAH Foundation Research Study; 2006.

12. Ulrich RS. Evidence-based health-care architecture. Lancet 2006;368(9554):S38.

13. Rashid M. A decade of adult intensive care unit design: a study of the physical design features of the best-practice examples. Crit Care Nurs Q 2006;29(4): 282–311.

14. Verderber S, Gray S, Suresh-Kumar S, et al. Intensive care unit built environments: a comprehensive literature review (2005-2020). Herd 2021;14(4):368–415.

15. Pati D, Evans J, Waggener L, et al. An exploratory examination of medical gas booms versus traditional headwalls in intensive care unit design. Crit Care Nurs Q 2008;31(4):340–56.

16. Fay L, Cai H, Real K. A systematic literature review of empirical studies on decentralized nursing stations. HERD: Health Environments Research & Design Journal 2018;12(1):44–68.

17. Hamilton D, Swoboda S, Lee J-T, et al. Decentralization: the corridor is the problem, not the alcove. Crit Care Nurs Q 2018;41:3–9.

18. Hamilton D, Swoboda S, Cadenhead C. Future ICU design: return to high visibility. ICU Management & Practice 2019;4:232–4.

19. Department of Health Education and Welfare. Coronary Care Unit. Washington, DC: US Gov't Printing Office; 1964.

20. Department of Health Education and Welfare. A facility designed for coronary care. Washington, DC: US Government Printing Office; 1965.

21. Barker J, Jones MV. The potential spread of infection caused by aerosol contamination of surfaces after flushing a domestic toilet. J Appl Microbiol 2005;99(2): 339–47.

22. Thompson DR, Hamilton DK, Cadenhead CD, et al. Guidelines for intensive care unit design. Crit Care Med. May 2012;40(5):1586–600.

23. Hamilton D, Shepley M. Design for critical care: an evidence-based approach. Milton Park, UK: Routledge; 2010.

24. Roemer MI. Hospital utilization under insurance. Hospitals 1959;33:36–7.

25. Zilm F. Four key decisions in the evolution of a critical care unit. Crit Care Nurs Q 1991;14(1):9–20.

26. Branca G, Capodanno D, Capranzano P, et al. Early discharge in acute myocardial infarction after clinical and angiographic risk assessment. J Cardiovasc Med 2008;9(8):858–61.

27. Hendrich AL, Fay J, Sorrells AK. Effects of acuity-adaptable rooms on flow of patients and delivery of care. Am J Crit Care 2004;13(1):35–45.

28. Carroll K, Frey-Moylan G. Nursing perspectives and knowledge with an acuity adaptable model. Nurs Sci Q. Apr 2020;33(2):128–31.

29. Chindhy SA, Edwards NM, Rajamanickam V, et al. Acuity adaptable patient care unit system shortens length of stay and improves outcomes in adult cardiac surgery: University of Wisconsin experience. Eur J Cardio Thorac Surg 2014;46(1): 49–54.

30. Emaminia A, Corcoran PC, Siegenthaler MP, et al. The universal bed model for patient care improves outcome and lowers cost in cardiac surgery. J Thorac Cardiovasc Surg 2012;143(2):475–81.

31. Bonuel N, Degracia A, Cesario S. Acuity-Adaptable patient room improves length of stay and cost of patients undergoing renal transplant: a pilot study. Crit Care Nurs Q 2013;36(2):181–94.
32. Kwan MA. Acuity-adaptable nursing care: exploring its place in designing the future patient room. Health Environments Research & Design Journal 2011;5(1):77–93.
33. Pati D, Cason C, Harvey TE, et al. An empirical examination of patient room handedness in acute medical-surgical settings. Health Environments Research & Design Journal 2010;4(1):11–33.
34. Reiling J. and culture 2007.
35. Pilosof NP, Barrett M, Oborn E, et al. Inpatient telemedicine and new models of care during COVID-19: hospital design strategies to enhance patient and staff safety. Int J Environ Res Publ Health 2021;18(16):8391.
36. Circular Nursing Division Runs Rings Around Rectangle, Modern Hospital, 1958, 91:5, p. 71.
37. Environmental Simulation, In: Marans R.W. and Stokols D., Research and Policy Issues, 1993, Plenum Press; New York and London, 327.

Afterword It Was a Different World Then... Ramblings from an Early Intensivist on Care and Quality Measures

INVENTING THE INTENSIVE CARE UNIT

My introduction, to what was to become Intensive Care, came in 1964 when I became the junior member of staff of the "Respiration Unit" in Oxford. The unit was part of the Neurology Department but was run, jointly, by John Spalding, a neurologist, and Alex Crampton Smith, an anesthetist. They had been working together for over 10 years and had distilled their research and experiences into *Clinical Practice and Physiology of Artificial Respiration*, one of the earliest books on Intensive Care.[1]

Ibsen's definitive demonstration of the efficacy and practicality of long-term intermittent positive pressure ventilation (IPPV), in patients with bulbar poliomyelitis in the early 1950s, encouraged clinicians all over the world to try the technique in a widening range of critical conditions. It quickly became apparent that attempting to manage artificially ventilated patients inside rooms off Nightingale wards, using oxygen from cylinders and looked after by terrified nurses experienced only in the use of sphygmomanometers and mercury thermometers, was disruptive and clinically unsatisfactory. The solution was to collect patients requiring this type of therapy into special areas with oxygen (and, later, suction) supplied to each bed, space for the bulky equipment, nursing staff who were familiar with its operation, and unprecedently high levels of medical and technical support. The Intensive Care Unit (ICU) was born.

The "Respiration Unit" was Oxford's first ICU. Lord Nuffield's Charitable Foundation had been persuaded in the mid-1950s to fund the Unit to care for patients with neurologic conditions that impaired their ability to breathe (eg, polio, polyneuritis, and tetanus). The six-bed ward was in the center of a WW2 military hospital, a brick building set among the Nissen huts.

EARLY LIMITATIONS

It is, perhaps, useful to remember what was *not* available at that time.

There were few plastic cannulas; most were made of steel. Syringes were made of glass, and endotracheal tubes were made of rubber. All had to be cleaned, packed, and autoclaved between uses. The central sterilization facility was one of the largest technical departments in every hospital. Single-use, plastic equipment only became widely available in the mid-1960s.

Bedside monitoring was initially carried out using unwieldy research equipment. Infusions were managed by eye and finger because the syringe driver did not appear until a decade later.

Crit Care Clin 39 (2023) xiii–xvii
https://doi.org/10.1016/j.ccc.2023.03.009
0749-0704/23/© 2023 Published by Elsevier Inc.

Oxford University had ONE computer; it filled a building and was much less powerful than a modern smartphone. Clinical calculations were carried out using slide rules and logarithmic tables.

The Internet was a science-fiction concept, so communication of research and developments took place by letter, by telephone, and through scientific society meetings and journals.

Although artificial ventilation was in regular use in operating theaters in the 1950s, employing the technique continuously for days or weeks had thrown up several problems. Tracheostomy tubes were traditionally curved and made from silver with an inner sleeve. The absence of an inflatable cuff made them unsuitable for IPPV, and they did not connect easily with a ventilator. The curved shape of an endotracheal tube lent itself to sliding down beyond the tracheal bifurcation, and to slipping out of the trachea during care procedures. The rubber, from which most endotracheal tubes were made, was satisfactory during surgery, but toxic chemicals leached out and damaged the tracheal mucosa during more-prolonged use. The right-angled Radcliffe tracheostomy tube, made from inert siliconized rubber, was the local solution to these problems. Devising a method for connecting the ventilator to the tube in the patient's airway tested the ingenuity of the early intensivists; the connection had to be airtight and robust enough to hold together during IPPV, nursing activity, and limited patient movement, yet easily detachable to allow for the aspiration of secretions. The need to compensate for the humidification of the inspired air by the bypassed upper airway had been tackled by passing inspired gases over a tank of heated water.

In the "Respiration Unit," patients were ventilated by mechanical bag-squeezers, which, repeatedly, lifted a weight to compress a bellows and push air into the patient's lungs (it was fitted with a handle to wind if the power failed). The Unit had a laboratory, and, in it, there was one of the very few systems for measuring blood gases in clinical use at that time. Blood was taken using metal needles (which had, hopefully, been sharpened before being autoclaved) attached to heparinized glass syringes, which were placed in icy water to slow metabolism before analysis. Each of the three components of the blood-gas analysis was measured on its own electrode. These had to be calibrated before the blood sample was introduced and recalibrated afterward. Readings were corrected for "drift" between the two calibrations, for the length of time between collection and analysis and for the patient's temperature. Oxygen in inspiratory and expiratory gas collections was measured using the oxygen electrode (with similar precautions), but, at this time, carbon dioxide gas was measured chemically using the Lloyd-Haldane apparatus (**Fig. 1**).[2] Nomograms of correction factors and the oxy-hemoglobin dissociation curve were provided and pasted onto hardwood boards, and calculations were made using a slide rule. It took over an hour to complete and check a "Riley analysis" (measurement of venous admixture and physiologic dead space), used to monitor the patient's lung function.

JUMPING FORWARD A DECADE OR TWO …

The practice of intensive care spread steadily and, by the end of the 1970s, very few acute hospitals did not have an ICU. In the United Kingdom, most had three to six beds and were housed in converted wards, but others were purpose-built. Hospitals, chronically starved of resources by economically challenged and uncomprehending governments, struggled to provide the equipment and staff—medical, nursing, and technical—and success depended very much on the drive and persuasiveness of dedicated individuals. Because patients who could benefit from intensive care came with a wide variety of conditions, the normal boundaries between specialties

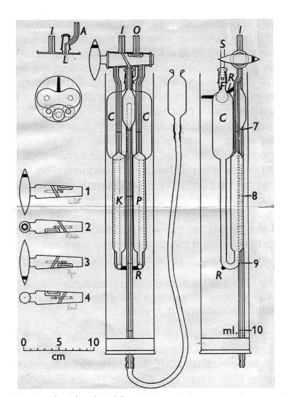

The Lloyd-Haldane Apparatus for measuring oxygen and carbon dioxide in gas mixtures. (Lloyd B.B. A development of Haldane's gas analysis apparatus. J Physiol 143, 5-6P, 1958)

Oxygen was absorbed into a pyrogallol solution (P) and carbon dioxide into potassium hydroxide (K). A sequence of 14 actions (either moving the reservoir, turning the tap or taking a reading) was required to set up the apparatus to receive a sample, and a further 16 to absorb the two gases.

Incidentally, the amount of carbon dioxide in air at that time (1960's) was 0.03%; it is now over 0.04%.

Fig. 1. The Lloyd Haldane apparatus.

had to be breached, and problems about who would be responsible for their care needed to be resolved. This was not always an easy process!

At this time, there were few clinicians who dedicated all their time to intensive care, and most units were run by a group of anesthetists who shared the responsibility for medical care. This came about because much of the novel equipment being deployed in ICUs was being used, routinely, by anesthetists in the operating theater. Their understanding of the physiology and pharmacology of the respiratory and cardiovascular systems, required to maintain patients during surgery, was also applicable during intensive care. Anesthetic departments were relatively large and organized to provide around-the-clock emergency cover across the whole range of surgical specialties. They also employed technicians who specialized in equipment maintenance. These factors, plus their exposure to a wide variety of acute clinical conditions, led anesthetists to take the lead in the organization and staffing of ICUs in many hospitals.

THE QUEST FOR QUALITY

In these exciting, individualistic circumstances, it was not surprising that little attention was paid to the quality of the care that was being provided. At the unit level, decisions had to be made about how to record, display, and utilize the unprecedented amount of information generated about each patient. Basic information was recorded about patients, usually in a unit logbook, which made retrieval for statistical analysis tedious and difficult. The amount of data collected differed from unit to unit, and the only variable with a standardized definition was the unit fatality rate.

Along with the ability to treat came the question of who to treat. Experience showed that the sicker and older the patient, the less likely they were to survive, and some conditions proved resistant to the new therapies provided in ICU. Experience also showed that artificial ventilation could not reverse chronic obstructive pulmonary disease, and referrals of such patients for intensive care declined fairly quickly. As ICUs admitted patients with a wide variety of diseases, the numbers with each condition tended to be small, making the build-up of expertise a slow process.

To overcome these limitations, far-sighted individuals realized that experiences with the new technologies should be described, shared, and discussed. The Intensive Care Society (ICS) in the United Kingdom was founded in 1970 and began holding meetings, twice a year, at different centers around the United Kingdom. The First World Congress of Intensive Care was held in London in 1974. Journals dealing specifically with intensive care topics appeared: *Critical Care Medicine* in 1973, and *Intensive Care Medicine* a year later.

Early in the 1980s, the ICS Council recognized that there could be benefits in pooling experience and that tools to measure the quality of the care provided were lacking. A research subcommittee was set up whose terms of reference included:

To encourage and coordinate research in intensive care with particular emphasis on multicentre cooperation, [and] To explore and research those areas of value in producing useful predictive information and clinical guidelines.

In the United States, Knaus and colleagues[3] were reporting multicenter studies in which they "scored" a patient's sickness severity and linked this to the outcome of their care. They showed using data from several US ICUs that there was a statistical relationship between a patient's Acute Physiology and Chronic Health Evaluation (APACHE) score and their likelihood of survival over a wide range of conditions.

In 1985, the ICS Council invited an independent Oxford research team to carry out a study to determine whether the APACHE methodology would work in the United Kingdom. (The independent research team consisted of the Professor of Public Health [Martin Vessey], a senior statistician [Klim Macpherson], and an intensive care consultant [the author]. The research study was coordinated and conducted by a doctoral research fellow [Kathryn Rowan]. Two additional intensivists [Drs Alastair Short and Ed Major] later joined the team.) Within the Society, there was anxiety about whether the method would be used to deny patients treatment and whether sufficient ICUs could be recruited since the research study data collection requirements were daunting. To be statistically valid, each participating ICU had to collect a large and complete set of data, from every patient, from the initial 24-hour period of the ICU admission. The data set required included the lowest and highest value for 12 physiologic parameters, which would subsequently be weighted (scored) depending on their greatest deviance from the normal range, plus information about the patient's age, chronic health conditions, and their survival status at hospital discharge. In the days of paper charts and records, this was a major undertaking for ICU staff. But, in practice, the most difficult information to collect was the survival data.

THE BIRTH OF THE INTENSIVE CARE NATIONAL AUDIT AND RESEARCH CENTRE

From 1987, some 26 ICUs, both large and small and geographically selected from across the United Kingdom and Ireland, completed the study and contributed data on nearly 9000 patients over the following 4 years. Following detailed analysis and publication of the encouraging results,[4,5] initial, government, pump-priming funds helped to establish the Intensive Care National Audit and Research Centre (ICNARC) as an independent, scientific, not-for-profit organization in 1994, to continue monitoring and evaluation of intensive care.

In the subsequent decades, ICNARC steadily expanded, and its Case Mix Programme now pools and validates data on all admissions from every ICU across England, Wales, and Northern Ireland. The accurate data on more than 3 million admissions have allowed statisticians to improve risk prediction for the critically ill, epidemiologists to describe critical illness (including rare conditions), and a platform for evaluation of new and existing interventions. These data have been essential to monitoring the care delivered and in finding ways to improve that care.

During the COVID-19 pandemic, ICNARC established a rapid reporting mechanism to generate daily numbers and a weekly overview of the number, characteristics, and outcomes for patients admitted to ICU with COVID-19. The widely available on-line report grew to be over 100 pages long and, ultimately, contained information on over 50,000 admissions. It was eagerly awaited, each week, by government, senior health care managers, researchers, and the general and scientific media.

The progression, in just my lifetime, has been from learning to treat individual critically ill patients to assessing and evaluating outcomes for millions of patients. It *is* now a very different world!

John H. Kerr, MA, DM (Oxon), FFARCS
Retired Consultant Anaesthetist
Nuffield Department of Anaesthetics
University of Oxford
Radcliffe Infirmary
Oxford, United Kingdom

E-mail address:
johnh.kerr@btinternet.com

REFERENCES

1. Spalding JMK, Smith AC. Clinical practice and physiology of artificial respiration. Blackwell Scientific; 1963.
2. Lloyd BB. Adevelopment of Haldane's gas analysis apparatus. Blackwell Scientific Publications. Oxford. J Physiol. 143, 1958, 5-6P
3. Knaus WA, Draper EA, Wagner DP, et al. APACHE II: a severity of disease classification system. Crit Care Med 1985;13(10):818–29.
4. Rowan KM, Kerr JH, Major E, et al. Intensive Care Society's APACHE II study in Britain and Ireland—I: variations in case mix of adult admissions to general intensive care units and impact on outcome. BMJ 1993;307(6910):972–7.
5. Rowan KM, Kerr JH, Major E, et al. Intensive Care Society's APACHE II study in Britain and Ireland—II: outcome comparisons of intensive care units after adjustment for case mix by the American APACHE II method. BMJ 1993;307(6910):977–81.

Moving?

Make sure your subscription moves with you!

To notify us of your new address, find your **Clinics Account Number** (located on your mailing label above your name), and contact customer service at:

Email: **journalscustomerservice-usa@elsevier.com**

800-654-2452 (subscribers in the U.S. & Canada)
314-447-8871 (subscribers outside of the U.S. & Canada)

Fax number: **314-447-8029**

Elsevier Health Sciences Division
Subscription Customer Service
3251 Riverport Lane
Maryland Heights, MO 63043

*To ensure uninterrupted delivery of your subscription, please notify us at least 4 weeks in advance of move.

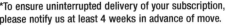
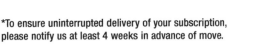

ELSEVIER

9780323940115